PHOTODYNAMIC THERAPY

PROCEDURES IN COSMETIC DERMATOLOGY

PROCEDURES IN COSMETIC DERMATOLOGY

Series Editors:

Jeffrey S. Dover, MD, FRCPC
Murad Alam, MD, MSCI, MBA

Recently published volumes:

2025

Scar Management
Second edition
Jessica G. Labadie, MD
Murad Alam, MD, MSCI, MBA
Jeffrey S. Dover, MD, FRCPC
ISBN 978-0-443-24590-9

2024

Cosmeceuticals
Fourth edition
Zoe Diana Draelos, MD
ISBN 978-0-443-11808-1

Cosmetic Procedures in Skin of Color
First edition
Andrew F. Alexis, MD
ISBN 978-0-323-83144-4

2023

Surgical Lifting
First edition
Hooman Khorasani, MD
Eyal Levit, MD
ISBN 978-0-323-67326-6

Soft Tissue Augmentation
Fifth edition
Jean Carruthers, MD, FRCS(C), FRC(Ophth)
Alastair Carruthers, MA, BM, BCh, FRCPC, FRCP(Lon)
Jeffrey S. Dover, MD, FRCPC
Murad Alam, MD, MSCI, MBA
Omer Ibrahim, MD
ISBN 978-0-323-83075-1

Botulinum Toxin
Fifth edition
Alastair Carruthers, MA, BM, BCh, FRCPC, FRCP(Lon)
Jean Carruthers, MD, FRCS(C), FRC(Ophth)
Jeffrey S. Dover, MD, FRCPC
Murad Alam, MD, MSCI, MBA
Omer Ibrahim, MD
ISBN 978-0-323-83116-1

Forthcoming volumes:

2025

Treatment of Leg Veins
Third edition
Murad Alam, MD, MSCI, MBA
Sirunya Silapunt, MD, FAAD
ISBN 978-0-443-25011-8

Body Contouring
Second edition
Anne Chapas, MD
Omar A. Ibrahimi, MD, PhD
Nazanin Saedi, MD
ISBN 978-0-443-26192-3

PROCEDURES IN COSMETIC DERMATOLOGY

PHOTODYNAMIC THERAPY

THIRD EDITION

Editor

Macrene Alexiades, MD, PhD, FAAD, FASLMS

Associate Clinical Professor
Department of Dermatology
Yale University School of Medicine
New Haven, Connecticut

Founder and Director
Dermatology and Laser Surgery Center of New York
New York, New York

Adjunct Professor
Department of Dermatology
Syggros Hospital
Athens, Greece

Series Editors

Jeffrey S. Dover, MD, FRCPC
Director
SkinCare Physicians
Chestnut Hill, Massachusetts

Associate Clinical Professor
Department of Dermatology
Yale University School of Medicine
New Haven, Connecticut

Clinical Professor
Department of Surgery
Dartmouth Medical School
Hanover, New Hampshire

Adjunct Associate Professor
Department of Dermatology
Brown Medical School
Providence, Rhode Island

Murad Alam, MD, MSCI, MBA
Professor
Departments of Dermatology, Otolaryngology, and Surgery
Chief, Section of Cutaneous and Aesthetic Surgery
Northwestern University
Chicago, Illinois

ELSEVIER

Elsevier
1600 John F. Kennedy Blvd.
Ste 1800
Philadelphia, PA 19103-2899

PROCEDURES IN COSMETIC DERMATOLOGY SERIES: PHOTODYNAMIC THERAPY, THIRD EDITION ISBN: 978-0-443-10689-7

Content Strategist: Jessica McCool
Senior Content Development Specialist: Sneha Kashyap
Publishing Services Manager: Deepthi Unni
Project Manager: Nandhini Thanga Alagu
Design Direction: Patrick Ferguson

Printed in India

Last digit is the print number: 9 8 7 6 5 4 3 2 1

This textbook is dedicated to my children, Sophia and Anthony, my reason for being and the source of my inspiration.

CONTRIBUTORS

Macrene Alexiades, MD, PhD
Associate Clinical Professor
Department of Dermatology
Yale University School of Medicine
New Haven, Connecticut
Founder and Director
Dermatology and Laser Surgery Center of New York
New York, New York
Adjunct Professor
Department of Dermatology
Syggros Hospital
Athens, Greece

Ron R. Allison, MD
Director
Department of Radiation Oncology
Federal Medical Center
Durham, North Carolina

Rox Anderson
Department of Dermatology
Massachusetts General Hospital
Laser and Cosmetic Center
Boston, Massachusetts
Wellman Center for Photomedicine
Massachusetts General Hospital
Wang Ambulatory Care Center
Boston, Massachusetts

Gabriela E. Beraja, MS
Medical Student
Lincoln Memorial University-DeBusk College of Osteopathic Medicine
Harrogate, Tennessee

Joi B. Carter, MD
Associate Professor
Department of Dermatology
Dartmouth Hitchcock Medical Center
Lebanon, New Hampshire

Rajeev Chavda, MD, DBM
Galderma SA
Geneva, Switzerland

Alexander A. Daoud
Associate Professor
Department of Dermatology and Surgery
Florida International University College of Medicine
Miami, Florida

Mary Dick, MD
Resident
Department of Dermatology
Vanderbilt
Nashville, Texas

William Driscoll, BSc
Clinical Research Fellow
Department of Dermatology
University of California, Irvine
Irvine School of Medicine
Irvine, California

Daphne G. Eckembrecher, MD, MPH
Resident Physician
Dr. Phillip Frost Department of Dermatology and Cutaneous Surgery
University of Miami Miller School of Medicine
Miami, Florida

Francelia J. Eckembrecher, MD, MPH
Resident Physician
Dr. Phillip Frost Department of Dermatology and Cutaneous Surgery
University of Miami Miller School of Medicine
Miami, Florida

Rachel Elsanadi, BS
Medical Student
Department of Dermatology
University of California, Irvine
Irvine, California

Nicole M. Golbari, MD, MPH
Surgical Fellow
Department of Dermatology
University of California, Irvine
Irvine, California

ACKNOWLEDGMENTS

It is an honor to edit the singular textbook on photodynamic therapy for cutaneous applications. I would like to thank Dr. Thomas Fitzpatrick posthumously for being a pivotal influence and advisor during his dermatology course at Harvard Medical School. While pursuing my BA, MD, and PhD at Harvard, Drs Jeffrey Dover and Kenneth Arndt were the first to suggest I become a dermatologist and continued to play a major role in my research and professional career for over 35 years. I thank my parents, Gregory and Sophie, for instilling in me the joys and honor of intellectual scholarship, and my children, Sophia and Anthony, both Harvard graduates themselves, for sacrificing time with their mother so that I could continue to strive toward academic excellence. Finally, I thank my colleagues in dermatology, medicine, and science who have become my extended family and whose genuine dedication to our field demonstrate that humanity, kindness, service, and community are the keys to a fulfilled life.

CONTENTS

Part I PDT for Follicular Disorders

Part II PDT for Pre-Cancer and Prevention

SECTION I PDT for Actinic Keratosis

SECTION II PDT for High-Risk Patients

Part III PDT for Neoplasia/Skin Cancer

Part IV PDT for Rejuvenation

Part V PDT for Infections

PART I

PDT for Follicular Disorders

1

Photodynamic Therapy for *Acne vulgaris*

Fernanda H. Sakamoto, Rox Anderson

KEY POINTS

- Photodynamic therapy (PDT) has been employed in the management of acne vulgaris for several decades.
- PDT targets sebaceous glands through selective uptake of a photosensitizer, followed by light activation, leading to gland destruction and decreased sebaceous activity.

OBJECTIVES

- Describe the mechanism of action of PDT in reducing acne and sebaceous gland activity.
- Review established PDT treatment protocols and evaluate reported clinical outcomes.
- Assess the current role of PDT within the broader acne treatment algorithm.

Photodynamic therapy (PDT) for acne was first demonstrated in 2000 by Hongcharu and colleagues[1] using topical aminolevulinic acid (ALA), a natural precursor of porphyrin synthesis, and high-dose red light (633 nm, 150 J/cm^2) irradiation given 3 hours after application of the ALA. Since then, numerous articles, but mainly reviews have been published with various protocols and results. In this chapter, we critically examine this work and the use of PDT for acne treatment.[2]

Acne is the most common disease in dermatology, affecting about 80% of patients seeking dermatologic care.[3] The pathophysiology of acne is complex, involving sebum production, hormones, innate and humoral immune responses, and bacterial proliferation, which creates hyperkeratosis with follicular obstruction, local inflammation, and destruction of sebaceous follicles, often leading to scarring. It is an inflammatory condition of sebaceous hair follicles, with the presence of natural porphyrins mainly produced by local *C. acnes* bacteria, a facultative anaerobe. Porphyrins are potent photosensitizers, triggered maximally by blue light. Even without the addition of a photosensitizing drug, acne improves temporarily after exposure to sufficient amounts of blue light.[4]Since 2000 PDT for acne has been explored in clinical studies using a wide range of study designs, light sources, dosimetry, and timing for both the drug and light exposure. For simplicity, in this chapter, we will focus mostly on porphyrin-precursor drugs: ALA and methyl aminolevulinic acid (MAL).

Fundamentally, PDT requires three elements: a photosensitizer, light, and oxygen. Upon absorption of a photon, the photosensitizer is excited to a reactive state capable of transferring energy to oxygen, creating reactive oxygen species (singlet oxygen and others). The reactive oxygen attacks biomolecules, including proteins and lipids, potentially overwhelming cellular function, leading to cell death. For acne treatment by ALA-PDT, irreversible damage to sebaceous glands appears to be a central mechanism for long-term improvement, evidenced by lower sebum output and long-term miniaturization of the glands.[1]

Different photosensitizers have been studied for acne treatment, but the most commonly used are porphyrin-precursor drugs, such as ALA and its esters, especially the methyl-ester of ALA (MAL). The ester drugs are widely used and approved for the treatment of acne in Europe and Asia, while in the United States, ALA is the most common drug available. Applied topically, both ALA and its esters can lead to high concentrations of porphyrins, notably protoporphyrin IX, in sebaceous follicles.

Regarding the level of evidence of the use of porphyrin-derivative photosensitizers for acne, and grading of recommendations assessment, to assess the quality of evidence (QoE),[5] analyzing 71 randomized clinical trials (RCTs) with 4211 participants (median sample size 31), a single study ($n = 266$, low QoE) showed little or no difference in effectiveness on participants' assessment of improvement between blue light 20% ALA-PDT versus vehicle plus blue light. Pooled data from three studies ($n = 360$, moderate QoE) showed that red light MAL-PDT, had a similar effect on changes in lesion counts versus placebo cream with red light. Most studies reported adverse effects, but inadequately; with scarring reported as absent, and blistering only in studies on intense pulsed light, infrared light, and PDT (very low QoE).[5] Similarly, Tang and colleagues[6] ran a systematic review and meta-analysis on 13 RCTs with 701 subjects and found very heterogeneous studies, concluding that PDT had a certain effect on acne vulgaris in terms of the outcomes of MPRILC (MD: 15.97, 95% CI: 11.93–20.00, $p < 0.00001$) and TER (RR: 1.55, 95% CI: 1.38–1.74, $p < 0.00001$). When comparing intense pulse light (IPL) versus red light (RL) versus long-pulsed dye laser (LPDL), and non-ablative fractional laser, the pooled results of different light types revealed that PDT outstandingly improved the clinical efficacy for acne (MD = 15.97; 95% CI = 11.93–20.00; $p < 0.00001$), and there was significant heterogeneity ($p = 0.0005$; $I2 = 72\%$). However, there was no subgroup difference among the four visible light sources ($p = .62$; $I2 = 0$).[6] Their overall recommendation was that PDT is beneficial for improving the clinical efficacy of inflammatory acne vulgaris, which can be widely recommended for clinical use.

The value of such reviews and meta-analyses is limited because the published studies vary tremendously in design, dosimetry, and important methodology, for example, the drug used, skin preparation, time of incubation, light source, wavelength(s), fluence, and irradiance. Despite those wide variations, it is notable that PDT never caused scarring and was deemed effective as a treatment for inflammatory acne. The practical application of PDT for acne treatment is well served by a thorough understanding of how PDT works, of the relative advantages and limitations of different light sources, and of practical advantages and pitfalls of this modality of treatment.

THE THEORY BEHIND PDT FOR ACNE

Hongcharu's pivotal work was a well-controlled prospective human study with both quantitative, qualitative, and histological endpoints. It used 20% ALA in ethanol, applied for 3 hours under occlusion, followed by irradiation of 150 J/cm^2 red light from a filtered lamp. Unlike shorter wavelengths, red light penetrates well to the level of sebaceous glands. There was moderate to strong pain during light exposure. Control sites in each subject received light alone, drug alone, and no treatment, in quadrants on the back. Moderate to severe acne on the back in 22 male subjects were included. They also compared the effects of a single treatment session versus. 4 treatment sessions. The endpoints were acne severity, serial quantitative measures of sebum output, porphyrin fluorescence microscopy, and histology evaluated for 6 months post-treatment. Interestingly, there was strong preferential porphyrin synthesis in sebaceous follicles (Fig. 1.1). Only PDT caused significant changes, as neither red light nor drug application alone were effective. Four treatment sessions produced significantly greater acne improvement than 1 treatment session. There was significant suppression of sebum output, and significant

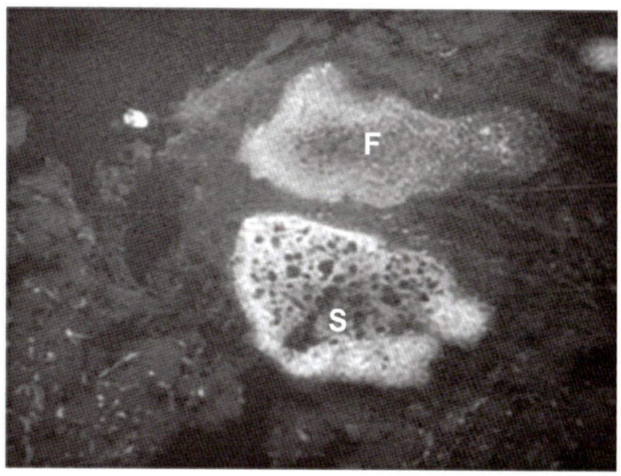

Fig. 1.1 Fluorescence microscopy showing greater PpIX accumulation in the sebaceous glands (S) than hair follicles (F). (From Hongcharu W, Taylor CR, Chang Y, Aghassi D, Suthamjariya K, Anderson RR. Topical ALA-photodynamic therapy for the treatment of acne vulgaris. *J Invest Dermatol*. 2000;115(2):183–192. doi:10.1046/j.1523–1747.2000.00046.x).

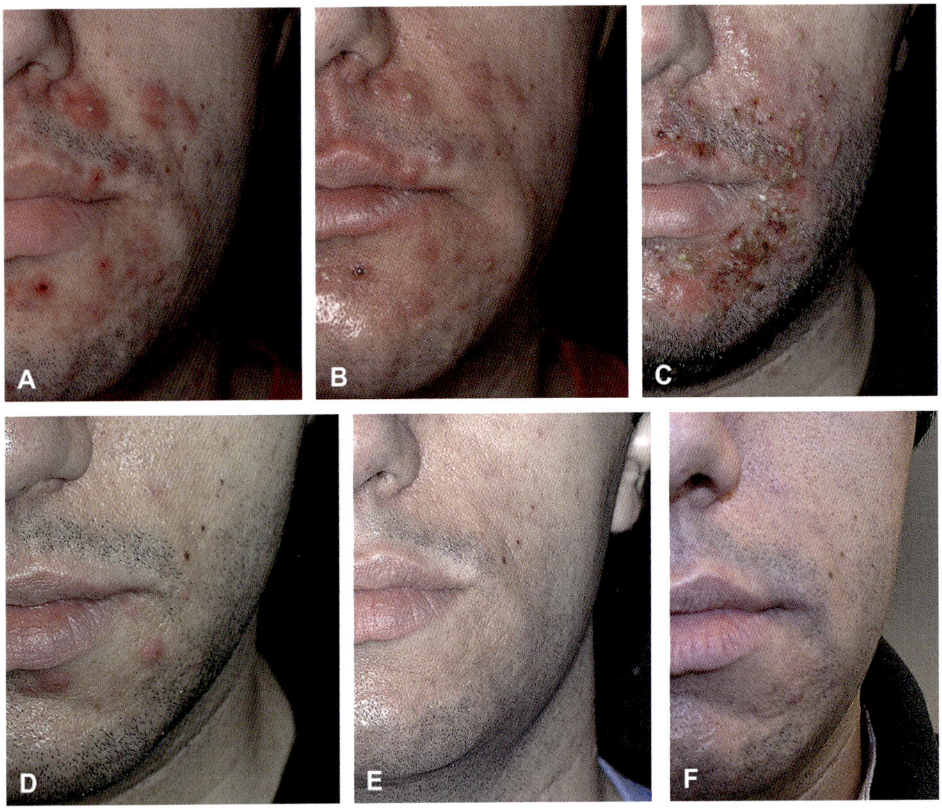

Fig. 1.2 Improvement of inflammatory acne and cicatricial lesions after topical application of 20% 5-aminolevulinic acid (ALA) for 3 hours of incubation under occlusion and 200 J/cm^2 of 633 nm red light (Omnilux; PhotoTherapeutics, Cheshire, UK) at 100 mW/cm^2. (A) Before treatment. (B) Immediately after the first session. (C) Two days after the first session. (D) Seven months after the first session and before the second session. (E) Ten months after the first session, 3 months after the second session. (F) One year and 2 months after the first session, after total of four sessions. Note the important inflammatory reaction after high dose red light ALA photodynamic therapy, with no long-lasting side effects. (Courtesy R. Rox Anderson, MD.)

acne improvement for a long period of time (greater than 6 months after PDT). The treatment caused intense inflammatory reaction (folliculitis) with evidence of direct sebaceous gland destruction, observed in histological samples.[1] Similar results were obtained using methyl-ester of ALA in combination with high fluence red light exposure from 630 nm LED array sources,[7,8] Wiegell and colleagues showed a reduction in inflammatory acne in 68% of patients, but not in comedones.[9] These studies established that "high-dose, red light" treatment protocols are highly effective for acne.[2]

Despite its efficacy and safety, high-dose red light PDT is painful, requires hours to perform, and is followed by days of treatment-induced folliculitis (Fig. 1.2). These drawbacks led to testing many other protocols with different degrees of success, using a lower drug concentration and/or shorter time between application of the drug and light and/or alternative light sources already present in dermatology. We have called these modalities "low-dose PDT".[2]

MECHANISM OF ACTION

Despite speculation, there is no evidence that high-dose red light PDT works through an antibiotic effect. In contrast, there is strong evidence for partial destruction of sebaceous glands, followed by prolonged reduction of sebum output, reduction of follicular obstruction, and hyperkeratosis. In addition, PDT modulates immune mechanisms with reduction of infiltrating inflammatory cells within acne lesions. PDT increases the expression of toll-like receptor TLR-2, which has been implicated in the inflammatory response against acne-related sebocytes. HSP-70 released from PDT-treated cells may directly mediate TLR-2 signaling.[10] Cosmetic changes in skin texture are observed after PDT for acne. PDT also stimulates metalloproteinases MMP-1 and MMP-3, thereby stimulating dermal collagen remodeling.[10–13]

Recently, Zhang and colleagues' *in vitro* study suggested that the mechanism of action of ALA-PDT for acne involves a cascade of inflammatory response created by reactive oxygen species (ROS) induction, leading to an increase in NLRP3 inflammasome, therefore heightening caspase-1 activation and IL-1β secretion.[14]

VARIABLES AFFECTING EFFICACY FOR PDT FOR ACNE

Drugs

PDT using porphyrin-inducing prodrugs is a complex photochemical reaction. Several variables can influence the ultimate clinical outcomes, including: 1. target tissue characteristics, 2. ALA formulation and methods of drug delivery, and 3. skin temperature,[15,16] and 4. the interaction between the drug and light.[2]

The penetration of visible light into the dermis is strongly wavelength-dependent, with longer (red) wavelengths penetrating far deeper than shorter (blue) wavelengths. ALA-PDT is extensively used for treatment of actinic keratosis, a very superficial epidermal lesion, with either blue or red wavelength excitation. In contrast, sebaceous glands are located in the mid-dermis between about 0.5–2.0 mm deep, largely beyond the reach of blue light. Ideally, the best treatment protocol should allow enough time for the porphyrin-inducing drug to be metabolized into porphyrin, followed by the irradiation with light that penetrates deep enough to destroy the sebaceous glands, with minimal side effects.

ALA is a naturally occurring amino acid. Soon after ALA-PDT began, the search for patentable PDT drugs was achieved by the simple conversion of the ALA carboxyl group to an ester linkage. In general, tissue and cellular esterases rapidly cleave the ester linkage, yielding ALA. Depending on the length of a hydrocarbon chain at the ester linkage, the molecule could be more lipophilic, potentially increasing drug absorption and concentration within the lipid-rich sebaceous glands. However, as the hydrocarbon length increases, molecular weight and size increases, which limit drug penetration. Both ALA and methyl-ALA (MAL) are small hydrophilic molecules, making them functionally similar for PDT.[2]

In a split-face clinical study comparing ALA-PDT with MAL-PDT, similar efficacy was observed in both modalities, but more severe and prolonged side effects were noted on the ALA side.[17]

The hexyl-ester of ALA, was tested in healthy volunteers, showing transient reduction of *C. acnes* after a single treatment session in a short follow-up time (14 days).[18] In theory, the hexyl-ester is much more lipophilic and might accumulate well inside the sebaceous glands; unfortunately, no commercial version is available for clinical use at this time.

ALA Concentration

Most of the clinical trials using PDT for acne have utilized either 20% ALA or 16.8% MAL. Another study ($n = 180$) comparing red light PDT at different ALA concentrations, found that 20% ALA-PDT showed similar results as 15% ALA-PDT but better than 10% and 5% ALA-PDT.[5] When comparing different drug concentrations, higher ALA concentrations (>10%) show long-term acne improvement but are also associated with more side effects.[19]

PDT with a newly developed nanoemulsion formulation containing 10% aminolaevulinic acid hydrochloride (BF-200 ALA) followed by red light exposure, approved for actinic keratosis, has been under investigation for the treatment of acne, pending results (ClinicalTrials.gov Identifier: NCT05080764).[20]

ALA and Light Delivery Factors

Time of Incubation

Interestingly, even when ALA is injected intraperitoneally in a mice model, porphyrins are accumulated in the sebaceous glands, making porphyrin prodrugs very attractive for the treatment of sebaceous gland conditions.[21] After the application of the prodrug, usually ALA or MAL, the peak of porphyrin production is reached at 12 hours. In order to reduce the treatment time, various protocols have been suggested, varying from 0 to 3 hours of incubation. Based on previous studies, in a porcine model that is very similar to human skin, when topically applied, ALA takes time to be metabolized and accumulate porphyrins at different histological targets. To reach the sebaceous glands, it takes about 60 min for the fluorescence to start within the glands.[2]

Short-contact protocols have been published with light irradiation applied 15–30 min after drug application. However, the results are limited due to very short follow-ups, lack of controls, and small sample sizes.[5,22]

Light Wavelength

While porphyrins are primarily absorbed within the blue spectrum at 410 nm, blue light has limited penetration depth, which may affect its ability to destroy sebaceous glands located about 1–2 mm deep. Other wavelengths with smaller peaks of porphyrins absorption (also called the Q-bands) at 505, 540, 580, and 630 nm have been used for acne treatment.

Blue light alone is moderately effective for treating inflammatory acne,[4] but its results are limited. When comparing blue light plus 20% ALA with blue light alone, PDT is no more effective than blue light alone after a short incubation time (45 min).[5]

In a split-face study, two sessions of red light (635 nm, 37 J/cm^2, 68 mW/cm^2) alone were compared to red light MAL-PDT, showing MAL-PDT's superiority in reducing inflammatory lesions (20% for red light vs. 54% for MAL-PDT), with no significant reduction in non-inflammatory lesions (20% for red light and 40% for MAL-PDT).[7]

Red light PDT followed by a long incubation period (3 hours) has shown more consistent results for both ALA and MAL.[1,7–9,17,22–24]

The use of common pulsed light sources like intense pulsed light (IPLs or flashlamps) or pulsed-dye lasers at 585–595 nm is very attractive to clinicians due to their broad availability and ability to produce less pain with fast light irradiation. In 20 acne subjects, Hong and colleagues[25] compared conventional MAL-PDT (red 635 nm 22 J/cm^2 at 34 mW/cm^2) with IPL-MAL-PDT (530 and 750 nm, 8–10 J/cm^2). Red light activation produced faster results at 4 weeks with more side-effects, but at 8 weeks both treatments produced similar reduction of lesions with no statistical significance. However, only very small studies with short follow-ups (4–8 weeks) have been reported, providing limited data about longevity of the results.

In an exploratory pilot study, long-pulsed dye laser PDT was studied in 14 patients with mild to severe acne. A PDL at 595 nm (7.0–7.5 J/cm^2 fluence, 10-ms pulse duration, 10-mm spot size, and dynamic cooling spray of 30 ms with a 30-ms delay) was applied after short incubation of ALA (45 min). One hundred percent of the subjects reported improvement of the acne with a mean follow-up time of 6 months after treatment and 2.9 sessions were necessary to achieve results (77% acne clearance). Post-treatment cosmesis was favorable, with concurrent resolution of erythematous acne scars following PDL-PDT.[26] Daylight PDT using a novel 1.5% 3-butenyl 5-aminolevulinate gel formulation has reported a reduction of 58% of inflammatory lesions and 34% of non-inflammatory lesions by 12 weeks.[27] In a split-face non-randomized clinical trial comparing DL-PDT versus conventional ALA-PDT for acne (2-hours incubation, 630 nm, 75 J/cm^2), Slutsky and colleagues found similar efficacy, with a substantial reduction in side effects and pain on the DL-PDT side at 12 weeks.[28]

However, this treatment modality is limited by weather conditions in different parts of the country/world. In a very small study with a short follow-up, laser-assisted drug delivery using a non-ablative 1550 nm laser (50 spots/cm^2 at 20 mJ/cm^2) followed by the application of ALA and activation with daylight showed superiority compared to DL-PDT alone (52% vs. 36% reduction in inflammatory acne at 8 weeks).[29]

SIDE-EFFECTS

When using high-dose PDT, pain, acute inflammatory skin reactions, and transient skin tanning are the most common side effects of ALA- or MAL-PDT. Pain is typically more severe at the beginning of light irradiation and can be alleviated with analgesics, cooling fans, and cold water spritzers. However, the pre-application of topical lidocaine should be avoided, as it often and unpredictably enhances PDT response (unpublished observations).

The metabolism of ALA into porphyrins continues for 12 hours or more after ALA application; so, in practice, once the drug is applied, it continues to produce the photosensitizer. This can cause persistent photosensitivity for up to 48 hours. Since porphyrins absorb light in the visible spectrum, common sunscreens that block UVA and UVB do not protect light-exposed areas after treatment. Patients should be advised to avoid direct sunlight, medical light exposure, and to use protective clothing, broad-brimmed hats, and stay indoors after treatment. These are additional restrictions to the practice of PDT for acne treatment.

Allergic reactions to ALA derivatives are rare; however, MAL contains a peanut oil component that may be a potential allergen source.

Pain can be intense and a limiting factor for this modality of treatment. Immediately after the light exposure, inflammatory response resembling a sunburn (mild to moderate edema and erythema) is observed.

PDT causes direct apoptosis of the sebaceous glands, leading to a sterile pustular reaction, followed by oozing and crusting typically about 24–72 hours after treatment. The complete resolution of this reaction can take up to 10 days, followed by transient tanning and post-inflammatory hyperpigmentation. There are no reports of PDT causing scarring under any treatment conditions; in contrast, both acne and surgical scars improve after ALA-PDT.[22,30] This improvement in post-treatment acne scar resolution may be explained by PDT's favorable effects on wound healing.[31]

PDT AND CONVENTIONAL THERAPIES

In a blind, randomized, and controlled trial of moderate acne, ALA-PDT was found to be superior to adapalene gel plus oral doxycycline.[32]

ALA-PDT in association with oral isotretinoin has been shown to decrease the duration of treatment and provide safe and faster results.[33]

Finally, when comparing ALA-PDT versus oral isotretinoin (total dose 90 mg/kg), there was no difference in efficacy; however, ALA-PDT provided much faster results than oral isotretinoin.[34] While this study shows promising results, the total isotretinoin dose used in this study was lower than the recommended total dose for acne treatment (150 mg/kg).

OTHER PDT DRUGS FOR ACNE

Other PDT drugs that do not induce porphyrin synthesis have been utilized for acne treatment. In a pilot trial, indocyanine green (in a 0.1% lotion) has shown some success for moderate acne after 3–5 sessions, but not for nodulo-cystic acne, when activated by a diode laser following a 30-min incubation period.[35] In a retrospective chart review, Park and colleagues found excellent response after 3–5 sessions using indocyanine green followed by IPL in 40% of their patients with the remaining cohort reporting minimal to moderate response.[36] Similarly, indole-3-acetic acid (IAA-PDT) followed by a 520 nm irradiation also showed a reduction in inflammatory lesions after a 3-month follow-up.[37] These drugs are rarely used due to the lack of FDA clearance, and/or not available on the market.

FINAL REMARKS

Despite clear evidence that high-dose red light PDT is highly effective, safe, and can lead to histological miniaturization of sebaceous glands, resulting in prolonged remission of acne, the various protocols can be confusing for clinicians trying to use PDT for acne. High-dose PDT with a long incubation period (3 hours) and higher drug concentration (>10% ALA), activated by deeper-penetrating red light, can yield much better results but also has more side effects. Clinical efficacy similar to those achieved with oral isotretinoin is common; however, the effort involved, as well as inflammatory and pigmentation side effects, are a significant impediment to high-dose red light PDT treatment.

The variety of treatment techniques for PDT for acne also makes it difficult for systematic reviews and meta-analyses. They cannot be grouped as the same type of treatment, as they differ enough from each other to produce completely different results. Indeed, there is a limitation in good quality studies with large groups of patients and long follow-ups.

The lack of regulatory approval in the US for acne specifically, also limits access to this treatment modality for a larger group of patients. New developments to optimize PDT for acne, minimize its side effects, and provide rational combinations with other treatments should be encouraged.

REFERENCES

1. Hongcharu W, Taylor CR, Chang Y, Aghassi D, Suthamjariya K, Anderson RR. Topical ALA-photodynamic therapy for the treatment of acne vulgaris. *J Invest Dermatol.* 2000;115(2):183–192. doi:10.1046/j.1523-1747.2000.00046.x.
2. Sakamoto FH, Lopes JD, Anderson RR. Photodynamic therapy for acne vulgaris: a critical review from basics to clinical practice: part I. Acne vulgaris: when and why consider photodynamic therapy? *J Am Acad Dermatol.* 2010;63(2):183–193. doi:10.1016/j.jaad.2009.09.056; quiz 193–194.
3. Bickers DR, Lim HW, Margolis D, et al. The burden of skin diseases: 2004 a joint project of the American academy of dermatology association and the society for investigative dermatology. *J Am Acad Dermatol.* 2006;55(3):490–500. doi:10.1016/j.jaad.2006.05.048.
4. Elman M, Slatkine M, Harth Y. The effective treatment of acne vulgaris by a high-intensity, narrow

band 405–420 nm light source. *J Cosmet Laser Ther.* 2003;5(2):111–117.
5. Barbaric J, Abbott R, Posadzki P, et al. Light therapies for acne: abridged Cochrane systematic review including GRADE assessments. *Br J Dermatol.* 2018;178(1):61–75. doi:10.1111/bjd.15495.
6. Tang X, Li C, Ge S, Chen Z, Lu L. Efficacy of photodynamic therapy for the treatment of inflammatory acne vulgaris: a systematic review and meta-analysis. *J Cosmet Dermatol.* 2020;19(1):10–21. doi:10.1111/jocd.13197.
7. Hörfelt C, Stenquist B, Larkö O, Faergemann J, Wennberg AM. Photodynamic therapy for acne vulgaris: a pilot study of the dose-response and mechanism of action. *Acta Derm Venereol.* 2007;87(4):325–329. doi:10.2340/00015555-0243.
8. Pollock B, Turner D, Stringer MR, et al. Topical aminolaevulinic acid-photodynamic therapy for the treatment of acne vulgaris: a study of clinical efficacy and mechanism of action. *Br J Dermatol.* 2004;151(3):616–622. doi:10.1111/j.1365-2133.2004.06110.x.
9. Wiegell SR, Wulf HC. Photodynamic therapy of acne vulgaris using 5-aminolevulinic acid versus methyl aminolevulinate. *J Am Acad Dermatol.* 2006;54(4):647–651. doi:10.1016/j.jaad.2005.12.033.
10. Hong SB, Lee MH. Topical aminolevulinic acid-photodynamic therapy for the treatment of acne vulgaris. *Photodermatol Photoimmunol Photomed.* 2005;21(6):322–325. doi:10.1111/j.1600-0781.2005.00181.x.
11. Bryld LE, Jemec GB. The bacterial flora of the skin surface following routine MAL-PDT. *J Dermatolog Treat.* 2006;17(4):222–223. doi:10.1080/09546630600830570.
12. Gozali MV, Yi F, Zhang JA, et al. Photodynamic therapy inhibit fibroblast growth factor-10 induced keratinocyte differentiation and proliferation through ROS in fibroblast growth factor receptor-2b pathway. *Sci Rep.* 2016;6:27402. doi:10.1038/srep27402.
13. Boen M, Brownell J, Patel P, Tsoukas MM. The role of photodynamic therapy in acne: an evidence-based review. *Am J Clin Dermatol.* 2017;18(3):311–321. doi:10.1007/s40257-017-0255-3.
14. Zhang J, Chang Y, Liu S, et al. ALA-PDT promotes IL-1β secretion from human SZ95 sebocytes via activation of the NLRP3 inflammasome. *Photodiagnosis Photodyn Ther.* 2024;46:104007. doi:10.1016/j.pdpdt.2024.104007.
15. Willey A, Anderson RR, Sakamoto FH. Temperature-modulated photodynamic therapy for the treatment of actinic keratosis on the extremities: a one-year follow-up study. *Dermatol Surg.* 2015;41(11):1290–1295. doi:10.1097/DSS.0000000000000512.
16. Willey A, Anderson RR, Sakamoto FH. Temperature-modulated photodynamic therapy for the treatment of actinic keratosis on the extremities: a pilot study. *Dermatol Surg.* 2014;40(10):1094–1102. doi:10.1097/01.DSS.0000452662.69539.57.
17. Wiegell SR, Wulf HC. Photodynamic therapy of acne vulgaris using methyl aminolaevulinate: a blinded, randomized, controlled trial. *Br J Dermatol.* 2006;154(5):969–976. doi:10.1111/j.1365-2133.2005.07107.x.
18. Yung A, Stables GI, Fernandez C, Williams J, Bojar RA, Goulden V. Microbiological effect of photodynamic therapy (PDT) in healthy volunteers: a comparative study using methyl aminolaevulinate and hexyl aminolaevulinate cream. *Clin Exp Dermatol.* 2007;32(6):716–721. doi:10.1111/j.1365-2230.2007.02472.x.
19. Zhang J, Zhang X, He Y, et al. Photodynamic therapy for severe facial acne vulgaris with 5% 5-aminolevulinic acid vs 10% 5-aminolevulinic acid: a split-face randomized controlled study. *J Cosmet Dermatol.* 2020;19(2):368–374. doi:10.1111/jocd.13038.
20. Steinecke A. Study to evaluate the safety and efficacy of BF-200 ALA (Ameluz®) and BF-RhodoLED® in the treatment of moderate to severe acne vulgaris with photodynamic therapy in adults. Biofrontera Bioscience GmbH.
21. Divaris DX, Kennedy JC, Pottier RH. Phototoxic damage to sebaceous glands and hair follicles of mice after systemic administration of 5-aminolevulinic acid correlates with localized protoporphyrin IX fluorescence. *Am J Pathol.* 1990;136(4):891–897.
22. Sakamoto FH, Torezan L, Anderson RR. Photodynamic therapy for acne vulgaris: a critical review from basics to clinical practice: part II. Understanding parameters for acne treatment with photodynamic therapy. *J Am Acad Dermatol.* 2010;63(2):195–211. doi:10.1016/j.jaad.2009.09.057; quiz 211–212.
23. Itoh Y, Ninomiya Y, Tajima S, Ishibashi A. Photodynamic therapy of acne vulgaris with topical delta-aminolaevulinic acid and incoherent light in Japanese patients. *Br J Dermatol.* 2001;144(3):575–579. doi:10.1046/j.1365-2133.2001.04086.x.
24. Pariser DM, Eichenfield LF, Bukhalo M, Waterman G, Jarratt M, Group PS. Photodynamic therapy with methyl aminolaevulinate 80 mg g(-1) for severe facial acne vulgaris: a randomized vehicle-controlled study. *Br J Dermatol.* 2016;174(4):770–777. doi:10.1111/bjd.14345.
25. Hong JS, Jung JY, Yoon JY, Suh DH. Acne treatment by methyl aminolevulinate photodynamic therapy with red light vs. intense pulsed light. *Int J Dermatol.* 2013;52(5):614–619. doi:10.1111/j.1365-4632.2012.05673.x.
26. Alexiades-Armenakas M. Long-pulsed dye laser-mediated photodynamic therapy combined with topical therapy for mild to severe comedonal, inflammatory, or cystic acne. *J Drugs Dermatol.* 2006;5(1):45–55.
27. Kwon HH, Moon KR, Park SY, Yoon JY, Suh DH, Lee JB. Daylight photodynamic therapy with 1.5% 3-butenyl 5-aminolevulinate gel as a convenient, effective and safe

therapy in acne treatment: a double-blind randomized controlled trial. *J Dermatol.* 2016;43(5):515–521. doi:10.1111/1346-8138.13191.

28. Slutsky-Bank E, Artzi O, Sprecher E, Koren A. A split-face clinical trial of conventional red-light photodynamic therapy versus daylight photodynamic therapy for acne vulgaris. *J Cosmet Dermatol.* 2021;20(12):3924–3930. doi:10.1111/jocd.14359.
29. Kim TI, Ahn HJ, Kang IH, Jeong KH, Kim NI, Shin MK. Nonablative fractional laser-assisted daylight photodynamic therapy with topical methyl aminolevulinate for moderate to severe facial acne vulgaris: results of a randomized and comparative study. *Photodermatol Photoimmunol Photomed.* 2017;33(5):253–259. doi:10.1111/phpp.12312.
30. Sakamoto FH, Izikson L, Tannous Z, Zurakowski D, Anderson RR. Surgical scar remodelling after photodynamic therapy using aminolaevulinic acid or its methylester: a retrospective, blinded study of patients with field cancerization. *Br J Dermatol.* 2012;166(2):413–416. doi:10.1111/j.1365-2133.2011.10576.x.
31. Oyama J, Fernandes Herculano Ramos-Milaré Á, Lopes Lera-Nonose DSS, et al. Photodynamic therapy in wound healing in vivo: a systematic review. *Photodiagnosis Photodyn Ther.* 2020;30:101682. doi:10.1016/j.pdpdt.2020.101682.
32. Nicklas C, Rubio R, Cárdenas C, Hasson A. Comparison of efficacy of aminolaevulinic acid photodynamic therapy vs. adapalene gel plus oral doxycycline for treatment of moderate acne vulgaris-A simple, blind, randomized, and controlled trial. *Photodermatol Photoimmunol Photomed.* 2019;35(1):3–10. doi:10.1111/phpp.12413.
33. Liu L, Liu P, Wei G, Meng L, Zhang C. Combination of 5-Aminolevulinic acid photodynamic therapy and isotretinoin to treat moderate-to-severe acne. *Photodiagnosis Photodyn Ther.* 2021;34:102215. doi:10.1016/j.pdpdt.2021.102215.
34. Zhang L, Yang Y, Wang B, et al. Modified red light 5-aminolevulinic acid photodynamic therapy versus low-dose isotretinoin therapy for moderate to severe acne vulgaris: a prospective, randomized, multicenter study. *J Am Acad Dermatol.* 2023;89(6):1141–1148. doi:10.1016/j.jaad.2023.07.1023.
35. Seo HM, Min HG, Kim HJ, et al. Effects of repetitive photodynamic therapy using indocyanine green for acne vulgaris. *Int J Dermatol.* 2016;55(10):1157–1163. doi:10.1111/ijd.13258.
36. Park KY, Kim JY, Hyun MY, et al. 1,213 Cases of treatment of facial acne using indocyanine green and intense pulsed light in Asian skin. *Biomed Res Int.* 2015;2015:596161. doi:10.1155/2015/596161.
37. Jang MS, Doh KS, Kang JS, Jeon YS, Suh KS, Kim ST. A comparative split-face study of photodynamic therapy with indocyanine green and indole-3-acetic acid for the treatment of acne vulgaris. *Br J Dermatol.* 2011;165(5):1095–1100. doi:10.1111/j.1365-2133.2011.10472.x.

2

Photodynamic Therapy for Hidradenitis Suppurativa

Gabriela E. Beraja, Michael H. Gold

KEY POINTS

- There is no current cure for hidradenitis suppurativa (HS) and more treatment options are needed.
- Photodynamic therapy (PDT) may be employed in recalcitrant cases or when alternative modalities are unavailable.
- PDT minimizes disease activity and provides better therapeutic control over HS.
- PDT side effects must be considered during treatment implementation.
- Larger and more controlled clinical trials are needed to standardize our approach to treating our HS patients.

OBJECTIVES

- To understand the incidence and prevalence of hidradenitis suppurativa (HS) and the factors associated with the disease.
- To understand the proper staging of HS.
- To understand the current treatment landscape with the biologic group of medicines.
- To understand the history and role of photodynamic therapy in the treatment of HS.

INTRODUCTION

The chronic and relapsing nature of hidradenitis suppurativa (HS) and the negative impact on patient quality of life make it a therapeutic priority. HS commonly affects apocrine gland-bearing skin in the axillary, groin, perianal, perineal, and inframammary regions resulting from different genetic, environmental, and immunologic responses. Also known as *acne inversa*, HS affects the follicular epithelium and manifests clinically as painful inflammatory papules, nodules, or abscesses.[1] These lesions give rise to sinus tracts that act as a nidus for perpetual inflammation in the body. Early lesions of HS are often misdiagnosed for another disorder, making prompt recognition imperative to minimize progression.

This chronic inflammatory disorder has an estimated prevalence ranging from 0.05% to 4.1% with up to 42% of patients reporting a family history.[1,2] In European and North American populations, females are three times more likely to be affected, with over half of females reporting a flare with their menstrual cycle.[3] Between puberty and menopause is the most common timeframe for HS to arise.[4]

The etiology of HS is influenced by genetic, behavioral, and environmental factors. A smoking history has been linked to many HS cases along with obesity, polycystic ovarian syndrome (PCOS), and metabolic syndrome.[4,5]

Disclosures: Dr. Gold has worked in the past with several of the companies in the PDT space but has no current or recent disclosures to report.

TABLE 2.1 The Hurley Stages of HS

Hurley Stage I	Mild	Presence of single lesion or multiple abscess formation with or without sinus tracts and cicatrization
Hurley Stage II	Moderate	Recurring single or multiple abscesses in multiple areas with limited sinus tract and cicatrization
Hurley Stage III	Severe	Multiple interconnected lesions, with extensive sinus tract formation and scaring across an entire area

HS begins when a defective hair follicle becomes occluded and ruptures, inducing an inflammatory response that leads to abscess formation and the destruction of the pilosebaceous unit and adjacent structures.[6] These lesions give rise to sinus tracts that act as a nidus for perpetual inflammation in the body.

HS lesions affect skin in the axillary, groin, perianal, perineal, and inframammary regions. The impact of skin color in clinical presentation is important to note and can even be one of the reasons contributing to misdiagnosis. In light skin colors, erythema of papules and nodules are apparent, while those of darker skin colors may range from red-brown to dark brown, violaceous, or even gray. What remains constant is the firmness and tenderness of these lesions that may drain malodorous pus. Post-inflammatory hyperpigmentation tends to persist in darker skin colors but is still noticeable in light skin tones.

The Hurley staging system grades HS based on severity (Table 2.1): abscess (single or multiple) without skin tunnels and scaring (Stage I), recurrent widely separated abscess (single or multiple) with skin tunnels and scarring (Stage II), and diffuse skin tunnels and abscesses (Stage III).[4]

TREATMENT

Treatment modalities are aimed at reducing new inflammatory lesions from forming, treating current lesions, and avoiding psychologic impairment. Regardless of stage, patient education, support, and proper management of pain and comorbidities are imperative.

Hurley Stage I/Mild Disease

Topical clindamycin is typically tried on patients in early uncomplicated cases first before escalating to oral agents. Oral agents such as tetracyclines, antiandrogenic agents, and metformin can be used if initial therapy fails. The anti-inflammatory properties associated with antibiotics such as tetracycline help reduce bacterial load.[7] Patients with menstrual flares or who have PCOS may benefit from antiandrogenic drugs (i.e., oral contraceptives, spironolactone, and finasteride), while metformin may benefit patients with comorbid obesity.[8] Other options for mild HS include intralesional corticosteroid injections, punch debridement, and topical resorcinol, but data on the efficacy of these interventions is limited.[4] Incision and drainage of lesions may paradoxically promote recurrence and should be used sparingly.

Hurley Stage II or III/Moderate-to-Severe Disease

Unlike Hurley Stage I, oral antibiotics are used initially for moderate-to-severe disease with the addition of clindamycin and rifampin thereafter; however, long-term benefits are short-lived after treatment cessation.[9] Those patients with moderate disease who still do not reach satisfactory results can add oral retinoids, dapsone, metformin, oral contraceptives, and spironolactone. The use of biologics or performing wide excision is reserved for patients with a severe and refractory disease process.[4]

BIOLOGICS

TNF-Inhibitors

Adalimumab (HUMIRA)

Adalimumab (ADA) is the only biologic approved for the treatment of moderate-to-severe HS in adults and adolescents by the Food and Drug Administration and European Medicines Agency. This is ADA's ninth indication for its use in the United States, a commonly used human monoclonal antibody that targets soluble and transmembrane TNF-α.[10] In 2016 Kimball and colleagues[11] demonstrated its efficacy through two Phase III trials, PIONEER I and PIONEER II, followed by

Zouboulis and colleagues[12] in 2019 presenting the long-term efficacy and safety of ADA.

Infliximab (REMICADE)

In 2010 Grant and colleagues conducted the first assessment of infliximab, a chimeric monoclonal antibody that targets soluble and transmembrane TNF-α, for moderate-to-severe HS.[10] This randomized, double-blind, placebo-controlled crossover trial did not show a significant difference between the treatment and placebo groups after 8 weeks (i.e., there was not a ≥50% decrease in disease severity score); however, it did show statistically significant improvements in patient quality of life, pain, and physician global assessment scores.[13] Other studies include prospective studies,[14–16] pilot studies,[17,18] retrospective studies,[19–25] case series,[26–28] and case reports[29–52] that described the use of infliximab in patients with HS.

IL-12/23 Inhibitor

Ustekinumab (STELARA)

Positive data with the use of ustekinumab, a human monoclonal antibody that binds with high affinity to the p40 subunit of IL-12 and IL-23, is available in the form of prospective studies,[53,54] case review studies,[31,55–58] and small series.[56,59–64] In 2016 Blok and colleagues conducted an uncontrolled study involving 17 patients with moderate-to-severe HS. At week 40, this study found a 37% reduction in the modified Sartorius score in six patients, and a 47% reduction in the modified Sartorius score in eight patients after receiving 45 or 90 mg of ustekinumab at weeks 0, 4, 16, and 28.[54]

IL-23 Inhibitor

Guselkumab (TREMFYA)

Guselkumab, a human monoclonal antibody that targets the p19 protein subunit of extracellular IL-23, has shown efficacy in a proof-of-concept study, retrospective study, case series, and case reports in patients with HS.[65–71] On the other hand, a study in 2020 reported poor results.[72]

IL-1 Receptor Antagonist

Anakinra

Anakinra's success in the treatment of HS has been reported in a number of cases.[73–76] In a 24-week randomized trial of 20 adults with moderate-to-severe HS, six out of nine patients in the anakinra group (100 mg injections daily for 12 weeks) saw reductions in disease activity and prolongation of time between new exacerbations compared to only two out of ten patients in the placebo group showing improvement (100 mg identical placebo syringes for 12 weeks).[75] Anakinra's failure has been reported in a number of trials[77–79] and there are also reports of patients switching to anti-TNF due to relapse.[80]

IL-17 Inhibitors

Secukinumab

Secukinumab (SEC) is a human monoclonal antibody that inhibits IL-17A. In 2019 an open-label study reported that 67% of patients achieved Hidradenitis Suppurativa Clinical Response (HiSCR) endpoint; they were administered SEC 300 mg weekly for 5 weeks and then every 4 weeks for a total of 24 weeks.[81] Similarly, a 28-week open-label trial of 20 patients received SEC at weekly 300 mg doses followed by repeat doses either every 4 weeks or every 2 weeks with 70% of all patients achieving the HiSCR endpoint (i.e., at least a 50% reduction in the number of abscesses and inflammatory nodules and no increase in draining fistula or abscess count relative to baseline) after 24 weeks.[82] There were no serious adverse events in either study. SEC has also been reported to induce HS in a patient with psoriasis.[83]

Bimekizumab

The results from a phase 2 randomized trial suggest bimekizumab, which inhibits both IL-17A and IL-17F, to be of value for patients with moderate-to-severe HS. This study is the first to use a placebo control and an active reference arm of ADA and show a higher (57%) HiSCR than the placebo group (26%).[84] A number of other drugs such as PDE-4 inhibitors, C5A-inhibitors, and JAK inhibitors used for HS are outlined in another review.[85]

PHOTODYNAMIC THERAPY

HS varies clinically, and its multifactorial disease process makes the reaction to treatment heterogeneous, further increasing the need to search for new therapies. Photodynamic light therapy (PDT) has been demonstrated to be safe and variably effective for HS's acute and chronic phases. The combination of topical 5-aminolevulinic acid (ALA) or the methyl ester of ALA (methyl

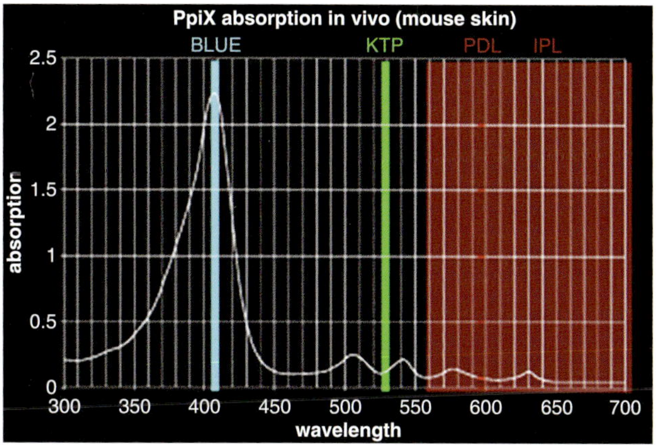

Fig. 2.1 PpIX absorption spectrum.

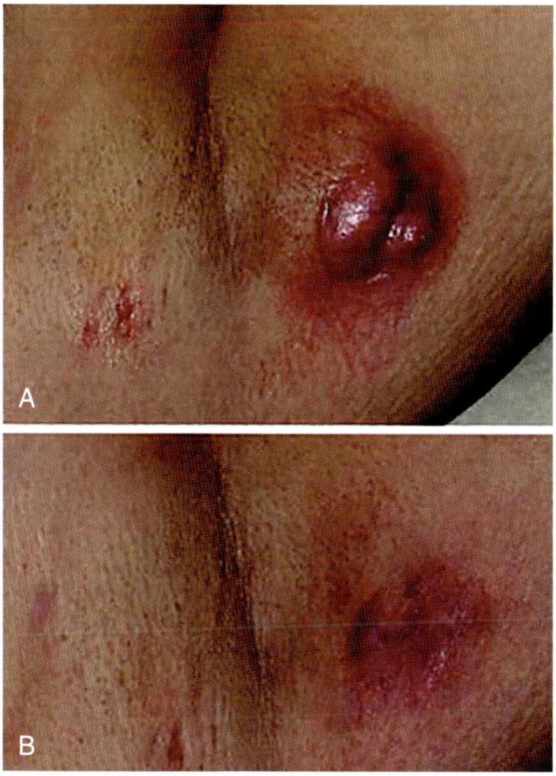

Fig. 2.2 Patient treatment with PDT for HS.

aminolevulinate hydrochloride [MAL]), coupled with the proper light source in the presence of oxygen has been shown to minimize the disease process.[86]

In 1990 Kennedy and colleagues presented the first porphyrin derivative, ALA. Once topically applied, this prodrug penetrates the stratum corneum, is absorbed by the pilosebaceous unit, and is then converted into its active form called protoporphyrin IX (PpIX). PpIX is photoactivated by lasers and light sources, which is the essence of PDT.[87,88] Fig. 2.1 shows the PpIX Absorption Spectrum.

Levulan Kerastick (Dusa Pharmaceuticals, a Sun Pharma company, Princeton, NJ) is available in the US, while Metvix (PhotoCure ASA, Oslo, Norway) and Metvixia (Galderma, Dallas, TX) are not.[87] Levulan Kerastick is the 20% 5-ALA solution, while Metvix and Metvixia are the 16.8% MAL solution. Levulan Kerastick is paired with a blue light illuminator, while Metvix and Metvixia are paired with a red light for activation. Both ALA and MAL have FDA approval for the treatment of nonhyperkeratotic actinic keratoses; all other uses are considered off label. Ameluz (Biofrontera) is another FDA-approved drug for AKs but has not been studied in HS.[86]

The first reported case of ALA and its success for HS was in 2004. Gold and colleagues observed the effectiveness of PDT therapy with a short-contact ALA and a blue light source in four patients who were not responding to standard therapy. The drug incubation time was between 15 and 30 min and roughly 18 min for blue light exposure. After three to four treatments at 1–2-week intervals, clearance was noted in 75%–100% of a total of four patients at the 3-month mark (Figs. 2.2 and 2.3).[86,89]

Two subsequent reports of ALA-PDT for HS showed inconsistent and variable efficacy. In 2005 Straus and colleagues reported their findings on four patients with

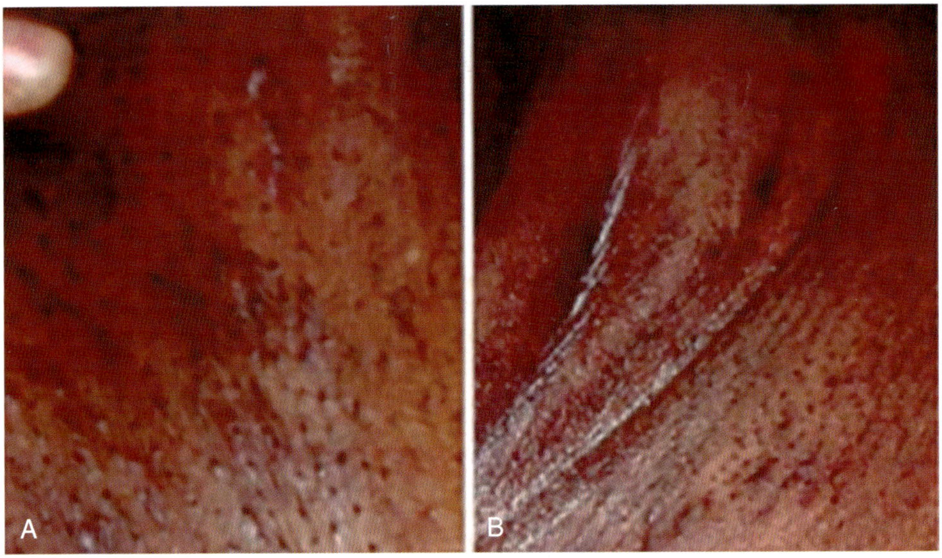

Fig. 2.3 Patient treatment with PDT for HS.

refractory HS. Topical ALA was incubated for 4 h, and local anesthesia was given to each site prior to light treatment. A CeramOptec diode laser (633 nm) was used in three patients and a broadband light source (570–640 nm) for one patient. Patients received three weekly treatments with an 8-week follow-up period. One of the patients received three treatments, two received two treatments with improvement in one but worsening in the other, and one patient did not complete the therapy due to severe burning and stinging reactions. These results were not enough to conclude PDT is useful for HS cases.[86,90] Sotiriou and colleagues also did not find significant improvement in HS lesions using ALA with red light after 3-h incubation of four treatments at 2-week intervals. The authors believe the permanent and deep scarring seen in long-standing HS may affect the penetration of topical ALA.[91]

Positive outcomes were reported by Rivard and Ozog in 2006 in two patients with HS treated with ALA and blue light. Topical ALA was incubated for approximately 1 h followed by blue light exposure. Either glycolic peels or vascular lasers were used in combination; the authors noted their patients improved but were not cured with PDT.[86,92]

In 2010 Guglielmetti and colleagues published a case report showing a decrease in inflammation and exudate between 90% and 100% after two sessions separated by 10 days using PDT-MAL with a red light source. These impressive effects were maintained at the 4-month follow-up with mild relapse in some treated areas at the 12-month follow-up.[93,94] In a similar case, Saraceno and colleagues observed the efficacy of PDT-MAL in the first case report of HS associated with pilonidal cysts. MAL was incubated for 3 h on the affected areas and then a red light source was applied. This method was repeated every 15 days for a total of nine applications and after a 6-month follow-up there was almost complete clinical remission.[95]

In 2011 Schweiger and colleagues reported their experience with ALA on 12 patients in an open-label, non-blinded study. Topical ALA was incubated for 45 min and then either a blue light (415 nm or 417 nm) or IPL (560–1200 nm) was utilized. Only nine patients completed the once-weekly PDT-ALA treatments for 4 weeks and followed up after another 4 weeks. The majority of patients noticed an improvement in their HS symptoms and three patients specifically noted complete clearing. Mean lesion size reduced by half at 4 weeks and around 30% by the 8-week follow-up; Global Severity Scores and Dermatology Life Quality Index scores also declined. Blue light therapy was better tolerated compared to IPL.[86,96]

In 2014 Navarrete and colleagues studied five patients with moderate-to-severe HS treated with PDT-ALA and a 635 nm light source. ALA was applied for 1.5 h followed by red light exposure for a total of four sessions at 1–2-week intervals with assessments at 4 and 8 weeks. This study supported the safety and efficacy of PDT for HS, as disease severity and quality of life considerably improved.[97]

Most recently, in 2018 Zhang and colleagues published a case report on the use of ALA and a 635 nm light source. After a total of nine treatments at a 10–15 day interval, the patient achieved resolution of skin lesions, ulcer healing, and disappearance of related symptoms.[98]

Intralesional treatments in HS are also utilized and are discussed in a recent systematic review.[99]

CONCLUSION

HS is a difficult disorder to treat as there is no current cure. ALA-PDT and MAL-PDT may be used when other therapies fail or may not be accessible. The studies discussed show that HS can be minimized and better controlled with PDT. Long drug incubation periods, local anesthesia, and red light therapy, however, are painful and can cause significant side effects when receiving treatments. The short-contact blue light therapy resulted in significant resolution of HS without discomfort.[100] Larger and more controlled clinical trials are needed to standardize our approach to treating our HS patients.

ACKNOWLEDGMENT

Editorial assistance provided by Angela Brown.

REFERENCES

1. Ingram JR. The epidemiology of hidradenitis suppurativa. *Br J Dermatol.* 2020;183:990.
2. Pink A, Simpson M, Desai N, et al. Mutations in the gamma-secretase genes NCSTN, PSENEN and PSEN1 underlie rare forms of hidradenitis suppurativa (Acne Inversa). *Br J Dermatol.* 2012;166:e32.
3. Wiltz O, Schoetz Jr DJ, Murray JJ, Roberts PL, Coller JA, Veidenheimer MC. Perianal hidradenitis suppurativa. The Lahey clinic experience. *Dis Colon Rectum.* 1990;33(9):731–734.
4. Mohammadi S, Gholami A, Hejrati L, Rohani M, Rafiei-Sefiddashti R, Hejrati A. Hidradenitis suppurativa; classification, remedies, etiology, and comorbidities; a narrative review. *J Family Med Prim Care.* 2021;10(11):4009–4016. doi:10.4103/jfmpc.jfmpc_795_21.
5. Breitkopf C, Bockhorst J, Lippold A. Pyodermia fistulans sinifica (akne inversa) und eachgewohnheiten. *Z Haut.* 1995;70:332–334.
6. van der Zee HH, Laman JD, Boer J, Prens EP. Hidradenitis suppurativa: viewpoint on clinical phenotyping, pathogenesis and novel treatments. *Exp Dermatol.* 2012;21(10):735–739.
7. Nazary M, van der Zee HH, Prens EP, et al. Pathogenesis and pharmacotherapy of hidradenitis suppurativa. *Eur J Pharmacol.* 2011;672:1.
8. Alikhan A, Sayed C, Alavi A, et al. North American Clinical Management Guidelines for hidradenitis suppurativa: a publication from the United States and Canadian hidradenitis suppurativa foundations: part II: topical, intralesional, and systemic medical management. *J Am Acad Dermatol.* 2019;81:91.
9. Caposiena Caro RD, Cannizzaro MV, Botti E, et al. Clindamycin versus clindamycin plus rifampicin in hidradenitis suppurativa treatment: clinical and ultrasound observations. *J Am Acad Dermatol.* 2019;80:1314.
10. Goldburg SR, Strober BE, Payette MJ. Hidradenitis suppurativa: current and emerging treatments. *J Am Acad Dermatol.* 2020;82:1061–1082.
11. Kimball AB, Okun MM, Williams DA, et al. Two phase 3 trials of adalimumab for hidradenitis suppurativa. *N Engl J Med.* 2016;375:422–434.
12. Zouboulis CC, Okun MM, Prens EP, et al. Long-term adalimumab efficacy in patients with moderate-to-severe hidradenitis suppurativa/acne inversa: 3-year results of a phase 3 open-label extension study. *J Am Acad Dermatol.* 2019;80:60.
13. Grant A, Gonzalez T, Montgomery MO, et al. Infliximab therapy for patients with moderate to severe hidradenitis suppurativa: a randomized, double-blind, placebo-controlled crossover trial. *J Am Acad Dermatol.* 2010;62:205–217.
14. Ghias MH, Johnston AD, Kutner AJ, et al. High-dose, high-frequency infliximab: a novel treatment paradigm for hidradenitis suppurativa. *J Am Acad Dermatol.* 2020;82(5):1094–1101.
15. Paradela S, Rodriguez-Lojo R, Fernandez-Torres R, et al. Long-term efficacy of infliximab in hidradenitis suppurativa. *J Dermatol Treat.* 2012;23(4):278–283.
16. Lesage C, Adnot-Desanlis L, Perceau G, et al. Efficacy and tolerance of prolonged infliximab treatment of moderate-to-severe forms of hidradenitis suppurativa. *Eur J Dermatol.* 2012;22(5):640–644.
17. Montaudie H, Seitz-Polski B, Cornille A, et al. Interleukin 6 and high-sensitivity C-reactive protein are potential predictive markers of response to infliximab in hidradenitis suppurativa. *J Am Acad Dermatol.* 2017;76(1):156–158.

18. Dini V, Oranges T, Rotella L, et al. TNF-alpha inhibitors and hidradenitis suppurativa: our clinical experience. *J Am Acad Dermatol.* 2016;74(suppl 5 1):AB9.
19. Kamal N, Cohen BL, Buche S, et al. Features of patients with Crohn's disease and hidradenitis suppurativa. *Clin Gastroenterol Hepatol.* 2016;14(1):71–79.
20. Van Rappard DC, Leenarts MF, Meijerink-Van't Oost L, et al. Comparing treatment outcome of infliximab and adalimumab in patients with severe hidradenitis suppurativa. *J Dermatol Treat.* 2012;23(4):284–289.
21. Sullivan TP, Welsh E, Kerdel FA, et al. Infliximab for hidradenitis suppurativa. *Br J Dermatol.* 2003;149(5):1046–1049.
22. Fardet L, Dupuy A, Kerob D, et al. Infliximab for severe hidradenitis suppurativa: transient clinical efficacy in 7 consecutive patients. *J Am Acad Dermatol.* 2007;56:624–628.
23. Fernandez Vozmediano JM, Armario Hita JC. Infliximab for the treatment of hidradenitis suppurativa. *Dermatology.* 2007;215:41–44.
24. Delage M, Samimi M, Atlan M, et al. Efficacy of infliximab for hidradenitis suppurativa: assessment of clinical and biological inflammatory markers. *Acta Derm Venereol.* 2011;91:169–171.
25. Oskardmay AN, Miles JA, Sayed CJ. Determining the optimal dose of infliximab for treatment of hidradenitis suppurativa. *J Am Acad Dermatol.* 2019;81(3):702–708.
26. Usmani N, Clayton TH, Everett S, et al. Variable response of hidradenitis supparativa to infliximab in four patients. *Clin Exp Dermatol.* 2007;32:204–205.
27. Moriarty B, Jiyad Z, Creamer D. Four-weekly infliximab in the treatment of severe hidradenitis suppurativa. *Br J Dermatol.* 2014;170:986–987.
28. Fougerousse AC, Reguiai Z, Roussel A, et al. Hidradenitis suppurativa management using tumor necrosis factor inhibitors in patients younger than 18 years: a series of 12 cases. *J Am Acad Dermatol.* 2020;83(1):199–201.
29. Ozer I, Karacin C, Adisen E, et al. Two diseases one remedy? Systemic amyloidosis secondary to hidradenitis suppurativa: treatment with infliximab. *Dermatol Ther.* 2017;30(2):e12445.
30. Groleau PF, Grossberg AL, Gaspari AA. Hidradenitis suppurativa and concomitant pyoderma gangrenosum treated with infliximab. *Cutis.* 2015;95(6):337–342.
31. Martin-Ezquerra G, Masferrer E, Masferrer-Niubo M, et al. Use of biological treatments in patients with hidradenitis suppurativa. *J Eur Acad Dermatol Venerol.* 2015;29(1):56–60.
32. Blazquez I, Gonzalez-Lama Y, Roustan G. Crohn's disease and hidradenitis suppurativa. An uncommon association that responds to infliximab. *J Crohn's Colitis.* 2013;7:e717–e718.
33. Bruzzese V. Pyoderma gangrenosum, acne conglobata, suppurative hidradenitis, and axial spondyloarthritis: efficacy of anti-tumor necrosis factor alpha therapy. *J Clin Rheumatol.* 2012;18(8):413–415.
34. Kozub P, Simaljakova M. Hidradenitis suppurativa treated with combination of infliximab and dapsone. *Bratisl Lek Listy.* 2012;113(5):319–323.
35. Von Preussen AC, Flux K, Hartschuh W, et al. Acne inversa successfully treated with infliximab. *Int J Dernatol.* 2012;51(8):1011–1013.
36. Husein-ElAhmed H, Fernandez-Pugnaire MA, Ruiz-Carrascosa JC. Severe hidradenitis suppurative in an HIV-positive male: use of multiple treatment modalities, including tumor necrosis factor blockade. *Aids Patient Care ST.* 2011;25(9):507–508.
37. Alecsandru D, Padilla B, Izquierdo JA, et al. Severe refractory hidradenitis suppurativa in an HIV- positive patient successfully treated with infliximab. *Arch Dermatol.* 2010;146(12):1343–1345.
38. Poulin Y. Successful treatment of hidradenitis suppurativa with infliximab in a patient who failed to respond to etanercept. *J Cutan Med Surg.* 2009;13(4):221–225.
39. Montes-Romero JA, Callejas-Rubio JL, Sanchez-Cano D, et al. Amyloidosis secondary to hidradenitis suppurativa. Exceptional response to infliximab. *Eur J Intern Med.* 2008;19(6):e32–e33.
40. Mekkes JR, Bos JD. Long-term efficacy of a single course of infliximab in hidradenitis suppurativa. *Br J Dermatol.* 2008;158(2):370–374.
41. Goertz RS, Konturek PC, Naegel A, et al. Experiences with a long-term treatment of a massive gluteal acne inversa with infliximab in Crohn's disease. *Med Sci Monit.* 2008;14(9):CS14–CS18.
42. Thielen A, Barde C, Saurat J, et al. Infliximab (REMICADE): a new treatment alternative for severe hidradenitis suppurativa. *J Invest Dermatol.* 2007;127(7):1813.
43. Thielen AM, Barde C, Saurat JH. Long-term infliximab for severe hidradenitis suppurativa. *Br J Dermatol.* 2006;154:1105–1107.
44. Rosi YL, Lowe L, Kang S. Treatment of hidradenitis suppurativa with infliximab in a patient with Crohn's disease. *J Dermatol Treat.* 2005;16:58–61.
45. Stipho S, Welch R, Feller E, et al. *Hidradenitis Suppurativa in Crohn's Disease Responding to Infliximab.* American College of Gastroenterology 69th Annual Scientific Meeting; 2004.
46. Lee CT, Dempsey J, Miller J, et al. *Hidradenitis Suppurativa: Response to Treatment with Infliximab.* American Academy of Dermatology 62nd Annual Scientific Meeting; 2004.
47. Massarotti E, Sobell J. *TNF-? Blockers for Hidradenitis Suppurativa.* American College of Rheumatology Annual Scientific Meeting; 2004.

48. Lebwohl B, Sapadin AN. Infliximab for the treatment of hidradenitis suppurativa. *J Am Acad Dermatol.* 2003;49(5):S275–S276.
49. Adams DR, Gordon KB, Devenyi AG, et al. Severe hidradenitis suppurativa treated with infliximab infusion. *Arch Dermatol.* 2003;139(12):1540–1542.
50. Roussomoustakaki M, Dimoulios P, Chatzicostas C, et al. Hidradenitis suppurativa associated with Crohn's disease and spondyloarthropathy: response to anti-TNF therapy. *J Gastroenterol.* 2003;38(10):1000–1004.
51. Katsanos K, Christodoulou D, Tsianos E, et al. Axillary hidradenitis suppurativa successfully treated with infliximab in a Crohn's disease patient. *Am J Gastroenterol.* 2002;97(8):2155–2156.
52. Martinez F, Nos P, Benlloch S, et al. Hidradenitis suppurativa and Crohn's disease: response to treatment with infliximab. *Inflamm Bowel Dis.* 2001;7(4):323–326.
53. Sánchez-Martínez EM, García-Ruiz R, Moneva-Léniz LM, et al. Effectiveness and safety of ustekinumab in patients with hidradenitis suppurativa using intravenous induction. *Dermatol Ther.* 2020;33(6):e14054.
54. Blok J. Ustekinumab in hidradenitis suppurativa: clinical results and a search for potential biomarkers in serum. *Br J Dermatol.* 2016;174(4):839–846.
55. Romaní J, Vilarrasa E, Martorell A, et al. Ustekinumab with intravenous infusion: results in hidradenitis suppurativa. *Dermatology.* 2020;236(1):21–24.
56. Montero-Vilchez T, Pozo-Román T, Sánchez-Velicia L, Vega-Gutiérrez J, Arias-Santiago S, Molina-Leyva A. Ustekinumab in the treatment of patients with hidradenitis suppurativa: multicenter case series and systematic review. *J Dermatolog Treat.* 2022;33(1):348–353. doi:10.1080/09546634.2020.1755008.
57. Valenzuela-Ubiña S, Jiménez-Gallo D, Villegas-Romero I, Rodríguez-Mateos ME, Linares-Barrios M. Effectiveness of ustekinunumab for moderate-to-severe hidradenitis suppurativa: a case series. *J Dermatolog Treat.* 2022;33(2):1159–1162. doi:10.1080/09546334.2020.1776208.
58. Gulliver WP, Jemec GBE, Baker KA. Experience with ustekinumab for the treatment of moderate to severe hidradenitis suppurativa. *J Eur Acad Dermatol Venereol.* 2012;26:911–914.
59. Sharon VR, Garcia MS, Bagheri S, et al. Management of recalcitrant hidradenitis suppurativa with ustekinumab. *Acta Derm Venereol.* 2012;92:320–321.
60. Santos-Pérez MI, García-Rodicio S, Del Olmo-Revuelto MA, et al. Ustekinumab for hidradenitis suppurativa: a case report. *Actas Dermosifiliogr.* 2014;105:720–722.
61. Eisen DB. Ustekinumab, another biologic with potential to help patients with hidradenitis suppurativa? *Br J Dermatol.* 2016;174:718–719.
62. Scholl L, Hessam S, Garcovich S, et al. High-dosage ustekinumab for the treatment of severe hidradenitis suppurativa. *Eur J Dermatol.* 2019;29:659–661.
63. Takeda K, Kikuchi K, Kanazawa Y, et al. Ustekinumab treatment for hidradenitis suppurativa. *J Dermatol.* 2019;46:1215–1218.
64. Cline A, Pichardo RO. Successful treatment of hidradenitis suppurativa in the setting of Crohn disease with combination adalimumab and ustekinumab. *Dermatol Online J.* 2019;25:13030.
65. Research Janssen, Development LLC. A phase 2, multicenter, randomized, placebo-controlled, double- blind, proof-of-concept study to evaluate guselkumab for the treatment of subjects with moderate to severe hidradenitis suppurativa. *ClinicalTrials.gov.* National Library of Medicine (US); 2000. https://www.clinicaltrials.gov/ct2/show/study/NCT03628924.
66. Casseres RG, Kahn JS, Her MJ, et al. Guselkumab in the treatment of hidradenitis suppurativa: a retrospective chart review. *J Am Acad Dermatol.* 2019;81(1):265–267.
67. Kovacs M, Podda M. Guselkumab in the treatment of severe hidradenitis suppurativa. *J Eur Acad Dermatol Venereol.* 2018;33(3):e140–e141.
68. Berman HS, Villa NM, Shi VY, et al. Guselkumab in the treatment of concomitant hidradenitis suppurativa, psoriasis, and Crohn's disease. *J Dermatol Treat.* 2021;32(2):261–263.
69. Kearney N, Byrne N, Kirby B, et al. Successful use of guselkumab in the treatment of severe hidradenitis suppuativa. *Clin Exp Dermatol.* 2020;45(5):618–619.
70. Jorgensen AHR, Holm JG, Thomsen SF. Guselkumab for hidradenitis suppurativa in a patient with concomitant Crohn's disease: report and systematic literature review of effectiveness and safety. *Clin Case Rep.* 2020;8(12):2873–2876.
71. Burzi L, Repetto F, Ramondetta A, et al. Guselkumab in the treatment of severe hidradenitis suppurativa, a promising role? *Dermatol Ther.* 2021;34(3):e14930.
72. Montero-Vilchez T, Martinez-Lopez A, Salvador-Rodriguez L, et al. The use of guselkumab 100 mg every 4 weeks on patients with hidradenitis suppurativa and a literature review. *Dermatol Ther.* 2020;33(3):e13456.
73. Hsiao JL, Antaya RJ, Berger T, et al. Hidradenitis suppurativa and concomitant pyoderma gangrenosum: a case series and literature review. *Arch Dermatol.* 2010;146:1265–1270.
74. Leslie KS, Tripathi SV, Nguyen TV, et al. An open-label study of anakinra for the treatment of moderate to severe hidradenitis suppurativa. *J Am Acad Dermatol.* 2014;70:243.
75. Tzanetakou V, Kanni T, Giatrakou S, et al. Safety and efficacy of anakinra in severe hidradenitis suppurativa: a randomized clinical trial. *JAMA Dermatol.* 2016;152:52.

76. Zarchi K, Dufour DN, Jemec GB. Successful treatment of severe hidradenitis suppurativa with anakinra. *JAMA Dermatol.* 2013;149:1192.
77. van der Zee HH, Prens EP. Failure of anti-interleukin-1 therapy in severe hidradenitis suppurativa: a case report. *Dermatology.* 2013;226:97.
78. Menis D, Maroñas-Jiménez L, Delgado-Marquez AM, et al. Two cases of severe hidradenitis suppurativa with failure of anakinra therapy. *Br J Dermatol.* 2015;172:810.
79. Russo V, Alikhan A. Failure of anakinra in a case of severe hidradenitis suppurativa. *J Drugs Dermatol.* 2016;15:772.
80. André R, Marescassier H, Gabay C, et al. Long-term therapy with anakinra in hidradenitis suppurativa in three patients. *Int J Dermatol.* 2019;58:e208–e209.
81. Prussick L, Rothstein B, Joshipura D, et al. Open-label, investigator-initiated, single-site exploratory trial evaluating secukinumab, an anti-interleukin-17A monoclonal antibody, for patients with moderate-to-severe hidradenitis suppurativa. *Br J Dermatol.* 2019;181:609.
82. Casseres RG, Prussick L, Zancanaro P, et al. Secukinumab in the treatment of moderate to severe hidradenitis suppurativa: results of an open-label trial. *J Am Acad Dermatol.* 2020;82:1524.
83. Marasca C, Megna M, Balato A, et al. Secukinumab and hidradenitis suppurativa: friends or foes? *JAAD Case Rep.* 2019;5:184–187.
84. Glatt S, Jemec GBE, Forman S, et al. Efficacy and safety of bimekizumab in moderate to severe hidradenitis suppurativa: a phase 2, double-blind, placebo-controlled randomized clinical trial. *JAMA Dermatol.* 2021;157:1279.
85. Amat-Samaranch V, Agut-Busquet E, Vilarrasa E, Puig L. New perspectives on the treatment of hidradenitis suppurativa. *Ther Adv Chronic Dis.* 2021;12. doi:10.1177/20406223211055920.
86. Gold Michael H. *Photodynamic Therapy in Dermatology.* Springer; 2011.
87. Gold MH. Photodynamic therapy: indications and treatment. *Aesthet Surg J.* 2008;28(5):545–552. doi:10.1016/j.asj.2008.08.007.
88. Kennedy JC, Pottier RH, Pross DC. Photodynamic therapy with endogenous protoporphyrin IX: basic principles and present clinical experience. *J Photochem Photobiol B.* 1990;6:143–148.
89. Gold M, Bridges TM, Bradshaw VL, Boring M. ALA-PDT and blue light therapy for hidradenitis suppurativa. *J Drugs Dermatol.* 2004;3(1 Suppl):S32–S35.
90. Strauss RM, Pollock B, Stables GI, et al. Photodynamic therapy using aminolaevulinic acid does not lead to clinical improvement in hidradenitis suppurativa. *Br J Dermatol.* 2005;152:803.
91. Sotiriou E, Apalla Z, Maliamani F, Ioannides D. Treatment of recalcitrant hidradenitis suppurativa with photodynamic therapy: report of five cases. *Clin Exp Dermatol.* 2009;34(7):e235–e236. doi:10.1111/j.1365-2230.2008.03094.x.
92. Rivard J, Ozog D. Henry Ford Hospital dermatology experience with Levulan Kerastick and blue light photodynamic therapy. *J Drugs Dermatol.* 2006;5(6):556–561.
93. Scheinfeld N. The use of photodynamic therapy to treat hidradenitis suppurativa a review and critical analysis. *Dermatol Online J.* 2015;21(1) 13030/qt62j7j3c1.
94. Guglielmetti A, Bedoya J, Acuna M, et al. Successful aminolevulinic acid photodynamic therapy for recalcitrant severe hidradenitis suppurativa. *Photodermatol Photoimmunol Photomed.* 2010;26:110.
95. Saraceno R, Teoli M, Casciello C, Chimenti S. Methyl aminolaevulinate photodynamic therapy for the treatment of hidradenitis suppurativa and pilonidal cysts. *Photodermatol Photoimmunol Photomed.* 2009;25(3):164–165. doi:10.1111/j.1600-0781.2009.00428.x98.
96. Schweiger ES, Riddle CC, Aires DJ. Treatment of hidradenitis suppurativa by photodynamic therapy with aminolevulinic acid: preliminary results. *J Drugs Dermatol.* 2011;10:381.
97. Andino Navarrete R, Hasson Nisis A, Parra Cares J. Effectiveness of 5-aminolevulinic acid photodynamic therapy in the treatment of hidradenitis suppurativa: a report of 5 cases. *Actas Dermosifiliogr.* 2014;105(6):614–617. doi:10.1016/j.ad.2013.10.016.
98. Zhang Y, Yang Y, Zou X. Photodynamic therapy for hidradenitis suppurativa/acne inversa: case report. *Photodiagnosis Photodyn Ther.* 2018;22:251–252. doi:10.1016/j.pdpdt.2018.04.014.
99. Cuenca-Barrales C, Montero-Vílchez T, Sánchez-Díaz M, et al. Intralesional treatments in hidradenitis suppurativa: a systematic review. *Dermatology.* 2022;238:1084–1091. doi:10.1159/000524121.
100. Gold MH. Aminolevulinic acid photodynamic therapy for hidradenitis suppurativa. *Dermatol Clin.* 2007;25(1):67–73. doi:10.1016/j.det.2006.09.002.

PART II

PDT for Pre-Cancer and Prevention

3

Conventional Photodynamic Therapy for Actinic Keratosis

Macrene Alexiades

KEY POINTS

- Topical photodynamic therapy (PDT) is approved for the treatment of actinic keratosis (AK) in the United States and European Union.
- Approved photosensitizers, including aminolevulinic acid (ALA) and methyl aminolevulinate (MAL), and light sources, including blue, red, and daylight are covered.
- Use as first-line therapeutic option for field cancerization is discussed.
- Off-label protocols including pretreatment with topical medications or procedures, short photosensitizer incubation, and alternative light sources are covered.

OBJECTIVES

- Learn the approved PDT protocols for AK.
- Understand the pre- and post-operative preparations, side effects, and complications.
- Recognize off-label PDT protocols and methods.
- Acquire knowledge of the relative therapeutic efficacy among PDT protocols and as compared to other approved treatments for AK.

INTRODUCTION

Photodynamic therapy (PDT) is the application of a light-absorbing compound photosensitizer, which selectively targets a subset of cells or tissues, followed by illumination with a paired highly absorbed wavelength, triggering a reaction that destroys the target. The term "photodynamic reaction" was used in 1900 to describe the effect of acridine orange dye plus light exposure triggering cell death in *Paramecia*.[1,2] The PDT reaction additionally requires the presence of oxygen; reactive oxygen species are generated leading to apoptosis and necrosis in the target.

Numerous photosensitizers and light sources have been used to photodynamically treat cutaneous and mucosal disorders. Systemic photosensitizers, mainly hematoporphyrin,[3] and broadband red and blue light have been utilized to treat cutaneous tumors.[4] The first FDA-approved photosensitizer was porfimer sodium in 1995 to treat esophageal carcinoma.[4] In 1999 the first topical photosensitizer, 5-aminolevulinic acid (ALA) was approved for cutaneous use, eliminating the adverse event of generalized cutaneous photosensitivity.[5]

The clinical efficacy of PDT as monotherapy, field cancerization, combined with topical therapies, laser assisted, and combined with various light sources such as daylight will be covered.[6–18] Meta-analyses have assessed the relative efficacy of PDT as compared to other approved treatment modalities, including cryotherapy, topical 5-fluorouracil, topical imiquimod, and topical diclofenac.[9–18] The clearance rates and efficacy of PDT are comparable to other approved modalities, maintaining its position as a first-line therapeutic option for AK.[6–18]

PRINCIPLES OF PDT

Light Absorption

To activate the PDT reaction, the absorption spectrum of the photosensitizer is matched to the wavelength of light. The penetration depth of the wavelength is matched to the target cells' location within the tissue. In the photosensitizer class generally employed in PDT, the porphyrin precursors to hemoglobin absorb light maximally from 360 nm to 400 nm (the Soret band) with smaller absorption peaks at 500 nm and 635 nm (the Q bands).[19,20] Once within the target cells, ALA is converted to protoporphyrin IX (PpIX) with two main absorption peaks at 417 nm (blue) and 650 nm (red). Tissue penetration depth increases in direct proportion to wavelength across the visible spectrum. The 50% penetration depth for 355 nm is 80 mm and for 694 nm is 1200 mm. Noncoherent light sources achieve less optical penetration due to scatter; however, they may achieve penetration up to 5 mm for 630-nm light and 1–2 cm for 700-nm to 800-nm light.[19,20] Broadband red and blue wavelengths are the main light sources used in PDT applications.

Photosensitizers

Topical ALA is typically paired with red and blue light, the latter FDA-approved for the treatment AK in 1999.[21] Multiple light sources and incubation methods have been utilized.[22,23] Methyl aminolevulinic acid (MAL) was approved with red light in the European Union (EU) in 2001 for the treatment of hyperkeratotic AK and basal cell carcinoma (BCC), and in the United States (US) in 2004 for the treatment of hyperkeratotic AK.[24,25] A nanoemulsion of ALA was approved with red light in the EU in 2011 for the treatment of AK and BCC[26] and FDA-approved in the US in 2016.[27]

Mechanism of Action

PDT involves the application of a topical photosensitizing agent over a target area, followed by light activation of the agent. The PDT reaction in the presence of oxygen generates reactive oxygen species, leading to apoptosis and necrosis due to irreversible oxidization.[28]

APPROVED PDT PROTOCOLS

The following are the current protocols approved for treatment of AK in the US and EU.

ALA Blue, Red, and Daylight Protocols

Topical ALA 20% solution with blue light is FDA-approved in the US for the treatment of AK on the face and scalp. ALA is applied to individual AK lesions, followed 14–18 h later by 10 J/cm^2 of blue light exposure with the Blu-U device.

Topical ALA 10% nanoemulsion gel with red light is FDA-approved in the US and licensed for use in the EU for the treatment of AK on the face and scalp. ALA is applied to AKs for 3 h followed by 37 J/cm^2 of red light exposure with the BF-RhodoLED lamp. In the EU it is also approved with 2 h of daylight.

The ALA 2 mg/cm^2 patch is licensed for use in the EU for the treatment of AK on face and scalp, applied for 4 h followed by 37 J/cm^2 of red light exposure with the BF-RhodoLED lamp.

MAL Red and Daylight Protocols

In the US, topical MAL 16.8% cream is FDA-approved for AK on the face and scalp following curettage with an incubation period of 3 h under occlusion with 37 J/cm^2 red light using the Aktilite, two sessions, 7 days apart.

In the EU, topical MAL 16.8% cream is licensed for AK of face/scalp following curettage of the lesion, cream application for 3 h incubation under occlusion with 37 J/cm^2 red light using the Aktilite, and two sessions, 7 days apart. It may also be illuminated with 2 h daylight.

Contraindications/Warnings/Precautions

Hypersensitivity to porphyrins or any component of the drug, porphyria, photodermatoses, and cutaneous photosensitivity at wavelengths used are contraindications. Safety in pregnancy is not generally established, and safety in pediatric populations 12 years and younger is not established.

Eye injury risk: Patients and healthcare providers must wear protective eyewear before operating light.

Photosensitivity: Protect treated lesions from sunlight exposure for 48 h post treatment.

Bleeding risk: Risk of bleeding may occur during lesion preparation in patients with coagulation disorders.

Ophthalmic adverse reactions: Avoid direct contact of photosensitizer drug with the eyes.

treatment sites to sunlight or bright indoor light during incubation.[31,32].

Step 5. Illumination. Remove the occlusive dressing, clean the area with saline and gauze. Position the lamp over the area to be illuminated so the distance between the LED panel and the lesion surface should be 50–80 mm (2–3.2 in).[34] The patient and operator should wear appropriate eye protection during illumination. The required illumination time (7–10 min) is calculated automatically, and remaining time displayed on the control panel. Each treatment field is limited to an area of 80 × 180 mm.

Step 6. Repeat treatment. Two treatment sessions should be administered 1 week apart.

Ameluz/Metvix(ia) and Daylight

Daylight is approved in the EU and Canada for AK with Metvix and additionally for field cancerization with Ameluz.[36] In these protocols, first sunscreen is applied and then lesion preparation and drug application are performed as aforementioned. Within 30 min of drug application, patients are exposed to daylight for 2 h.[36] Daylight is not FDA-approved in the US.

Step 1. Sunscreen application: Sunscreen is applied to the entire area to be treated. Wait for adsorption for approximately 15 min.

Step 2. Skin preparation: As above for Ameluz or Metvix.

Step 3. Drug application: As above for Ameluz or Metvix. Alert: No occlusion.

Step 4. Incubation: None or limited to maximum of 30 min.

Step 5. Illumination: Within 30 min of drug application, patients are exposed to daylight for 2 h.

Peri-operative Side Effects

Patients should be advised that transient pain, burning, or stinging at the target lesion sites may occur during the period of light exposure. The illumination may be paused and restarted.

Post-treatment Instructions

After light treatment, patients should wear a broad-brimmed hat and not expose themselves to sunlight or intense light for at least 48 h. Noncompliance can result in a severe phototoxic reaction.

Treated lesions that have not completely resolved after 8 weeks may be treated a second time with ALA photodynamic therapy. Regular patient follow-up is recommended.

Treatment Site Adverse Reactions

Levulan Blu-U: The most common local adverse reactions (AE) (incidence ≥10%) to Levulan and Blu-U are erythema, edema, stinging/burning, scaling/crusting, itching, erosion, hypo/hyperpigmentation, oozing/vesiculation/crusting, scaling, and dryness.

Ameluz and RhodoLED: Most common AEs include application site erythema, pain/burning, irritation, edema, pruritus, exfoliation, scab, induration, and vesicles.

Metvixia and Aktilite: The most common AEs (>1%) include skin burning/pain, erythema, scabbing/crusting/blistering/erosions, pruritus, edema, exfoliation, discharge, skin hemorrhage, skin tightness, hyperpigmentation.

Complications: Complications of photodynamic therapy include[37]:

- Short-term localized AEs, including pain, erythema, edema, pruritus, urticaria, contact dermatitis, erosive pustular dermatosis of the scalp, decreased delayed-type hypersensitivity responses.
- Systemic AEs, secondary to extensive ALA application including systemic absorption and systemic phototoxicity.
- Long-term AEs may include pigmentary changes and scarring including hyperpigmentation/hypopigmentation and rare incidences of bullous pemphigoid.
- Immunomodulation, including immunostimulatory and immunosuppressive effects, may be observed following PDT, which warrants further study.
- Carcinogenicity, including potential increased progression of keratoacanthomas, basal cell carcinoma, invasive squamous cell carcinoma, and melanomas, has been reported posttreatment with PDT.[36] The author reported a prevalence of biopsy-proven skin carcinoma in as high as 45% of non-responding lesions post-PDT, emphasizing the need to follow-up and perform evaluations on non-responding lesions.[22] The role of PDT in tumor progression has not been clearly defined and requires further elucidation.[37]

OFF-LABEL PROTOCOLS

AK

ALA Blue Light

Skin preparation variations. Skin may be prepared or degreased using a variety of methods to increase drug penetration or PDT efficacy. Acetone wipes, gentle curettage, pretreatment with urea, topical retinoids, or 5-fluorouracil have been tested and studied.

Light Dosimetry

- Levulan Kerastick: While the product labeling specifies a 14- to 18-h ALA incubation of ALA, this results in a greater incidence of unwanted AEs. Short incubation ALA was introduced by the author in 2003[22] and ultrashort incubation in 2017[38]; ALA incubations varying between 15 min and 3 h have been reported.[22,23,38] Short incubation has eliminated intense phototoxic reactions while maintaining satisfactory albeit lower AK clearance rates.[22,23,38]
- Ameluz: While the approved incubation time for this photosensitizer is 3 h, short incubation times of 1 h with red light and 30 min with daylight have been reported with satisfactory efficacy.[24]

Alternative Illumination Protocols

The application of alternative light sources to activate the PDT reaction includes lasers, intense pulsed light, broadband light sources, light-emitting diodes (LED), lamps, and fiber-optic illumination systems.[39] The most pertinent for the laser community include the following:

Intense pulsed light: IPL devices as a PDT light source have yielded significant results in patients with diffuse actinic damage.[40,41] When IPL is applied to PDT, short incubation of 1–3 h followed by long pulse duration and reduced fluence are recommended with improvements in AK clearance as well as photoaging, including telangiectasiae and lentigines.[39–41] Caution is recommended as post-treatment erythema and exfoliation are proportionate to the degree of actinic damage.

Pulsed dye laser: PDL has been used to activate PDT of AK, AC, acne, acne scars, lichen sclerosus, and vascular malformations.[19,20,42–46] Long-pulsed PDL (595 nm) is recommended at 10 ms pulse durations and moderate fluences of 5–7 J/cm^2 in two passes for actinic damage and acne/acne scars.[42] When using 585 nm PDL, shorter pulse durations of 1.5 ms have been employed (with purpura expected) for the treatment of vascular malformations such as port wine stains.[46,47]

Fractionated illumination: Discontinuous light exposure periods have been proposed to improve PDT efficacy by theoretically allowing for re-oxygenation between exposures. Published reports indicate superiority of fractionated illumination ALA-PDT for AK (94% vs. 85% at 1-year follow-up).[48] Interestingly, no difference in efficacy has been observed for MAL-PDT with fractionation, purportedly due to the differential localization of the drug.[24]

Daylight PDT (DL MAL-PDT, DL ALA-PDT)

Daylight PDT is performed with initial widespread application of sunscreen followed approximately 15 min later by lesion preparation, then nanoemulsion ALA or MAL to treatment area, without occlusion.[36]

Within 30 min of application, patients are exposed to daylight for 2 h with licensed approvals for AK and field cancerization.[36]

Alternative Clinical Applications

Actinic cheilitis: Approved PDT protocols of AC have demonstrated efficacy, as have variations with PDL and with the Alacare patch, which is available in the EU.[29,30] Long-term follow-up studies have shown a complete remission rate of 62% (3–30 months) and a histological cure of 47% (1.5–18 months) following PDT of AC.[49]

PUBLISHED CLINICAL DATA

Standard Protocols

The clearance rates for AKs of face and scalp using topical ALA or MAL-PDT-approved protocols of blue or red light range between 89% and 92% with quality of evidence I and strength of recommendation A.[6–9] Efficacy rates are lower for trunk and extremities and when using daylight PDT.[52] A photographic example of outcome for AK following ALA-PDT is shown for an individual AK lesion (Fig. 3.1) and as a field treatment (Fig. 3.2).

ALA Blue Light

PDT with topical 20% ALA at 14- to 18-h incubation times and blue light irradiation for the treatment of AK demonstrate complete response (CR) of 88% at 8-week follow-up; 89% at 3-month follow-up; and 78% after two treatments at 12-month follow-up.[6–8]

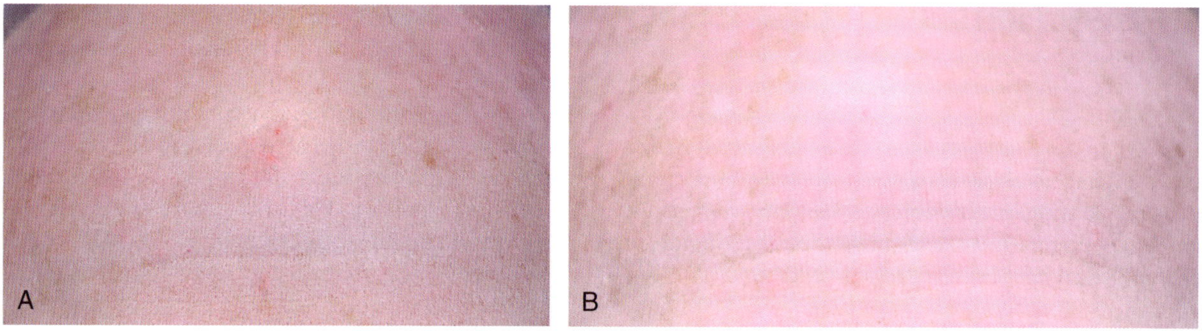

Fig. 3.1 Actinic keratosis treated with ALA-PDT. Patient prior to (A) and 8 weeks following (B) one session of ALA-PDT with Levulan and Blu-U. (Courtesy Macrene Alexiades MD, PhD.)

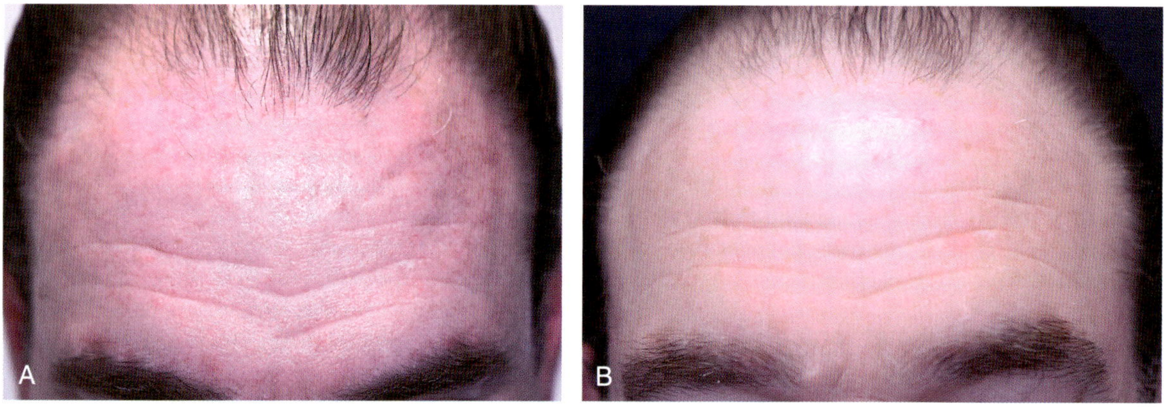

Fig. 3.2 Field treatment of AKs with ALA-PDT. Patient prior to (A) and 8 weeks following (B) ALA-PDT field treatment with Levulan and Blu-U. (Courtesy Macrene Alexiades MD, PhD.)

ALA versus MAL-PDT versus Cryotherapy versus Imiquimod

A meta-analysis of 2741 studies screened 15 independent randomized clinical trials with an overall sample size of 4252 patients and were analyzed.[9] Participant complete clearance, participant partial clearance, and lesion-specific clearance were the outcomes, with each assessed at least 12 months after the end of treatment. The outcome of participant complete clearance with ALA-PDT showed the most favorable risk ratio (RR) compared with placebo (RR 8.06; 95% CI, 2.07–31.37; grade, moderate), followed by imiquimod, 5% (RR, 5.98; 95% CI, 2.26–15.84; grade, very low), MAL-PDT (RR 5.95; 95% CI, 1.21–29.41; GRADE, low), and cryosurgery (RR 4.67; 95% CI, 1.36–16.66; GRADE, very low). Similarly, ALA-PDT had the highest RR for lesion-specific clearance (RR 5.08; 95% CI, 2.49–10.33; grade, moderate). This systematic review and network meta-analysis found that therapy including ALA-PDT, imiquimod, 5%, MAL-PDT, and cryosurgery was associated with significant long-term efficacy.[9]

Nanoemulsion ALA and MAL Red Light

A meta-analysis investigated PDT with BF-200 ALA and MAL by selecting eligible randomized controlled trials consisting of 5988 AKs, with a total of 2953 actinic keratosis lesions treated with BF-200 ALA and 3035 actinic keratosis lesions treated with MAL.[10] BF-200 ALA-PDT showed significantly higher overall complete clearance rates (RR 1.07, 95% confidence interval (CI) 1.02–1.12, $P = .01$) and 3-month complete clearance rates (RR

1.09, 95% CI 1.06–1.12, $P < .00001$) compared to MAL. A subgroup analysis was performed for BF-200 ALA-PDT, revealing increased complete clearance rates of grade II-III lesions in comparison with MAL (RR 1.24, 95% CI 1.05–1.46, $P = .01$). Compared with MAL, the pooled relative risk for the meta-analysis for recurrence was 0.67 (95% CI 0.48–0.92, $P = .01$) at 12 months after BF-200 ALA-PDT. PDT with BF-200 ALA was concluded to yield a 9% greater probability of complete clearance at 3 months and a 24% greater probability of complete clearance of grade II-III lesions after treatment as compared to MAL.[10]

PDT versus Cryotherapy, Imiquimod, and Diclofenac

A meta-analysis of PDT imiquimod, cryotherapy, and other methods compared treatment efficacy, adverse events, recurrence rates, cosmetic results, and complications.[11] Twenty-nine articles with 3850 participants and 24,747 lesions were included and quality of evidence was rated high. The efficacy of PDT was better in CR (lesions CR; RR 1.87; 95% CI 1.55–1.87/patient CR; RR 3.07; 95% CI 2.07–4.56), overall preference, and cosmetic results. Two groups showed no statistically significant differences in recurrence.[11]

A meta-analysis of PDT, cryotherapy, imiquimod, and diclofenac included eleven trials with a total sample size of $n = 4109$ AKs.[12] Three of the studies had an active-controlled design, while seven were single-armed. The lesion-specific clearance rate was only reported for PDT and was 74% (95% CI 56%–87%), which was lower than other reported trials.[12] Participant complete clearance following ALA-PDT was only reported for one trial at 33.6%, in contrast to 25.7% for cryotherapy, 23.5%–48.7% for diclofenac, 52.1% for imiquimod,[12] and 23.1% for diclofenac sodium 3% gel to 88.9% for ingenol mebutate 0.05% gel. The recurrence rate was lowest for ALA-PDT at 23.5%, and significantly higher for imiquimod at 82.6% and diclofenac at 90.7% (RR 1.10, 95% CI 1.02–1.1.8).[12]

PDT versus Cryotherapy

Only randomized PDT trials that used ALA or MAL with 10 or more participants were considered. Primary outcome measures were lesion response, cosmetic results, and patient satisfaction after the intervention. In total, 875 journal articles and meeting abstracts were screened and 13 studies were included in analysis, of which four were eligible for final meta-analysis. The only comparator for which meta-analysis was performed was cryotherapy; 641 participants, with a total of 2174 AKs treated with cryotherapy and 2170 AKs treated with PDT. Compared with cryotherapy, the pooled relative risk for the meta-analysis for complete lesion response was 1.14 (95% CI, 1.11–1.18) for PDT. Therefore PDT has a 14% greater likelihood of achieving complete lesion clearance than cryotherapy at 3 months after treatment for thin AKs on the face and scalp.[13]

PDT versus 5-Fluorouracil versus Imiquimod

A systematic literature review and meta-analysis to identify and qualitatively assess RCTsin immunocompetent patients with head AKs treated with field-directed, lesion-directed, and other therapies and quantitatively evaluate field-directed therapies (5-fluorouracil formulations, diclofenac sodium, imiquimod, ingenol mebutate, 5-aminolevulinic acid or methyl aminolevulinate plus photodynamic therapy) using complete clearance or partial clearance of actinic keratoses lesions, and adverse event-related withdrawals as a proxy of acceptability.

Of 2863 references identified, 75 trials reported in 151 publications were included. In summary, comparative network meta-analysis evaluation showed complete clearance rates of 16.59% for ALA-PDT; 8.71% for MAL-PDT; 22.58 and 22.84% for 5-fluorouracil 4% and 5%, respectively; 14.26%, 8.70%, and 6.93% for imiquimod; 5%, 3% and 2.5%, respectively; and 2.53% for diclofenac.[14] While 5-fluorouracil 4% and 5% formulations were the most efficacious, ALA-PDT ranked second and was superior to MAL-PDT and imiquimod.[14]

In a systematic review, 1186 studies were screened, of which 80 RCTs with 6748 patients were included in the analysis. The greatest degree of improvement was seen with PDT used adjunctively with other modalities, but was not significantly different compared to other treatments. PDT, cryotherapy, imiquimod, ingenol mebutate (IMB), 5-fluorouracil (5-FU), trichloroacetic acid (TCA), and ablative fractional laser (AFXL) were all non-inferior to one another in terms of percent clearance of AKs, but the lowest rates of clearance were seen with diclofenac sodium. When results were substratified by body site, 5-FU, combination PDT, and combination 5-FU with calcipotriol were the most beneficial for AKs on the head and neck, although they often caused the highest proportion of initial side effects.

Conventional versus Daylight PDT

A meta-analysis of RCTs to compare the efficacy and safety of daylight PDT versus conventional MAL-PDT in patients with AK included six RCTs with 369 patients and 5556 AK lesions for analysis.[16] The CR was not significantly different between the two groups (RR 0.93, $P = .07$). Subgroup analyses indicated that daylight PDT was non-inferior to MAL-PDT for CR in studies that only included grade III AK lesions (RR 0.97, $P = .41$), but less effective for CR in studies that also included grade III lesions (RR 0.87, $P < .001$). Daylight PDT was associated with a significantly reduced maximal pain score (mean difference = −4.51, $P < .001$) and lower risk of adverse events (RR 0.70, $P < .001$) as compared with MAL-PDT.[16]

Conventional versus Laser-Assisted PDT

Of 817 studies, seven RCTs were included in the qualitative analysis and four were included in the meta-analysis. Laser-assisted PDT showed significantly higher clearance rates than did PDT monotherapy (RR, 1.33; 95% CI, 1.24–1.42; $I^2 = 25\%$; $P < .01$).[14]

The author was the first to compare the safety and efficacy of ultrashort 15- and 30-min ALA incubations followed by blue light PDT with or without antecedent fractional CO_2 ($FxCO_2$) treatment in a split-face paired group comparison.[38] Ultrashort incubations yielded statistically significant AK CR of 69.23% after 15-min and 71.20% after 30-min ALA incubation. Pretreatment with $FxCO_2$ increased AK CR to 86.38% after 15-min and 89.78% after 30-min ALA incubation, with differences that were statistically significant as compared to paired controls. The findings reported here suggest that ultrashort incubations of 15 and 30 min followed by blue light are adequate for a PDT response and AK clearance; however, pretreatment with $FxCO_2$ greatly enhanced AK CR for both groups.[38]

PDT Combination Protocols

To investigate if PDT combined with a topical intervention is superior to monotherapy in terms of efficacy and tolerability, a systematic literature research was conducted of 1800 references initially identified; 10 RCTs with a total sample size of $n = 277$ were included. Four studies investigated a combination of PDT with imiquimod cream, three with 5-fluorouracil cream, and one each with ingenol mebutate gel, tazarotene gel, and calcipotriol ointment, respectively. Patients treated with a combination showed higher participant completion (RR 1.63; 95% CI 1.15–2.33; $P = .007$) and partial clearance rates (RR: 1.19; 95% CI 0.84–1.67; $P = .33$). Similarly, the lesion-specific clearance was higher for PDT plus topical intervention compared to monotherapy (RR 1.48; 95% CI 1.04–2.11; $P = .03$). A subgroup analysis was performed for PDT combined with imiquimod, revealing an increased participant complete clearance rate compared to monotherapy (RR 1.57, 95% CI 1.09–2.25, $P = .02$). The combination of PDT with another topical drug intervention did improve AK clearance rates compared to either monotherapy alone indicating that sequential application of two field-directed treatments represents a more effective approach in patients with multiple AK and field cancerization.

CONCLUSION

Topical PDT is a well-established and highly effective treatment modality for AK in the US and EU. Approved photosensitizers include ALA and MAL, while illumination options include blue light and red light in the US and additionally daylight in the EU. Off-label PDT protocols include skin preparation and incubation methods, including short incubation, and alternative illumination methods, including lasers, IPL, and fractionated exposures. PDT provides a well-tolerated option for field cancerization. Meta-analyses reveal comparable or higher lesional and complete clearance rates, and lower recurrence rates, as compared to alternative therapies such as cryotherapy and topical agents, supporting the classification of PDT as a first-line treatment of AK.

REFERENCES

1. Raab O. Ober die Wirkung fluorescierender stoffe auf infusoria. *Z Biol.* 1900;39:524–529.
2. Tappeiner HV, Jodlbauer A. Uber die wirkung der photodynamischen (fluoreszierenden) stoffe auf infusorien. *Dtsch Arch Klin Med.* 1904;80:427–487.
3. Meyer-Betz F. [Investigationofbiological(photodynamic) actions of hematoporphyrins and other derivatives of blood and bilirubin]. *Dtsch Arch Klin Med.* 1913;112:476 [In German].

4. Szeimies R-M, Dräger J, Abels C, Landthaler M. Chapter 1 history of photodynamic therapy in dermatology. In: Calzavara-Pinton P, Szeimies R-M, Ortel B, eds. *Comprehensive Series in Photosciences*. 2001;2:3–15.
5. Kennedy JC, Pottier RH, Pross DC. Photodynamic therapy with endogenous protoporphyrin IX: basic principles and present clinical experience. *J Photochem Photobiol B*. 1990;14:275–292.
6. Jeffes EW, McCullough JL, Weinstein GD, Kaplan R, Glazer SD, Taylor JR. Photodynamic therapy of actinic keratoses with topical aminolevulinic acid hydrochloride and fluorescent blue light. *J Am Acad Dermatol*. 2001;45:96–104.
7. Piacquadio DJ, Chen DM, Farber HF, et al. Photodynamic therapy with aminolevulinic acid topical solution and visible blue, light in the treatment of multiple actinic keratoses of the face and scalp— investigator-blinded, phase 3, multicenter trials. *Arch Dermatol*. 2004;140:41–46.
8. Tschen EH, Wong DS, Pariser DM, Dunlap FE, Houlihan A, Ferdon MB. Photodynamic therapy using aminolaevulinic acid for patients with nonhyperkeratotic actinic keratoses of the face and scalp: phase IV multicentre clinical trial with 12-month follow up. *Br J Dermatol*. 2006;155:1262–1269.
9. Steeb T, Wessely A, Petzold A, et al. Evaluation of long-term clearance rates of interventions for actinic keratosis: a systematic review and network meta-analysis. *JAMA Dermatol*. 2021;157(9):1066–1077.
10. Fu C, Kuang BH, Qin L, Zeng XY, Wang BC. Efficacy and safety of photodynamic therapy with amino-5-laevulinate nanoemulsion versus methyl-5-aminolaevulinate for actinic keratosis: a meta-analysis. *Photodiagnosis Photodyn Ther*. 2019;27:408–414.
11. Hu C, Luo X, Jiang C, Lei S, Sun Y. Efficacy and safety of photodynamic therapy for the treatment of actinic keratoses: a meta-analysis update of randomized controlled trials. *Dermatol Surg*. 2023;49(6):544–551.
12. Steeb T, Wessely A, Harlaß M, et al. A systematic review and meta-analysis of interventions for actinic keratosis from post-marketing surveillance trials. *J Clin Med*. 2020;9(7):2253.
13. Patel G, Armstrong AW, Eisen DB. Efficacy of photodynamic therapy vs. other interventions in randomized clinical trials for the treatment of actinic keratoses: a systematic review and meta-analysis. *JAMA Dermatol*. 2014;150(12):1281–1288.
14. Ezzedine K, Painchault C, Brignone M. Systematic literature review and network meta-analysis of the efficacy and acceptability of interventions in actinic keratoses. *Acta Derm Venereol*. 2021;101(1):1–8; adv00358.
15. Worley B, Harikumar V, Reynolds K, et al. Treatment of actinic keratosis: a systematic review. *Arch Dermatol Res*. 2023;315(5):1099–1108.
16. Mei X, Wang L, Zhang R, Zhong S. Daylight versus conventional photodynamic therapy for the treatment of actinic keratosis: a meta-analysis of randomized controlled trials. *Photodiagnosis Photodyn Ther*. 2019;25:23–28.
17. Steeb T, Schlager JG, Kohl C, Ruzicka T, Heppt MV, Berking C. Laser-assisted photodynamic therapy for actinic keratosis: a systematic review and meta-analysis. *J Am Acad Dermatol*. 2019;80(4):947–956.
18. Heppt MV, Steeb T, Leiter U, Berking C. Efficacy of photodynamic therapy combined with topical interventions for the treatment of actinic keratosis: a meta-analysis. *J Eur Acad Dermatol Venereol*. 2019;33(5):863–873.
19. Alexiades-Armenakas MR. Laser-mediated photodynamic therapy. *Clin Dermatol*. 2006;24(1):16–25.
20. Alexiades-Armenakas MR. Aminolevulinic acid photodynamic therapy for actinic keratoses/actinic cheilitis/acne: vascular lasers. *Dermatol Clin*. 2007;25:25–33.
21. U.S. Food and Drug Administration. Label for NDA 020965, 2018; Supplement 016. Retrieved from https://www.accessdata.fda.gov/drugsatfda_docs/label/2018/020965s016lbl.pdf.
22. Alexiades-Armenakas MR, Geronemus G. Laser- mediated photodynamic therapy of actinic keratoses. *Arch Dermatol*. 2003;139(10):1313–1320.
23. Touma D, Yaar M, Whitehead S, Konnikov N, Gilchrest BA. A trial of short incubation, broad-area photodynamic therapy for facial actinic keratoses and diffuse photodamage. *Arch Dermatol*. 2004;140(1):33–40. doi:10.1001/archderm.140.1.33.
24. Morton C, Szeimies R-M, Basset-Seguin N, et al. European dermatology forum guidelines on topical photodynamic therapy 2019 part 1: treatment delivery and established indications – actinic keratoses, Bowen's disease and basal cell carcinomas. *J Eur Acad Dermatol Venereol*. 2019;33:2225–2238. doi:10.1111/jdv.16017.
25. U.S. Food and Drug Administration. (2018). Label: Levulan Kerastick, NDA 020965/S-016. U.S. Department of Health and Human Services. Retrieved from https://www.accessdata.fda.gov/drugsatfda_docs/label/2018/020965s016lbl.pdf.
26. U.S. Food and Drug Administration. (1999). Drug Label for Ameluz, NDA 020965. U.S. Department of Health and Human Services. Retrieved from https://www.accessdata.fda.gov/drugsatfda_docs/label/1999/20965lbl.pdf.
27. European Medicines Agency. (n.d.). Ameluz: EPAR – Authorisation Details. Retrieved from https://www.ema.europa.eu/en/medicines/human/EPAR/ameluz#authorisation-details-section.
28. Electronic Medicines Compendium. (n.d.). Ameluz: Summary of Product Characteristics (SmPC). Retrieved from https://www.medicines.org.uk/emc/product/3158/smpc/print.

29. Radakovic S, Dangl M, Tanew A. 5-Aminolevulinic acid patch (Alacare) photodynamic therapy for actinic cheilitis: data from a prospective 12-month follow-up study on 21 patients. *J Eur Acad Dermatol Venereol.* 2020;34(9):2011–2015. doi:10.1111/jdv.16247.
30. Electronic Medicines Compendium. (n.d.). Metvix: Summary of Product Characteristics (SmPC). Retrieved from https://www.medicines.org.uk/emc/product/6777.
31. U.S. Food and Drug Administration. (2005). Drug Label for Metvixia, NDA 021415/S-001. U.S. Department of Health and Human Services. Retrieved from https://www.accessdata.fda.gov/drugsatfda_docs/label/2005/021415s001lbl.pdf.
32. U.S. Food and Drug Administration. (n.d.). Blu-U: Premarket Approval (PMA) Supplement P990019C. U.S. Department of Health and Human Services. Retrieved from https://www.accessdata.fda.gov/cdrh_docs/pdf/P990019C.pdf.
33. Galderma. (2018). Aktilite product information sheet. Retrieved from https://www.galderma.com/se/sites/default/files/inline-files/Produktblad_Aktilite_DK-NO-eng-2018_0.pdf.
34. National Library of Medicine. (n.d.). Ameluz - Drug information. DailyMed. Retrieved from https://www.dailymed.nlm.nih.gov/dailymed/drugInfo.cfm?setid=650daa9f-aeec-49ce-95b9-5fa20b988afd.
35. Galderma. (n.d.). Metvix product monograph. Retrieved from https://www.galderma.com/sites/default/files/inline-files/Metvix-PM-E.pdf.
36. Borgia F, Giuffrida R, Caradonna E, Vaccaro M, Guarneri F, Cannavò SP. Early and late onset side effects of photodynamic therapy. *Biomedicines.* 2018;6(1):12. doi:10.3390/biomedicines6010012.
37. Alexiades M. Randomized, controlled trial of fractional carbon dioxide laser resurfacing followed by ultrashort incubation aminolevulinic acid blue light photodynamic therapy for actinic keratosis. *Dermatol Surg.* 2017;43(8):1053–1064. doi:10.1097/DSS.0000000000001117.
38. Kim MM, Darafsheh A. Light sources and dosimetry techniques for photodynamic therapy. *Photochem Photobiol.* 2020;96:280–294. doi:10.1111/php.13219.
39. Alam M, Dover JS. Treatment of photoaging with topical aminolevulinic acid and light. *Skin Therapy Lett.* 2004;9(10):7–9.
40. Piccolo D, Kostaki D. Photodynamic therapy activated by intense pulsed light in the treatment of nonmelanoma skin cancer. *Biomedicines.* 2018;6(1):18. doi:10.3390/biomedicines6010018.
41. Alexiades-Armenakas M. Long-pulsed dye laser-mediated photodynamic therapy combined with topical therapy for mild to severe comedonal, inflammatory, or cystic acne. *J Drugs Dermatol.* 2006;5(1):45–55.
42. Alexiades-Armenakas M. Laser-mediated photodynamic therapy of lichen sclerosus. *J Drugs Dermatol.* 2004;3(6 Suppl):S25–S27.
43. Passeron T, Lacour JP, Ortonne JP. Comparative treatment of extragenital lichen sclerosus with methylaminolevulinic acid pulsed dye laser-mediated photodynamic therapy or pulsed dye laser alone. *Dermatol Surg.* 2009;35(5):878–880. doi:10.1111/j.1524-4725.2009.01148.x.
44. Channual J, Choi B, Osann K, Pattanachinda D, Lotfi J, Kelly KM. Vascular effects of photodynamic and pulsed dye laser therapy protocols. *Lasers Surg Med.* 2008;40(9):644–650. doi:10.1002/lsm.20673.
45. Yuan KH, Li Q, Yu WL, Zeng D, Zhang C, Huang Z. Comparison of photodynamic therapy and pulsed dye laser in patients with port wine stain birthmarks: a retrospective analysis. *Photodiagnosis Photodyn Ther.* 2008;5(1):50–57. doi:10.1016/j.pdpdt.2007.12.001.
46. Zhang B, Zhang TH, Huang Z, Li Q, Yuan KH, Hu ZQ. Comparison of pulsed dye laser (PDL) and photodynamic therapy (PDT) for treatment of facial port-wine stain (PWS) birthmarks in pediatric patients. *Photodiagnosis Photodyn Ther.* 2014;11(4):491–497. doi:10.1016/j.pdpdt.2014.06.004.
47. Sotiriou E, Apalla Z, Chovarda E, Goussi C, Trigoni A, Ioannides D. Single vs. fractionated photodynamic therapy for face and scalp actinic keratoses: a randomized, intraindividual comparison trial with 12-month follow-up. *J Eur Acad Dermatol Venereol.* 2012;26(1):36–40. doi:10.1111/j.1468-3083.2011.04003.x.
48. Yazdani Abyaneh MA, Falto-Aizpurua L, Griffith RD, Nouri K. Photodynamic therapy for actinic cheilitis: a systematic review. *Dermatol Surg.* 2015;41:189–198.
49. Tampa M, Sarbu M, Matei C, et al. Photodynamic therapy: a hot topic in dermatooncology (review). *Oncol Lett.* 2019;17:4085–4093.

4

Daylight Photodynamic Therapy for Actinic Keratosis

Nicole M. Golbari, William Driscoll, Christopher B. Zachary

KEY POINTS

- Daylight photodynamic therapy (dPDT) provides a convenient, well-tolerated, almost pain-free alternative to conventional PDT (cPDT).
- Randomized trials have demonstrated that dPDT protocols for the treatment of thin to moderate actinic keratoses (AKs) have similar efficacy when compared to cPDT protocols.
- "Painless PDT" protocols can be used in areas where dPDT is not as feasible year-round.
- While dPDT is most commonly used in the treatment of AKs and superficial non-melanoma skin cancers, it can be used in the treatment of acne, actinic cheilitis, and photoaging, and possibly in infectious diseases and more.

OBJECTIVES

- To describe the mechanism and uses of daylight PDT compared to conventional PDT.
- To outline the protocols approved for daylight PDT.
- To review the available data and reported uses for daylight PDT.

BACKGROUND

Since photodynamic therapy (PDT) was first approved by the United States Food and Drug Administration (US FDA) for the treatment of esophageal cancer in 1994, PDT indications have expanded to include not only other solid organ malignancies, but also precancerous actinic keratoses (AKs) and cutaneous field cancerization.[1] Indeed, PDT has been found to be very useful in the management of both malignant and benign dermatologic diseases and has been used in the treatment of acne, psoriasis, vitiligo, and even infectious conditions, such as verruca, tinea, and leishmaniasis.[2]

PDT requires the use of a chemical photosensitizer (5-aminolaevulinic acid [ALA] or its methylated ester [MAL]) which, once absorbed into the skin and converted to protoporphyrin IX (PpIX), interacts with light and oxygen to form cytotoxic free radicals. These free radicals target rapidly diving precancerous and cancerous cells, inducing phototoxic apoptosis, potentiating immune response, and causing vascular compromise and tumor-targeted hypoxia.[3,4] PpIX has the largest absorption (Soret band) at 405 nm, but also has four smaller absorption peaks between 500 and 640 nm.

Traditional or conventional PDT (cPDT) protocols require the photosensitizer to be applied under occlusion for 3 h (for MAL) to 14–18 h (for ALA) prior to light exposure.[5] Thereafter, the area is cleansed and patients are placed under a fixed light source. In the US, the most commonly used light source is blue light (410 nm), while in Europe a red light source that utilizes the approximately 635 nm PpIX absorption peak is more commonly employed. While effective, this cPDT protocol is often limited by significant side effects including stinging, burning, erythema, edema, and blistering, which can be severe enough to cause nonadherence, discontinuation of treatment, and refusal for future treatment.[6]

While the exact mechanism for PDT-associated pain is yet to be elucidated, it is hypothesized that the pain is secondary to the free radical reactive oxygen species created in the phototoxic chemical reaction. These free radicals cause both local tissue hypoxia due to the oxygen consumption in the process of free radical formation as well as direct nociceptor activation not only around target mitochondria, but also surrounding normal tissues.[7] Studies comparing shorter photosensitizer incubation times (1–2 h) to cPDT protocols have found similar efficacy in the improvement of AKs with a reduction in patient discomfort.[8]

In recent years, daylight PDT protocols, which employ a much shorter photosensitizer incubation (typically 30 min) followed by 1–3 h of outside sunlight exposure have been introduced with similar efficacy in AK reduction and minimal associated discomfort.[9–12] As daylight is not specific and includes potentially damaging ultraviolet (UV) light, UV-blocking chemical sunscreens are employed prior to sun exposure. The UVA- and UVB-specific sunscreens still allow light from the visible light spectrum to activate the photosensitizers. It is suspected that the shorter incubation time still allows for adequate cutaneous delivery of the photosensitizer as well as sufficient mitochondrial accumulation of PpIX in precancerous lesions without excessive production of phototoxic precursors in the surrounding tissues.[7] The daylight protocols also allow for continuous and steady generation and activation of the PpIX over the treatment time, without the accumulation of large amounts of cytotoxic precursors.

As sun exposure is less controlled than a fixed light source, studies have attempted to identify the adequate threshold for effective light dose for the treatment of AKs.[13–15] These studies have demonstrated that there is likely a certain minimum dose threshold for which dPDT is effective and that there is no dose-dependent increased benefit over this threshold. This dose, or PpIX-weighted radiant exposure, is typically measured over the duration of treatment and has been found to be between 3.5 and 8 J/cm^2.[16–18]

Although dosimetry is not routinely used in dPDT treatment, one study examined the PpIX light dose across six different countries at various latitudes over the time period of 6 months and found that at most latitudes effective dose (8 J/cm^2) was achieved in 2 h during all sunny days between July and September.[13] At lower latitudes, minimum doses could be achieved all year round. In this study, Wiegell and colleagues recommended that treatment be conducted at temperatures of at least 10°C (50°F) both for the comfort of the patient as well as to maximize production of PpIX, which decreases at lower temperatures. Additionally, the authors found that the light dose achieved on rainy or overcast days was about half that of sunny or partially sunny days. Nevertheless, effective light dose was still achieved in 2 h on rainy days at the higher measured altitudes (59°55′N) during the summer months. While the UV Index may be helpful in determining if there might be adequate sunlight on a given day, the UV index is not precise, and it is instead suggested that clinicians use time of year, temperature, and weather to determine if dPDT would be appropriate on a given day.[13]

In environments or at latitudes where daylight PDT may be more difficult to perform year-round, "painless PDT" or "gentle PDT" protocols, wherein photosensitizer is applied with immediate direct illumination under fixed light source provide an equally effective alternative to dPDT protocols for the treatment of AKs.[19–21]

PROTOCOLS

Approved EU versus US

In the US, three photosensitizers have been approved for use with cPDT protocols for the treatment of AKs (Table 4.1): Ameluz (10% ALA gel) used in conjunction with BF-RhodoLED red light lamp, Levulan (20% ALA solution) used with BLU-U Blue Light illuminator, and Metvixia (16.8% MAL cream) with Aktilite CL128 red light lamp. While FDA approved in 2004, Metvixia production has since been discontinued in the US. All on-label FDA-approved protocols currently require use of a standard fixed light source.

In Europe, there are license approvals for dPDT with the use of Metvix for the treatment of mild to moderate AKs and Ameluz for the treatment of mild to moderate AKs of the face and scalp as well as field cancerization.[22] Both protocols require treatment to be performed on dry days with temperatures greater than 10°C. Treatment starts with the application of organic sunscreen until dry, followed by cleansing of lesions and removal of all scales and crusts. Then photosensitizer is applied

TABLE 4.1 **FDA-Approved Photosensitizers and their Indications**

Photosensitizer	Composition	Incubation Time	Light Source	Treatment Time	FDA Approved Indication
Ameluz	10% ALA gel	3 h	BF-RhodoLED red light lamp	10 min	actinic keratoses of mild-to-moderate severity on the face and scalp
Levulan	20% ALA solution	14–18 h for scalp or face 3 h for upper extremities, with occlusion	BLU-U Blue Light illuminator	A 1000 s (16 min 40 s)	minimally to moderately thick actinic keratoses of the face or scalp, or actinic keratoses of the upper extremities
Metvixia	16.8% MAL cream	at least 2.5 h, but no more than 4 h	Aktilite CL128 red light lamp	7–10 min	thin and moderately thick, non-hyperkeratotic, non-pigmented actinic keratoses of the face and scalp

TABLE 4.2 **Summary of Reported Daylight Photodynamic Therapy Protocols in the United States**

Location	Photosensitizer	Incubation Time	Daylight Exposure Time	3-Month Reduction in AK
Northern California[12]	20% ALA solution	15 min	1 h	61.8%
Southern California[23]	20% ALA solution	60 min	2 h	Not reported
Southern California[24]	20% ALA solution	30 min	2 h	81%

to treatment areas without occlusion and patients are exposed to 2 h of sunlight within 30 min of photosensitizer application.

Unapproved

Although not currently included in the FDA-approved protocol, use of dPDT has been reported in Northern and Southern California (Table 4.2).[12,23,24] Chemical sunscreen was applied after photosensitizer application, but prior to sun exposure in both Southern California reports. While incubation and daylight exposure time varied across the studies, all reported low pain, high satisfaction, and improvement in Aks (Fig. 4.1).

Although dPDT is employed widely across the international community, US clinicians appear to have more hesitation to adopt dPDT protocols. One reason may be due to the lack of direct supervision during treatment course and possible risk of light overexposure and phototoxicity (Fig. 4.2). Another reason may be due to a lack of available clear US consensus, guidelines, and FDA-approved protocol. Nevertheless, the authors in the US report low rates of nonadherence and adverse reactions associated with dPDT.[12]

CLINICAL RESULTS

Clinical trials comparing dPDT to cPDT have widely found dPDT to be as effective, yet significantly less painful and more tolerable than cPDT. All but one randomized study found dPDT to be non-inferior to cPDT

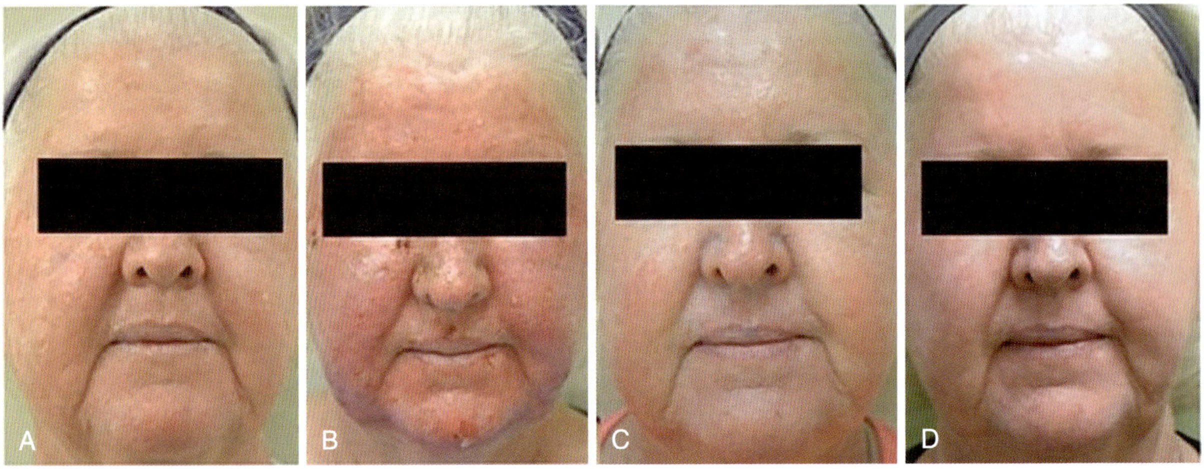

Fig. 4.1 Photographs of a patient at day 0 prior to dPDT treatment (A), day 3 (B), 1 month (C), and 3 months (D) after treatment.

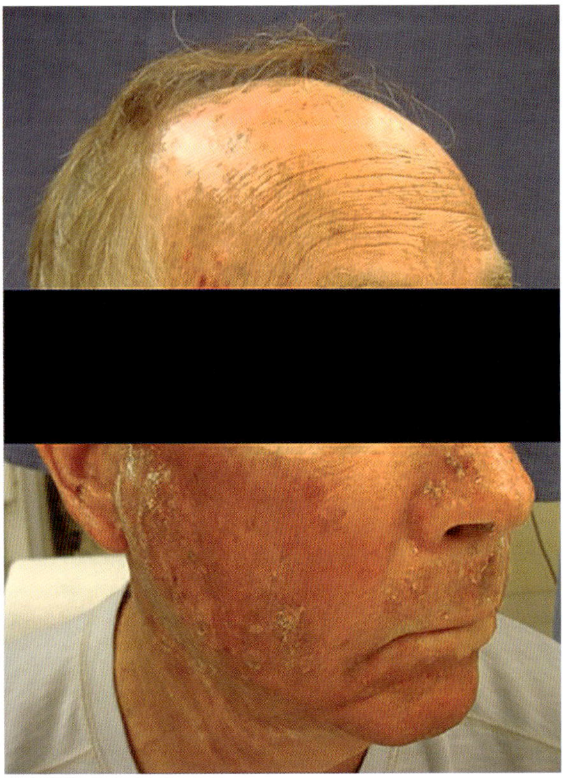

Fig. 4.2 Patient with exuberant reaction after dPDT treatment. Patient failed to follow instructions to avoid sunlight exposure 24–48 h after treatment.

with regard to lesion clearance (Table 4.3).[9–11,24–27] Some studies also found decreased rates of other local cutaneous response (e.g., edema, crusting) with dPDT as compared to cPDT.[28]

In one split-face head-to-head study comparing the efficacy of cPDT versus dPDT for the treatment of AKs on the scalp, it was found that there was no significant difference in the reduction of AK lesion count (79% vs. 71% reduction dPDT and cPDT, respectively).[27] While cPDT was associated with significantly more pain than daylight PDT, both protocols were associated with erythema and crusting post-treatment. The same group later compared daylight exposure times and found that 1.5 h was as effective as 2.5 h of exposure time.[29] However, the group did find that dPDT was not as effective for grade III and grade II thickness AKs as compared to grade I, or thin AKs (49.1%, 61.2%, and 75.9% AK clearance rate at 3 months, respectively).[15]

Unsurprisingly, one large multicenter study looking at not only outcomes, but also clinician and patient satisfaction with treatment found that 90.3% of clinicians and 80.4% of patients reported satisfaction with dPDT protocol with a 90.0% of patients reporting that they would consider using dPDT again in the future.[30] While multiple successive treatments have been suggested to improve efficacy of dPDT, one study comparing one versus two treatment(s) of dPDT separated 1 week apart found no significant

TABLE 4.3 Summary of Reported Trials Comparing Daylight and Conventional Photodynamic Therapy

Study	Location	Design	Photosensitizer	Incubation	Daylight Exposure	AK % Clearance	Pain Score
Zhu et al.[25]	Shanghai, China	Randomized, prospective	10% ALA Cream	30 min	2h (repeated every 2 weeks x3)	At 1 month: dPDT – 95.5% cPDT – 96.8%	dPDT – 1.7 cPDT – 5.2 $P < .05$
Lacour et al.[10]	Europe (multicenter)	RCT, split-person	16.8% MAL Cream	≤30 min	2 h	At 12 weeks dPDT – 70% cPDT – 74%	dPDT – 0.7 cPDT – 4.4 $P < .001$
Crow et al.[24]	San Francisco, USA	RCT	20% ALA Solution	15 min	1 h	At Day 84 dPDT – 63.9% cPDT – 61.8%	ΔVAS = –3.4 dPDT compared to cPDT $P < .0001$
Wiegell et al.[27]	Copenhagen, Denmark	RCT, split-person	16.8% MAL Cream	30 min	2.5 h	At 3 months dPDT – 79% cPDT – 71%	dPDT – 2.0 cPDT – 6.7 $P < .0001$
Rubel et al.[9]	Australia	RCT, split-person	16.8% MAL Cream	30 min	2 h	At 12 weeks dPDT – 89.2% cPDT – 92.8%	dPDT – 0.8 cPDT – 5.7 $P < .001$
Neittaanmäki-Perttu et al.[11]	Helsinki, Finland	Randomized, prospective	16.8% MAL Cream	30 min	2 h	At 6 months dPDT – 72.4% cPDT – 89.2% $p = 0.0025$	Not reported
Fargnoli et al.[26]	L'Aquila, Italy	Prospective, split-person	16.8% MAL Cream	30 min	2 h	At 3 months dPDT – 87% cPDT – 91%	ΔVAS = –2.2 dPDT compared to cPDT $P < .01$
Sotiriou et al.[28]	Greece	RCT, split-person	16.8% MAL Cream	30 min	2 h	At 3 months dPDT – 78% cPDT – 80.6%	dPDT – 1.14 cPDT – 6.06 $P = 0$

difference in AK clearance rate between a single versus multiple treatments (80.7% vs. 85.6%, respectively $P = .28$).[31] Studies comparing dPDT with ALA versus MAL have suggested that ALA may be more effective than MAL for the clearance of thin AKs.[32] One study found that clearance rates were higher for grade I AKs treated with ALA ($P = .027$), but similar resolution rates for higher grade AKs ($P = .564$).[11] No differences were reported in pain or adverse reactions. Another study found similar rates of clearance at 12 weeks, but higher rates of recurrence in MAL dPDT-treated patients (31.6%) as compared to ALA dPDT-treated patients (19.9%).

There have also been studies looking at combining dPDT with other treatments. One study evaluated the efficacy of MAL dPDT in combination with diclofenac 3% in 2.5% hyaluronic acid (DHA).[33] The study found no difference in AK clearance efficacy but reported that MAL dPDT + DHA had reduced inflammation and skin reaction scores as compared to the MAL dPDT alone group. Another study examined the effect of calcipotriol ointment pretreatment.[34] This split-face design study found that although pretreatment with 15 days of once-daily calcipotriol ointment was associated with better rates of clearance at 3 months (85% vs. 70%) with dPDT alone; patients experienced higher rates of erythema and desquamation, and overall, preferred dPDT alone to calcipotriol/dPDT. Lastly, another split-face study comparing dPDT pretreatment microdermabrasion and ablative fractional laser found that ablative fractional laser had higher rates of AK clearance, improved skin texture and dyspigmentation, and higher rates of patient satisfaction, despite also being associated with more immediate morbidity (more intense skin reaction and post-treatment infection rates).[35] Treatment of arms and legs is dramatically enhanced with fractionated Er:YAG laser prior to application of ALA; low-density scans of intraepidermal vaporization (20–30 μm) with 15- to 20-min incubation will increase the absorption of these topical agents thus increasing the efficacy of PDT, daylight or otherwise.

OTHER USES

Skin Cancer

While there are currently no approvals for the use of dPDT for the treatment of skin cancer, there have been studies of the use of dPDT to treat squamous cell carcinoma in situ (SCCis) and basal cell carcinoma (BCC). In one study of treatment of SCCis with dPDT, two treatment sessions were given 1 week apart, with each treatment session consisting of MAL administration followed by 2 h of sunlight.[36] The treatment yielded complete clinical response for 25% of lesions, with another 33% showing more than 75% partial response, and patients reporting minimal pain during treatment. There were, however, fewer cases of complete response versus cPDT, indicating that cPDT might still be generally preferred for SCCis.

This general recommendation for cPDT can be considered within the context of a particular clinical scenario, however, as shown in a case study of a SCCis patient with extensive erosive scalp lesions who requested dPDT rather than cPDT due to concerns about associated pain.[37] Three months after MAL dPDT treatment, the patient achieved complete healing with good cosmetic results, which persisted at a 9-month follow-up, indicating dPDT as an important and reasonable alternative to cPDT in cases of extensive lesions and/or patient preference.

A study of treatment of BCC with MAL dPDT showed response rates and recurrence rates comparable to cPDT, with pain-free results and good or excellent cosmetic outcomes.[38] At 3 months, 94% of lesions showed complete response, with a 21% recurrence rate at 12 months. The mean effective light dose was 10.8 J/cm^2 during 152 min of daylight exposure.

Additionally, dPDT can be considered in combination therapy for the treatment of non-melanoma skin cancer. One study compared the efficacy of MAL dPDT alone versus in combination with 5% topical imiquimod cream (TIC) for treating superficial BCCs.[39] Patients treated with MAL dPDT plus TIC showed a significantly higher clearance rate (91.3%) at 12 months compared to those treated with MAL dPDT alone (83.4%, $P = .01$). Furthermore, the combination therapy demonstrated superior efficacy in patients with multiple lesions and/or eroded lesions. However, combination treatments may be limited by side effect profile. Local skin reactions were generally mild with MAL dPDT alone, but increased with the addition of TIC, especially when the recommended interval between treatments was not observed. Female patients exhibited a better clinical response to the combined therapy ($P \leq .01$).

Photoaging

Photoaging due to chronic sun exposure is another possible use for dPDT. An international expert group defined the concept of actinic field damage as "photodamage associated with actinic epidermal dysplasia"—damage that can include wrinkles, telangiectasias, and erythema—and posited dPDT as a "complementary and convenient treatment option to already existing rejuvenation procedures for patients with actinic field damage."[40]

Multiple studies have evaluated the impact of dPDT on signs of non-AK photoaging, even as the primary purpose of the dPDT was the treatment of actinic keratoses. One found improvements to photodamage, mottled pigmentation, roughness, and sallowness—with additional improvements to fine lines, erythema, and coarse wrinkles in regions of skin treated with both MAL dPDT and microneedling.[41] Another noted a reduction in lentigines and other signs of aging in patients treated for AKs with either ALA or MAL dPDT.[23]

One study assessed the efficacy of dPDT specifically for non-AK photodamage, with results suggesting marked improvement for sallowness and tactile roughness, as well as some improvement to fine lines, mottled pigmentation, erythema, and coarse lines. cPDT has been reported to have similarly positive impacts on most of these features of photoaging, although not erythema, possibly due to differences in light source.[42]

Actinic Cheilitis

Multiple studies have also examined the use of dPDT in the management of actinic cheilitis (AC). In one study, 22 individuals with histologically confirmed AC underwent two sessions of MAL dPDT 1 week apart.[43] Results showed a complete clinical response in 80% of patients after 12 months, with 100% response rate observed for grade I AC and a 50% response rate for grade II AC. Adverse events were mild and transient, with no significant pain reported. A similar study repeated MAL dPDT sessions every 2–4 weeks until clinical remission was achieved or considered improbable.[44] The cure rate was 91%, and the median number of treatments to achieve remission was two.

A systematic review directly comparing cPDT (using MAL or ALA) with MAL dPDT interestingly found not only a higher number of patients reporting a painless experience (87.1% in the dPDT vs. 31.25% in the cPDT) and a lower incidence of local phototoxicity (0% in the dPDT vs. 47.78% in the cPDT), but also found superior complete clinical response rates for dPDT (76.74% vs. 65.14%).[45] The review only surfaced seven patients, however, who had dPDT responses confirmed with histopathology, versus 85 patients for cPDT.

Acne

As with cPDT, dPDT has also been shown to be effective in the treatment of acne vulgaris. Treatment for acne requires multiple treatments spaced 1–4 weeks apart (Fig. 4.3). *Cutibacterium acnes* produces endogenous porphyrins as part of normal metabolic and reproductive processes. PpIX photosensitizer accumulates in the pilosebaceous units and activation leads to the generation of reactive oxygen species, destruction of *C. acnes* cell wall lipids, and damage to the pilosebaceous unit. A double-blind randomized controlled trial, for example, found ALA dPDT to reduce the incidence of both inflammatory and noninflammatory acne lesions by 58.0% and 34.1%, respectively, after 12 weeks of treatment, suggesting its viability for acne therapy.[46] Another study showed similarly positive results, with a 69% reduction in inflammatory lesions at first follow-up.[47]

The results of a direct, split-face comparison between cPDT and dPDT for acne were in keeping with the theme of such comparisons for other conditions: Results were either similar or slightly in favor of dPDT for reductions in comedones, nodules, papules, and pustules, with dPDT offering superior tolerability and fewer adverse effects.[48] Concurrent treatment with a fractional, nonablative laser has been shown to improve results in dPDT for acne—with a lesion-count reduction of 51.8% versus 36.0% for dPDT alone in one comparative study—possibly due to increased absorption of the photosensitizing agent.[49]

Infections

Cutaneous infection treatment is another potential use for dPDT. In warts, for example, treatment with dPDT was compared to treatment with cPDT for the treatment of recalcitrant facial flat warts caused by HPV, with both treatment groups demonstrating similarly positive results (73.3% "excellent response" for cPDT vs. 80% for dPDT).[50] A similar success rate (65%) was

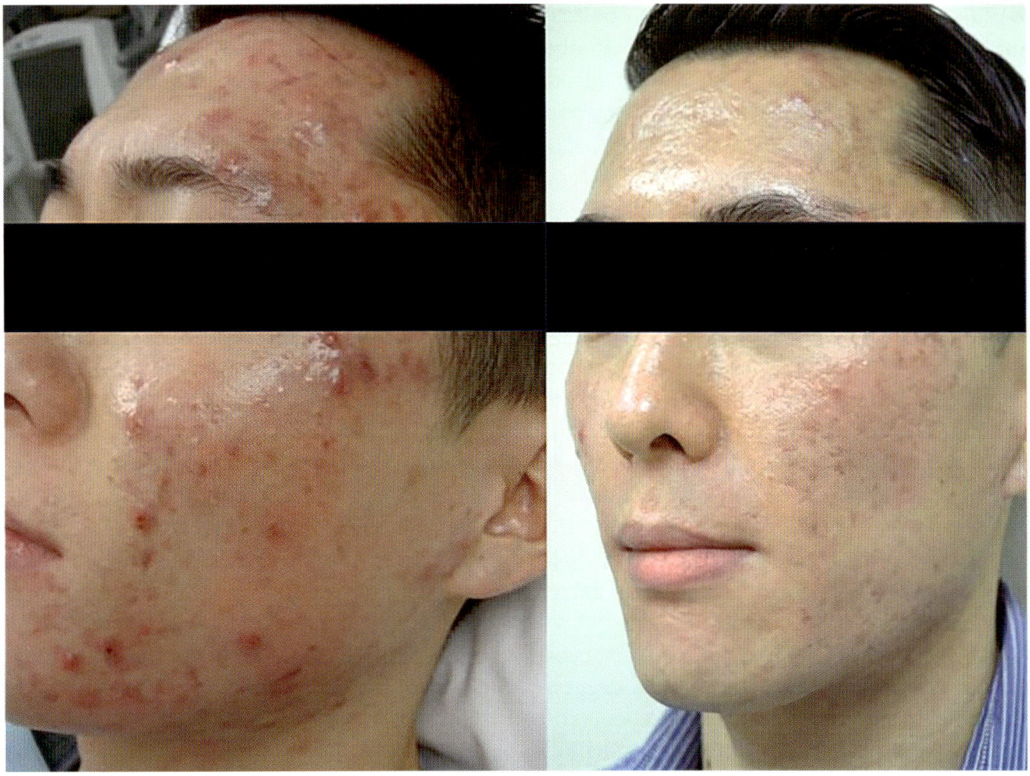

Fig. 4.3 Photographs of a patient treated with dPDT for acne prior to treatment and after six dPDT treatments given at 3- to 4-week intervals.

seen in a study of multiple plane warts treated with dPDT using 10% methylene blue gel as the photosensitizing agent.[51]

Treatment with dPDT has also been studied for cutaneous leishmaniasis (CL), an infection caused by intracellular parasites belonging to the Leishmania genus. Children are more commonly impacted due to their still-developing immune systems and greater exposure to sandflies. A case report of a 6-year-old boy with a nodule on his left cheek noted that three treatments of a 10% solution of ALA in polyethylene glycol ointment followed by 2 h exposed to daylight resulted in complete resolution of the lesion with only a small scar remaining after 6 months and only a mild burning sensation attested to during the light exposure.[52]

In a similar case of a 5-year-old boy with a CL lesion on his right ankle, treatment was initiated with ALA cDPT but discontinued due to pain during the light exposure.[53] Treatment was restarted with simulated daylight (sdPDT), and the lesion healed successfully, further suggesting dPDT as a preferable alternative for young children or pain-sensitive patients.

One multi-patient study did not compare cPDT to dPDT in the treatment of leishmaniasis but rather compared self-administered treatment at home versus supervised treatment in a hospital setting (in both cases the treatments were the same and consisted of MAL application and daylight exposure).[54] The study showed not only dPDT's effectiveness in treating leishmaniasis, with an overall cure rate of 89%, but also the lack of a difference in outcomes between the two treatment groups (92% for self-administered vs. 86% for hospital-based), implying an ease of self-administration.

Various fungal conditions have also been treated with dPDT. A 10-year-old boy exposed to *Microsporum canis* from a feral cat and presenting with tinea capitis was successfully treated with a total of 10 weekly sessions of MAL dPDT—along with 2% ketoconazole shampoo—after systemic treatment was refused and topical antifungals alone proved ineffective.[55] In a different case study, a man presented with an erythematous nodule suggestive of sporotrichosis caused by the *Sporothrix schenckii* fungus.[56] The patient refused oral treatment and so was instead given six treatments of intralesional 1% methylene blue injection followed by 30 min of occlusion and 2 h of daylight exposure. After six treatments, the lesion showed a complete clinical and microbiological response.[56]

Other

Inflammatory conditions may also be considered for treatment with dPDT. For example, there have been reported successful clinical applications of dPDT for the treatment of necrobiosis lipoidica, Darier disease, erosive pustular dermatosis, and atopic dermatitis.[57–60]

CONCLUSION

While there are many advantages of dPDT protocols over cPDT with similar outcomes, dPDT may not be practical all year round in certain rainy climates and at higher latitudes where there are fewer hours of adequate sunlight.[61] With weather conditions as a constraining factor for effective treatment, certain geographic locations may be limited to specific seasonal windows for dPDT treatment. However, there are year-round options for a more painless alternative to cPDT. Studies exploring the option of "indoor dPDT" have recently been reported using greenhouses or simulated daylight illumination sources with good efficacy in AK clearance.[62,63] Similarly, several "painless PDT" or "gentle PDT" protocols have been introduced, which revert to the use of a fixed blue or red light source, but with little to no incubation time (0–30 min) and varying lengths of irradiation (30–150 min).[20] These painless PDT protocols allow for similar treatment efficacy as cPDT and dPDT, but with reduced pain and no weather or latitudinal limitations.[19,21]

Despite the geographic constraints, the lack of associated pain, higher rates of satisfaction, and ease of implementation make dPDT an excellent option for the treatment of AKs and field cancerization in patients. dPDT is simpler and more convenient for patients. It can be performed at home, has short incubation times, and does not require occlusion. Additionally, without the limitations of a fixed light source, larger body surface areas can be targeted for treatment. Daylight PDT is also associated with lower rates of scarring and dyspigmentation as compared to cPDT.[9] Most importantly, dPDT appears to be at least as effective as cPDT for the treatment of AKs with minimal pain and less intense local skin response and offers a potential therapeutic option for the treatment of many other dermatologic conditions.

REFERENCES

1. Hamblin MR. Photodynamic therapy for cancer: what's past is prologue. *Photochem Photobiol.* 2020;96(3):506–516.
2. Buggiani G, Troiano M, Rossi R, Lotti T. Photodynamic therapy: off-label and alternative use in dermatological practice. *Photodiagnosis Photodyn Ther.* 2008;5(2):134–138.
3. Beiki D, Eggleston IM, Pourzand C. Daylight-PDT: everything under the sun. *Biochem Soc Trans.* 2022;50(2):975–985. doi:10.1042/BST20200822.
4. Busch TM. Local physiological changes during photodynamic therapy. *Lasers Surg Med.* 2006;38(5):494–499.
5. Braathen LR, Szeimies RM, Basset-Seguin N, et al. Guidelines on the use of photodynamic therapy for nonmelanoma skin cancer: an international consensus. International Society for Photodynamic Therapy in Dermatology, 2005. *J Am Acad Dermatol.* 2007;56(1):125–143.
6. Middelburg TA, Nijsten T, Neumann MH, de Haas ER, Robinson DJ. Red light ALA-PDT for large areas of actinic keratosis is limited by severe pain and patient dissatisfaction. *Photodermatol Photoimmunol Photomed.* 2013;29(5):276–278.
7. Borgia F, Giuffrida R, Caradonna E, Vaccaro M, Guarneri F, Cannavò SP. Early and late onset side effects of photodynamic therapy. *Biomedicines.* 2018;6(1):12.
8. Touma D, Yaar M, Whitehead S, Konnikov N, Gilchrest BA. A trial of short incubation, broad-area photodynamic therapy for facial actinic keratoses and diffuse photodamage. *Arch Dermatol.* 2004;140(1):33–40.
9. Rubel DM, Spelman L, Murrell DF, et al. Daylight photodynamic therapy with methyl aminolevulinate cream as a convenient, similarly effective, nearly painless alternative to conventional photodynamic therapy in actinic keratosis treatment: a randomized controlled trial. *Br J Dermatol.* 2014;171(5):1164–1171.
10. Lacour JP, Ulrich C, Gilaberte Y, et al. Daylight photodynamic therapy with methyl aminolevulinate cream is effective and nearly painless in treating actinic keratoses: a randomised, investigator-blinded, controlled, phase III study throughout Europe. *J Eur Acad Dermatol Venereol.* 2015;29(12):2342–2348.
11. Neittaanmäki-Perttu N, Karppinen TT, Grönroos M, Tani TT, Snellman E. Daylight photodynamic

therapy for actinic keratoses: a randomized double-blinded nonsponsored prospective study comparing 5-aminolaevulinic acid nanoemulsion (BF-200) with methyl-5-aminolaevulinate. *Br J Dermatol.* 2014;171(5):1172–1180.

12. Shive ML, Coakley BJ, Bierman DF, et al. Use of 5-aminolevulinic acid and daylight photodynamic therapy for the treatment of actinic keratoses. *Dermatol Surg.* 2019;45(4):529–535.
13. Wiegell SR, Fabricius S, Heydenreich J, et al. Weather conditions and daylight-mediated photodynamic therapy: protoporphyrin IX-weighted daylight doses measured in six geographical locations. *Br J Dermatol.* 2013;168(1):186–191.
14. Wiegell SR, Haedersdal M, Eriksen P, Wulf HC. Photodynamic therapy of actinic keratoses with 8% and 16% methyl aminolaevulinate and home-based daylight exposure: a double-blinded randomized clinical trial. *Br J Dermatol.* 2009;160:1308–1314.
15. Wiegell SR, Fabricius S, Gniadecka M, et al. Daylight-mediated photodynamic therapy of moderate to thick actinic keratoses of the face and scalp: a randomized multicentre study. *Br J Dermatol.* 2012;166:1327–1332.
16. Campbell CL, Wood K, Valentine RM, Brown CT, Moseley H. Monte Carlo modelling of daylight activated photodynamic therapy. *Phys Med Biol.* 2015;60:4059–4073.
17. O'Mahoney P, Khazova M, Eadie E, Ibbotson S. Measuring daylight: a review of dosimetry in daylight photodynamic therapy. *Pharmaceuticals (Basel).* 2019; 12(4):143.
18. Juzeniene A, Juzenas P, Kaalhus O, et al. Temperature effect on accumulation of protoporphyrin IX after topical application of 5-aminolevulinic acid and its methylester and hexylester derivatives in normal mouse skin. *Photochem Photobiol.* 2002;76:452–456.
19. Kaw U, Ilyas M, Bullock T, et al. A regimen to minimize pain during blue light photodynamic therapy of actinic keratoses: bilaterally controlled, randomized trial of simultaneous versus conventional illumination. *J Am Acad Dermatol.* 2020;82(4):862–868.
20. Heerfordt IM, Philipsen PA, Wulf HC. Bringing the gentle properties of daylight photodynamic therapy indoors: a systematic review of efficacy and safety. *Photodiagnosis Photodyn Ther.* 2022;39:102858.
21. Gandy J, Labadie B, Bierman D, Zachary C. Photodynamic therapy effectively treats actinic keratoses without pre-illumination incubation time. *J Drugs Dermatol.* 2017;16(3):275–278.
22. Morton CA, Szeimies RM, Basset-Seguin N, et al. European dermatology forum guidelines on topical photodynamic therapy 2019 part 1: treatment delivery and established indications - actinic keratoses, Bowen's disease and basal cell carcinomas. *J Eur Acad Dermatol Venereol.* 2019;33(12):2225–2238.
23. Lane KL, Hovenic W, Ball K, Zachary CB. Daylight photodynamic therapy: the Southern California experience. *Lasers Surg Med.* 2015;47(2):168–172.
24. Crow LD, Saylor D, Griffith-Bauer K, et al. Comparative tolerability and efficacy of daylight, conventional, and combination aminolevulinic acid photodynamic therapy for treatment of actinic keratosis. *J Am Acad Dermatol.* 2021;85(4):967–969.
25. Zhu L, Wang P, Zhang G, et al. Conventional versus daylight photodynamic therapy for actinic keratosis: a randomized and prospective study in China. *Photodiagnosis Photodyn Ther.* 2018;24:366–371.
26. Fargnoli MC, Piccioni A, Neri L, Tambone S, Pellegrini C, Peris K. Conventional vs. daylight methyl aminolevulinate photodynamic therapy for actinic keratosis of the face and scalp: an intra-patient, prospective, comparison study in Italy. *J Eur Acad Dermatol Venereol.* 2015;29(10):1926–1932.
27. Wiegell SR, Haedersdal M, Philipsen PA, Eriksen P, Enk CD, Wulf HC. Continuous activation of PpIX by daylight is as effective as and less painful than conventional photodynamic therapy for actinic keratoses; a randomized, controlled, single-blinded study. *Br J Dermatol.* 2008;158(4):740–746.
28. Sotiriou E, Evangelou G, Papadavid E, et al. Conventional vs. daylight photodynamic therapy for patients with actinic keratosis on face and scalp: 12-month follow-up results of a randomized, intra-individual comparative analysis. *J Eur Acad Dermatol Venereol.* 2018;32(4):595–600.
29. Wiegell SR, Fabricius S, Stender IM, et al. A randomized, multicentre study of directed daylight exposure times of 1½ vs. 2½ h in daylight-mediated photodynamic therapy with methyl aminolaevulinate in patients with multiple thin actinic keratoses of the face and scalp. *Br J Dermatol.* 2011;164(5):1083–1090.
30. Fargnoli MC, Ibbotson SH, Hunger RE, et al. Patient and physician satisfaction in an observational study with methyl aminolevulinate daylight photodynamic therapy in the treatment of multiple actinic keratoses of the face and scalp in six European countries. *J Eur Acad Dermatol Venereol.* 2018;32(5):757–762.
31. Gutiérrez García-Rodrigo C, Pellegrini C, Piccioni A, Tambone S, Fargnoli MC. Single versus two-treatment schedule of methyl aminolevulinate daylight photodynamic therapy for actinic keratosis of the face and scalp: an intra-patient randomized trial. *Photodiagnosis Photodyn Ther.* 2019;27:100–104.
32. Räsänen JE, Neittaanmäki N, Ylitalo L, et al. 5-aminolaevulinic acid nanoemulsion is more effective than

methyl-5-aminolaevulinate in daylight photodynamic therapy for actinic keratosis: a nonsponsored randomized double-blind multicentre trial. *Br J Dermatol.* 2019;181(2):265–274.
33. Cantisani C, Paolino G, Scarnò M, et al. Sequential methyl-aminolevulinate daylight photodynamic therapy and diclofenac plus hyaluronic acid gel treatment for multiple actinic keratosis evaluation. *Dermatol Ther.* 2018;31(6):e12710. doi:10.1111/dth.12710.
34. Galimberti GN. Calcipotriol as pretreatment prior to daylight-mediated photodynamic therapy in patients with actinic keratosis: a case series. *Photodiagnosis Photodyn Ther.* 2018;21:172–175. doi:10.1016/j.pdpdt.2017.11.019.
35. Wenande E, Phothong W, Bay C, Karmisholt KE, Haedersdal M, Togsverd-Bo K. Efficacy and safety of daylight photodynamic therapy after tailored pretreatment with ablative fractional laser or microdermabrasion: a randomized, side-by-side, single-blind trial in patients with actinic keratosis and large-area field cancerization. *Br J Dermatol.* 2019;180(4):756–764.
36. Martins CC, Bakos RM, Martins Costa M. Daylight photodynamic therapy for Bowen's disease. *An Bras Dermatol.* 2020;95(4):529–531. doi:10.1016/j.abd.2019.11.012.
37. Safar R, Alkhars A, Tallegas M, Korsaga-Some N, Machet L. Successful treatment for extensive Bowen's disease using daylight-mediated photodynamic therapy. *Acta Derm Venereol.* 2019;99(7):701–702.
38. Wiegell SR, Skødt V, Wulf HC. Daylight-mediated photodynamic therapy of basal cell carcinomas - an explorative study. *J Eur Acad Dermatol Venereol.* 2014;28(2):169–175.
39. Paolino G, Didona D, Scarnò M, et al. Sequential treatment of daylight photodynamic therapy and imiquimod 5% cream for the treatment of superficial basal cell carcinoma on sun exposed areas. *Dermatol Ther.* 2019;32(2):e12788.
40. Philipp-Dormston WG, Sanclemente G, Torezan L, et al. Daylight photodynamic therapy with MAL cream for large-scale photodamaged skin based on the concept of "actinic field damage": recommendations of an international expert group. *J Eur Acad Dermatol.* 2016;30:8–15.
41. Torezan L, Chaves Y, Niwa A, Sanches Jr JA, Festa-Neto C, Szeimies RM. A pilot split-face study comparing conventional methyl aminolevulinate-photodynamic therapy (PDT) with microneedling-assisted PDT on actinically damaged skin. *Dermatol Surg.* 2013;39(8):1197–1201.
42. Sanclemente G, Mancilla GA, Hernandez G. A double-blind randomized controlled trial to assess the efficacy of daylight photodynamic therapy with methyl-aminolevulinate vs. Placebo and daylight in patients with facial photodamage. *Actas Dermosifiliogr.* 2016;107(3):224–234.
43. Andreadis D, Pavlou A-M, Vakirlis E, et al. Daylight photodynamic therapy for the management of actinic cheilitis. *Arch Dermatol Res.* 2020;312(10):731–737.
44. Levi A, Hodak E, Enk CD, Snast I, Slodownik D, Lapidoth M. Daylight photodynamic therapy for the treatment of actinic cheilitis. *Photodermatol Photoimmunol Photomed.* 2019;35(1):11–16.
45. Yang Y, Shen S, Wang P, Wang X. Efficacy of photodynamic therapy in actinic cheilitis: a systematic review. *Photodiagnosis Photodyn Ther.* 2022;38:102782.
46. Kwon HH, Moon KR, Park SY, Yoon JY, Suh DH, Lee JB. Daylight photodynamic therapy with 1.5% 3-butenyl 5-aminolevulinate gel as a convenient, effective and safe therapy in acne treatment: a double-blind randomized controlled trial. *J Dermatol.* 2016;43(5):515–521.
47. Del Duca E, Manfredini M, Petrini N, et al. Daylight photodynamic therapy with 5-aminolevulinic acid 5% gel for the treatment of mild-to-moderate inflammatory acne. *Ital J Dermatol Venerol.* 2021;156(1):46–50.
48. Slutsky-Bank E, Artzi O, Sprecher E, Koren A. A split-face clinical trial of conventional red-light photodynamic therapy versus daylight photodynamic therapy for acne vulgaris. *J Cosmet Dermatol.* 2021;20(12):3924–3930.
49. Kim TI, Ahn HJ, Kang IH, Jeong KH, Kim NI, Shin MK. Nonablative fractional laser-assisted daylight photodynamic therapy with topical methyl aminolevulinate for moderate to severe facial acne vulgaris: results of a randomized and comparative study. *Photodermatol Photoimmunol Photomed.* 2017;33(5):253–259.
50. Borgia F, Macca L, Giuffrida R, et al. Recurrence after conventional versus daylight photodynamic therapy in children effected by multiple facial flat warts. *Photodiagnosis Photodyn Ther.* 2021;36:102579.
51. Fathy G, Asaad MK, Rasheed HM. Daylight photodynamic therapy with methylene blue in plane warts: a randomized double-blind placebo-controlled study. *Photodermatol Photoimmunol Photomed.* 2017;33(4):185–192.
52. Li Pomi F, Peterle L, Vaccaro M, Borgia F. Daylight photodynamic therapy for cutaneous leishmaniasis in a pediatric setting: a case report and literature review. *Photodiagnosis Photodyn Ther.* 2023;44:103800.
53. Hobelsberger S, Krauß MP, Bogdan C, Aschoff R. Erfolgreiche Therapie der kutanen Leishmaniose mit simulierter Tageslicht-photodynamischer Therapie [Successful treatment of cutaneous leishmaniasis with simulated daylight photodynamic therapy]. *Hautarzt.* 2022;73(5):376–378.
54. Enk CD, Nasereddin A, Alper R, Dan-Goor M, Jaffe CL, Wulf HC. Cutaneous leishmaniasis responds to

daylight-activated photodynamic therapy: proof of concept for a novel self-administered therapeutic modality. *Br J Dermatol.* 2015;172(5):1364–1370.

55. Aspiroz C, Melcon B, Cerro PA, Gilaberte Y. Tinea capitis caused by Microsporum canis treated with methyl-aminolevulinate daylight photodynamic therapy and ketoconazole shampooing. *Photodermatol Photoimmunol Photomed.* 2021;37(6):567–568.
56. García-Malinis AJ, Milagro Beamonte A, Torres Sopena L, García-Callen O, Puertolas-Villacampa P, Gilaberte Y. Cutaneous sporotrichosis treated with methylene blue-daylight photodynamic therapy. *J Eur Acad Dermatol Venereol.* 2018;32(3):e90–e91.
57. López Sanz P, Faura Berruga C, Guerrero Ramírez C, Manso Córdoba S, Alfaro Martínez ME, García Vázquez A. Daylight photodynamic therapy in necrobiosis lipoidica: a promising treatment? *Photodermatol Photoimmunol Photomed.* 2023;39(3):294–295.
58. Morelló-Vicente A, Antoñanzas J, Estenaga Á, Oteiza-Rius I, Salido-Vallejo R, España A. Refractory facial Darier's disease treated with daylight photodynamic therapy. *J Dtsch Dermatol Ges.* 2022;20(12):1633–1635.
59. Arteaga-Henriquez M, Gonzalez-Hernandez S, Garcia-Peris E. Conventional versus daylight photodynamic therapy in the treatment of erosive pustular dermatosis of the scalp. *Dermatol Ther.* 2020;33(2):e13220.
60. Kremer N, Sherman S, Lapidoth M, et al. Self-administered daylight-activated photodynamic therapy for the treatment of hand eczema: a prospective proof-of-concept study. *Dermatol Ther.* 2020;33(6):e14329.
61. Kotb I, Lesar A, O'Mahoney P, Eadie E, Ibbotson SH. Daylight photodynamic therapy for actinic keratosis: is it affected by the British weather? *Photodermatol Photoimmunol Photomed.* 2021;37(2):157–158. doi:10.1111/phpp.12610.
62. Mordon S, Vignion-Dewalle AS, Thecua E, et al. Can daylight-PDT be performed indoor? *G Ital Dermatol Venereol.* 2018;153(6):811–816.
63. Bai-Habelski JC, Medrano K, Palacio A, Reinhold U. No room for pain: a prospective study showing effective and nearly pain-free treatment of actinic keratosis with simulated daylight photodynamic therapy (SDL-PDT) using the IndoorLux® system in combination with BF-200 ALA (Ameluz®). *Photodiagnosis Photodyn Ther.* 2022;37:102692.

5

Photodynamic Therapy and Facilitated Delivery

Jill S. Waibel, Mary Dick, Rebecca L. Quiñonez, Alexander A. Daoud

KEY POINTS

- The skin's natural barrier limits transcutaneous absorption, with only 1%–5% of topical formulations penetrating, and smaller, semi-lipophilic molecules are more effective in skin penetration.
- For effective photodynamic therapy (PDT), photosensitizers like aminolevulinic acid (ALA) and methyl aminolevulinate (MAL) must penetrate the epidermis and reach the keratinocytes.
- ALA penetration depth depends on factors like incubation time and lesion type, with ALA penetrating up to 2.5–3.0 mm, and shorter incubation times (15–30 minutes) showing effective clearance of actinic keratoses (AKs).
- ALA's hydrophilicity and molecular weight make it challenging to cross the stratum corneum, requiring occlusion or large quantities for effective absorption.
- MAL, a more lipophilic photosensitizer, improves absorption, and ALA nanoemulsion, developed in 2013, enhances PDT by increasing stability and skin penetration.
- Laser-assisted techniques are used to improve the delivery and penetration of photosensitizers, enhancing PDT effectiveness for conditions like actinic keratosis, acne, and photodamage.
- This section emphasizes the critical role of photosensitizer penetration in PDT and explores advancements in formulation and delivery systems to overcome the limitations of the skin barrier, improving clinical outcomes.

OBJECTIVE

- To examine the mechanisms of penetration and effectiveness of photosensitizers in photodynamic therapy (PDT).
- Idenitfy the challenges of skin absorption
- Discuss strategies such as laser-facilitated delivery to enhance treatment outcomes for conditions like actinic keratosis and other dermatological conditions.

PDT- AND LASER-FACILITATED DELIVERY

Introduction

The skin is designed to be impenetrable to the outside world. Its protective barrier limits transcutaneous absorption ultimately minimizing topical absorption to as low as 1%–5%.[1] Topical formulations have varying properties pertaining to solubility and size that can hinder or allow for optimum penetration through the uppermost layers of the skin. Semi-lipophilic and a small molecular size allows for successful penetration through the stratum corneum and into the keratinocyte's lipid. Larger molecules are prevented by normal, intact skin; therefore they require more effective ways to penetrate or completely surpass the skin barrier. For photodynamic therapy (PDT) to be effective the photosensitizers

TABLE 5.1 Penetration of ALA

Skin Lesion	Effect of Penetration versus Normal Skin
AKs, abrasions, inflammation	ALA penetrates more readily versus normal skin
Thicker skin (often seen in ethnic groups such as Native Americans and Asians)	ALA less permeable versus normal skin
Heavily lentiginous skin	ALA penetrates in an irregularly dotted pattern versus normal skin
Superficial BCC and SCC	Due to abnormal keratin being more easily penetrated by ALA versus normal skin

TABLE 5.2 Photosensitizers Used in Dermatology for PDT

Class	Prodrug	Commercial Drug
Porphyrin	Hematoporphyrin derivative (HpD)	Photofrin Axcan Pharma, Canada
Porphyrin	5-Aminolevulinic acid	Ameluz Biofrontera, Germany
Porphyrin	5-Aminolevulinic acid	Levulan Kerastick DUSA, USA
Porphyrin	Methyl-5-amino-4-oxopentanoate (methyl aminolevulinate, MAL)	Metvix (QLT Phototherapeutics, Canada)
Porphyrin	Meta-tetra(hydroxyphenyl)chlorin (m-THPC)	Foscan Biolitec, Germany
Texafrin	Motexafin lutetium	Lutrin (clinical trial)

must penetrate to keratinocytes throughout the squamous layers and the basal layer.

Penetration of ALA Into the Skin

The effectiveness of PDT depends partly on how deeply and efficiently the photosensitizing agents penetrate the skin. The penetration of aminolevulinic acid (ALA) has been well studied and is influenced by several factors as reviewed in Table 5.1.

For cutaneous application, the photosensitizer ALA or methyl aminolevulinate (MAL) is applied to the skin. ALA applied to the skin penetrates the underlying epidermis where it is converted to protoporphyrin IX (PpIX), a photosensitive compound. PpIX is then taken up by both normal and rapidly dividing (malignant) cells but cleared less rapidly from neoplastic cells. Photosensitizers then are localized in and kill tumor cells by direct destruction by singlet oxygen, damage to blood vessels, and activations of an immune response. The rate that PpIX accumulates in cutaneous lesions is dependent on lesion type.[2] One major area of debate and study over the past few decades has been incubation times. It has been studied that ALA requires 3–15 h to penetrate 2.5–3.0 mm into various tissues.[3] It takes 60 min for ALA to penetrate into actinic keratoses (AKs).[3,4] More recent studies have been conducted to shorten ALA incubation times and have significant AK clearance with as little as 15–30 min incubation time.[5]

The epidermis ranges in depth from 47 to 105 mm depending on the anatomical body site. Whereas the dermis ranges in depth from 1961 to 1986 mm depending on the anatomical body sites.[6] Because ALA has a molecular weight of 168 Daltons and is hydrophilic and does not readily cross the stratum corneum, a large amount must be applied to the skin to assure adequate absorption for PDT (Table 5.2).[7] One form of ALA is alcohol based (Kerastick), and thus requires occlusion with Saran Wrap when applied to intact skin due to the significant risk of evaporation of the solution.

The development of a second photosensitizer came about due to the hydrophilic concerns of ALA. MAL was developed with lipophilic esters to promote better absorption. MAL is lipophilic and has a molecular weight of 181 Daltons, which favors absorption.[8]

Another improvement in photosensitizer precursors was the development in 2013 of ALA nanoemulsion.[9,10] The characteristics of the ALA nanoemulsion include average particle size below 50 nm, narrow particle size distribution, increased stability, and skin-neutral pH. During manufacturing of the ALA nanoemulsion, lipophilic active ingredients can be inserted into the core. Hydrophilic active ingredients can be dissolved in the dispersion media (water) and bind to the nanovesicle outer layer.

Challenges of PDT: Time and Inadequate Penetration

PDT is proven to be an effective treatment for superficial non-melanoma skin cancers, actinic keratoses, and acne.[8,9] Based on efficacy, PDT is cited to be one of the most successful treatments of actinic keratoses; however, several inherent issues exist in clinical practice. One problem that arises with PDT is the in-office procedure time required for ALA incubation. Conventional PDT requires the application of ALA on the areas of interest, followed by a 1-h incubation period. The patient is then exposed under the light for 16 min per treatment area. Patients who are being treated for multiple areas; for example, face and arms, may be looking at a 2-h appointment. For practitioners, this poses a limitation on how many patients can be scheduled for PDT, especially in a medical setting where rooms or staff are limited.

Another is the challenge of delivery of the photosensitizer to the target cells. Thicker lesions have shown to be more resistant to PDT due to the inadequate depth of penetration by topical photosensitizers.[11] Both challenges can be overcome by laser-assisted delivery (LAD).

Solution: Laser-Assisted Delivery

As previously discussed, the stratum corneum is the most significant barrier to percutaneous drug absorption. Several modalities have been developed to enhance the absorption of topically applied medications. These methods include chemical enhancers (carrier vesicular systems such as liposomes and modified liposomes), physical enhancers (sonophoresis, ionophoresis, iontophoresis, cryoelectrophoresis, hydroelectrophoresis, and lasers), ablative techniques (microdermabrasion,

Laser-Assisted Delivery Systems
Using Fractional Ablative Columns to Deliver ALA

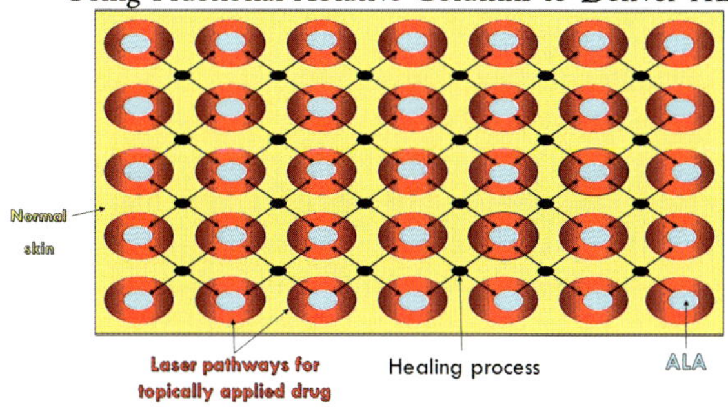

Fig. 5.1 Normal skin (yellow) undergoes ablation leaving columns (red areas) that are spaced apart to make channels in which ALA (blue) is delivered when applied to the skin. Bridges of normal skin allow for proper wound healing.

tape stripping, and lasers), agents to increase skin temperature, microarrays, microneedles, and biosynthetic agents. To date, the ablative techniques appear to be the most effective method for maximum topical absorption. Ablative fractional laser therapy is a unique modality that can destroy the stratum corneum and other cutaneous layers in a predictable and controlled manner, resulting in the potential for increased penetration of topically applied molecules such as ALA (Fig. 5.1).[5,12] The fractional ablative laser vaporizes the skin to create a channel or conduit for delivery. The location, diameter, depth, and other characteristics of these channels can be precisely controlled by the settings of the laser.

Types of Lasers

The erbium:yttrium-aluminum-garnet (Er:YAG) laser and the carbon dioxide (CO_2) laser are the two types of laser devices most commonly studied in regard to laser-assisted drug delivery. The Er:YAG laser has a wavelength of 2940 nm and is strongly absorbed by water in the epidermis. It exerts its ablation effect with minimal penetration depth and heat generation and therefore minimal thermal damage. The CO_2 laser has a wavelength of 10,600 nm and to achieve ablation exerts a greater thermal effect than the Er:YAG laser. Using heat to increase the permeability of the stratum corneum, the CO_2 laser results in a greater depth of ablation compared to the Er:YAG laser.

Traditionally, the conventional Er:YAG and CO_2 lasers were used to ablate the epidermis in a continuous fashion. Fractional lasers are a relatively recent modality, with the concept of fractional photothermolysis first described in 2004. Like conventional lasers, fractional lasers also ablate the skin; however, as their name suggests, they do so in fractions, splitting the laser beam into microbeams. These microbeams create microscopic vertical channels of ablation in the skin surrounded by thin layers of coagulated tissue referred to as the microscopic treatment zone (MTZ). The MTZ is surrounded by healthy, unabated, undamaged tissue. The creation of these MTZ channels theoretically provides access pathways for topically applied drug molecules that would otherwise be too large to traverse the epidermal layer, while minimizing the healing time that is necessary after continuous laser ablation. Both continuous ablation and fractional ablation have been used in drug delivery studies (Table 5.3).

TABLE 5.3 Parameters to Consider in LAD With PDT

Type of laser	Ablative Fractional Carbon Dioxide 10,600 nm Ablative Fractional Erbium:YAG 2,940 nm
Laser density	Number of channels per skin area – tunable by laser
Depth of laser channel	Tunable by pulse energy – in PDT targets are superficial
Coagulation zone	Zones where photosensitizer will be applied to directly penetrate to keratinocytes

Laser-Assisted Delivery in PDT

Laser pretreatment of the skin has been shown to increase the penetration of these photosensitizers. Fig. 5.2 demonstrates the step-by-step process in which patients are treated with LAD in PDT.

In an ex vivo porcine skin model, both continuous and fractional ablative Er:YAG lasers increased the penetration of topically applied ALA.[4] Another in vitro study showed that skin pretreatment with the fractional ablative Er:YAG laser increased the flux of ALA 27–124 fold in the nude mouse skin and 3–260 fold in the porcine skin.[13] These investigators suggested that laser pretreatment of the skin could potentially reduce the required dose of topically applied ALA by 20%, which may decrease side effects such as paresthesias and dyspigmentation.[13]

Current Applications: Protocols and Clinical Data

PDT-Facilitated Laser Delivery: Actinic Keratosis

The efficacy of ablative fractional laser (AFL)-PDT in the treatment of AKs has been described since 2012.

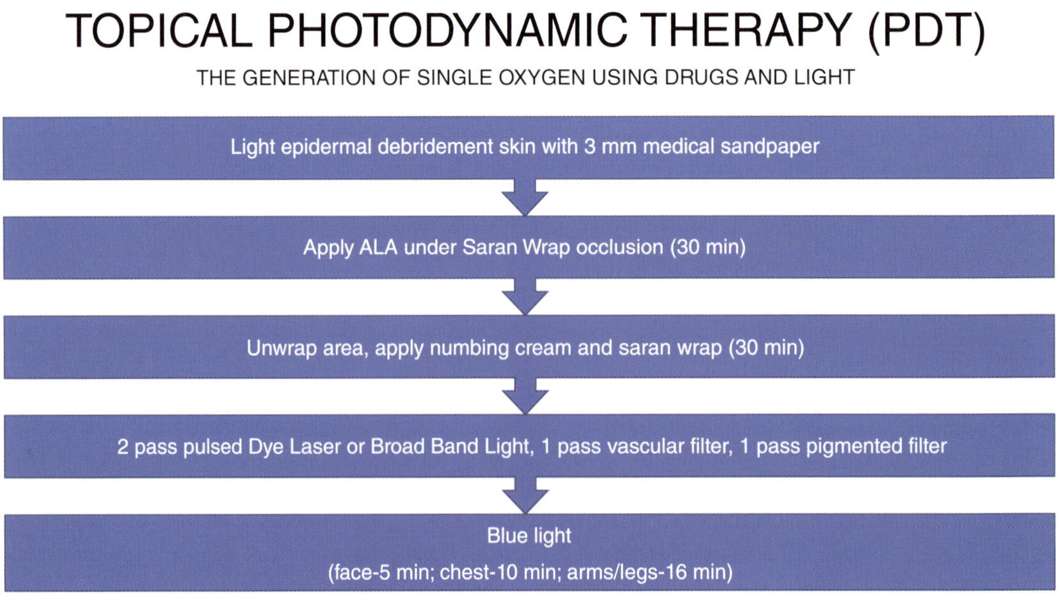

Fig. 5.2 Laser-assisted delivery in PDT.

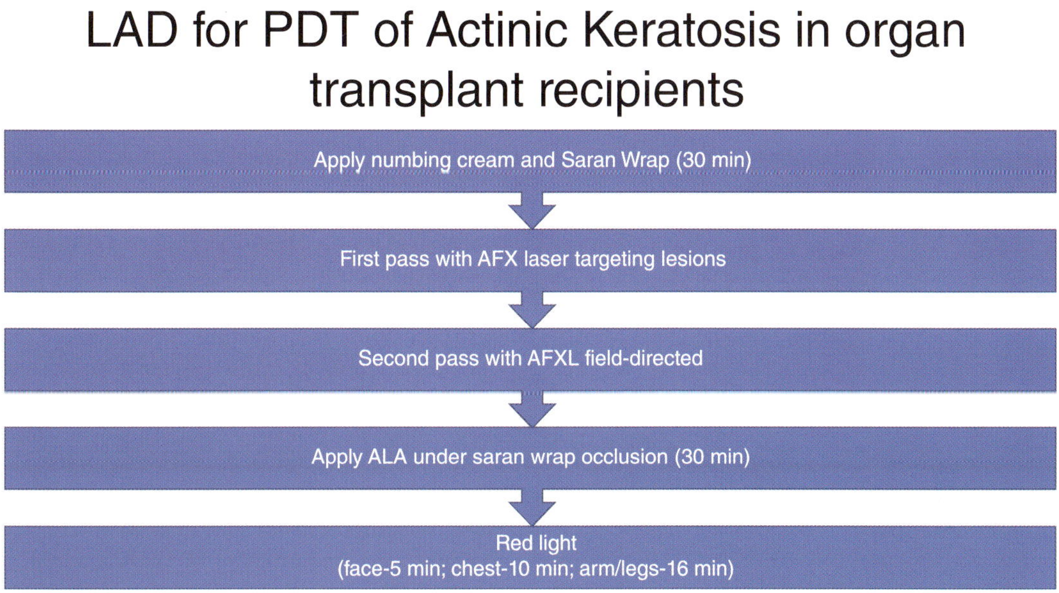

Fig. 5.3 A summary of the recommended steps for treatment of LAD for PDT of actinic keratosis in organ transplant recipients.

The approval by the FDA for the treatment of AKs with PDT in dermatology has provided patients with an effective treatment option, especially in larger surface areas. The improvement of treatment outcomes with laser-facilitated delivery is a logical next step. AKs in the setting of field cancerization are more efficaciously treated with field-directed therapies due to the multifocal dysplasia as opposed to lesion-directed therapies.[14] PDT efficacy is highly determined by lesion thickness with cure rates of up to 80%–90% in thin lesions and 39%–59% in moderate to very thick lesions. AFL pretreatment not only improves individual clearance of thin and thick AKs but decreases the rate of new actinic keratosis development. Togsverd and colleagues compared 109 AKs treated with conventional PDT to 103 AKs within identical treatment areas on the face and scalp. AKs with moderate to severe hyperkeratosis were curettaged and then randomized for conventional PDT with MAL under 3-h occlusion or AFL with CO_2 (12 mm spot size, 10 mJ per pulse, single pulse, 5% density) followed by conventional PDT. In the AFL group, 100% of thin AKs were cleared with a mean of 88% clearance rate in moderate-to-severe AKs. Conventional PDT cleared 88% of thin AKs and 59% of those that were moderate to severe thickness. At the 3-month follow-up the PDT-only group developed eight more AKs than those treated with AFL-PDT.[15]

The combination treatment of fractional CO_2 laser with PDT has also been used by Macrene for the treatment of AKs.[5] After the subjects were divided into four treatment groups (Group 1: ALA-PDT -15 min; Group 2: ALA-PDT -30 min; Group 3: +FxCO_2 ALA-PDT -15 min; Group 4: +FxCO_2 ALA-PDT -30 min) the authors concluded that both groups pretreated with fractional ablative resurfacing yielded significantly greater AK clearance at ultra-short ALA incubation times followed by blue light.[5]

PDT-Facilitated Laser Delivery: Acral Actinic Keratosis in Organ Transplant Recipients

PDT for AKs in organ transplant recipients (OTRs) has demonstrated to have lesser efficacy, specifically in the acral regions. Helsing and colleagues reported the use of AFXL with PDT to intensify therapy and response to treatment. Ten OTRs with a total of 680 AKs on the dorsal hands were targeted with AFXL followed by AFXL field treatment of both hands. The treatment regions were randomized to AFXL-PDT or no further treatment with laser. This study found that a single treatment with AFXL-PDT was highly effective at treatment of the lesions while leaving no scarring in the treated areas (Fig. 5.3 and Table 5.4).

TABLE 5.4 Recommended Setting for LAD With PDT for AKs in Organ Transplant Recipients

Ablative fractional CO_2 laser	10,600 nm 30 W 0.12-mm spot size
1st pass: lesion-targeted treatment of AKs	**Non-atrophic skin:** 160 mJ per pulse 6.25-ms pulse duration 5.3% coverage **Atrophic skin:** 140 mJ per pulse 5.65-ms pulse duration 5.2% coverage
2nd pass: field-directed pass settings	**Non-atrophic skin:** 6 0 mJ per pulse 2.06-ms pulse duration 5.2% coverage **Atrophic skin:** 40 mJ per pulse 1.32-ms pulse duration, 4.3% coverage

PDT-Facilitated Laser Delivery: Treatment of AKs and Prevention SCC in Organ Transplant Recipients

OTR have been reported to have a decreased response rate as compared to their non-transplant counterparts.[16] Lonsdorf and colleagues evaluated patients with AKs on the face and scalp in OTR who underwent both conventional PDT and AFL-low irradiance-PDT on opposing photodamaged sites. Conventional PDT with MAL and 3-h occlusion (intensity set to 100% with the corresponding irradiance of 61.67 mW/cm^2 and 10-min standard irradiation time) was completed on one side. On the contrasting side, curettage was followed with one pass of an Er:YAG laser and PDT with 3-h incubation (intensity set to 30% corresponding with an irradiance of 18.5 mW/cm^2 and standard irradiation time of 33 min and 20 s). The facilitated delivery arm of the study achieved a higher mean lesion response rate reduction of 77.3% ± 23.6% compared to (61.8% ± 21.4%; $p = 0.025$) in conventional PDT 3 months after treatment. There was no significant difference in pain between the two arms (Fig. 5.4).[17]

PDT-Facilitated Laser Delivery: Skin Cancers

Basal cell carcinoma. The synergistic efficacy in the treatment of basal cell carcinoma (BCC) with AFL-PDT was assessed by Wozniak and colleagues. Fifty-four histologically confirmed BCCs were stratified by subtype including superficial (36), nodular (6), infiltrating (4), sclerosing (2), and not specified (6)—all no deeper than 2 mm within the epidermis. The patient population included those who had previously undergone cryotherapy or surgical removal, surgically or aesthetically challenging locations, and/or clinically uncommon syndromes (i.e., Gorlin syndrome). BCCs were treated with superficial curettage, 20% 5-ALA under 4-h occlusion, and then illuminated (for photodynamic diagnostics at 405 nm to confirm protoporphyrin IX accumulation produced from 5-ALA) followed by PDT at 638 nm. The number of treatment sessions ranged from 1 to 4 treatments within a 2- to 4-week interval based on size, histologic subtype, and underlying genetic syndrome. Most patients received one total treatment. Complete response occurred in 97% of superficial BCCs, 67% of nodular BCCs, and 50% of infiltrating BCCs. No response was achieved in sclerosing BCCs. Large lesion size was associated with a lower cure rate and a need for an increased number of treatments. Follow-up was completed at 36 months.[18]

Smucler and colleagues also compared treatment refractory BCCs under a depth of 2 mm on the head and neck. The first group involved PDT with MAL applied to the lesion and 1 cm beyond the visible lesion edge incubated for 3 h before illumination. The treatment was repeated after 7 days. The second group involved short pulse Er:YAG (usually with 600–1000 mJ of energy at a frequency of 7 Hz) to the entire lesion. The final group initiated therapy with a combination of Er:YAG as above followed by one treatment of PDT. A histologic examination was completed at 12 months. At 1 year, there were no recurrences in the combined therapy group for 98.97% of patients compared with 91.75% of those treated only with Er:YAG and 94.85% in those treated with PDT alone.[19]

Squamous cell carcinoma. Squamous cell carcinomas have also been trialed with fractional laser-facilitated PDT. Kim and colleagues treated 84 squamous cell carcinoma in situ (SCCis) lesions on the lower extremities with a single treatment of AFL (ER:YAG, 550- to 600-μm ablation depth with level 1 coagulation, 22% treatment density, and a single pulse) and PDT with MAL compared to two treatments at 1-week intervals of classic PDT. The follow-up period was 5 years with recurrence with any clinically suspicious recurrence further evaluated with punch biopsy for histopathology. At 5 years, 9.3% of AFL-PDT

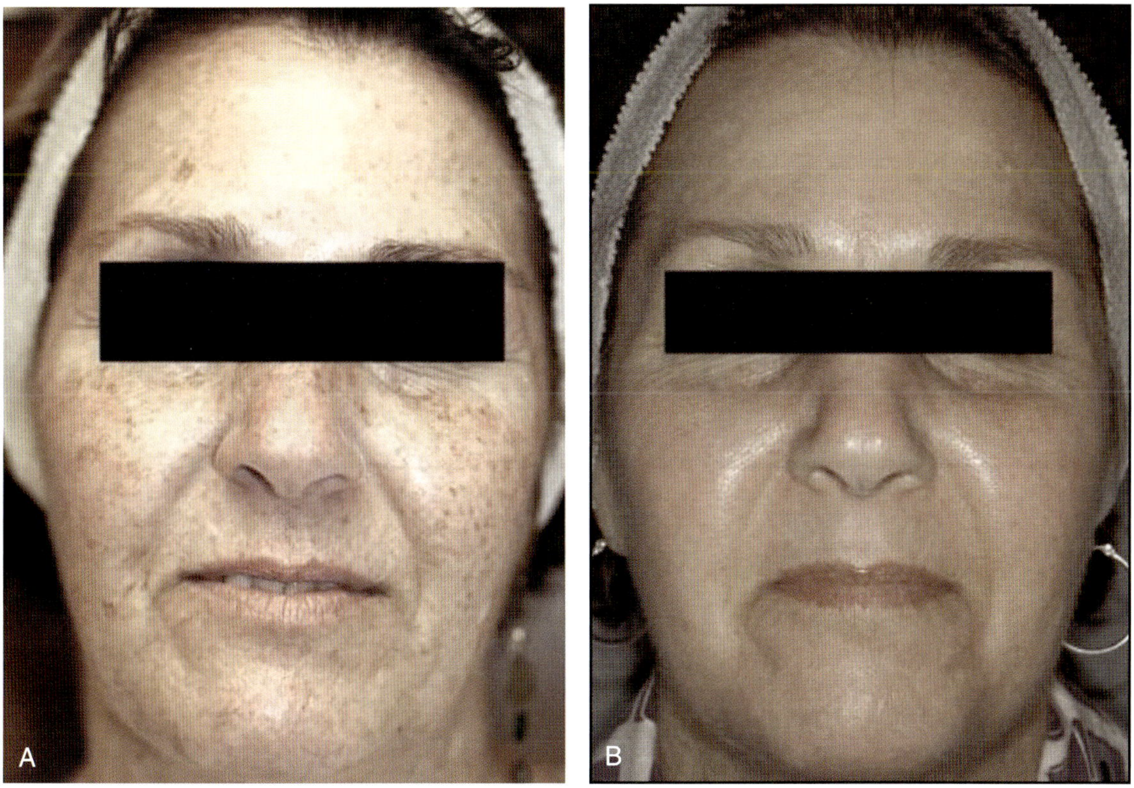

Fig. 5.4 A 55-year-old organ transplant recipient with multiple AKs, SKS, and lentigos before (A) and 3 months after (B) LAD with PDT.

squamous cell carcinomas in situ had recurred compared to 41.4% of those treated with classic PDT. Of those that recurred, 66% were over 20 mm in pretreatment size.[20] Cai and colleagues additionally studied 22 SCCis lesions, of an average 2.6 ± 0.9 cm in diameter, with either CO_2 AFL and PDT with ALA under 5-h incubation (light dose of 180 J/cm^2 and a fluence rate of 100 mW/cm^2) or CO_2 laser alone (power ranging between 2 and 3 W). Treatment was repeated for a total of three sessions after which patients were referred to surgery if they did not achieve complete lesion resolution. Follow-up was completed at 6 months. Of those treated with laser-facilitated delivery, 72.7% responded after one to three treatment sessions with maintained clearance at 6 months in 90.1%. Of those treated with CO_2 laser alone, 63.6% achieved a complete response with maintained clearance in only 45.5% of patients (Fig. 5.5).[21]

Melanoma: nonsurgical candidates. The use of PDT-facilitated delivery and melanoma must be approached with caution. The current gold standard treatment for any melanoma is surgical excision. The first prospective trial utilizing AFL-PDT for lentigo maligna was completed by Marini and colleagues in 2019. This study may provide support for laser-facilitated PDT in those with superficial melanomas for which the gold standard of surgical excision is contraindicated or in the setting of patients who refuse surgery. In this study, 10 biopsy-proven lentigo malignas, without known invasive components, were treated (including 5.0 mm margins) three times bimonthly with an ablative fractional CO_2 laser (density level of 5, depth level of 7, and pulse duration of 700 ms, corresponding to a distance of 0.8 mm between the laser pores and calculated pulse energy of 84 mJ per pore) followed by ALA over the lesion and margins with 3-h occlusion and with a 630 nm wavelength red light LED (dose of 90 J/cm^2). Four weeks after treatment, all lesions were surgically removed with wide-local excision for histopathology. Seventy percent of the lesions had complete, confirmed histologic clearance without any clinically apparent scar (Fig. 5.6).[22]

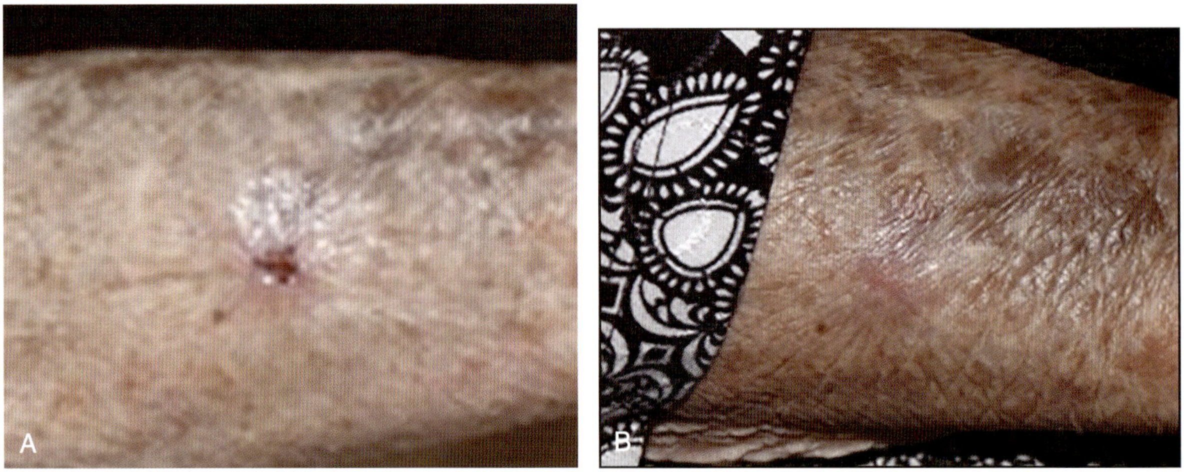

Fig. 5.5 An 89-year-old female patient with a recurring SCC of right left forearm before (A) and 1 month after (B) treatment with LAD with PDT.

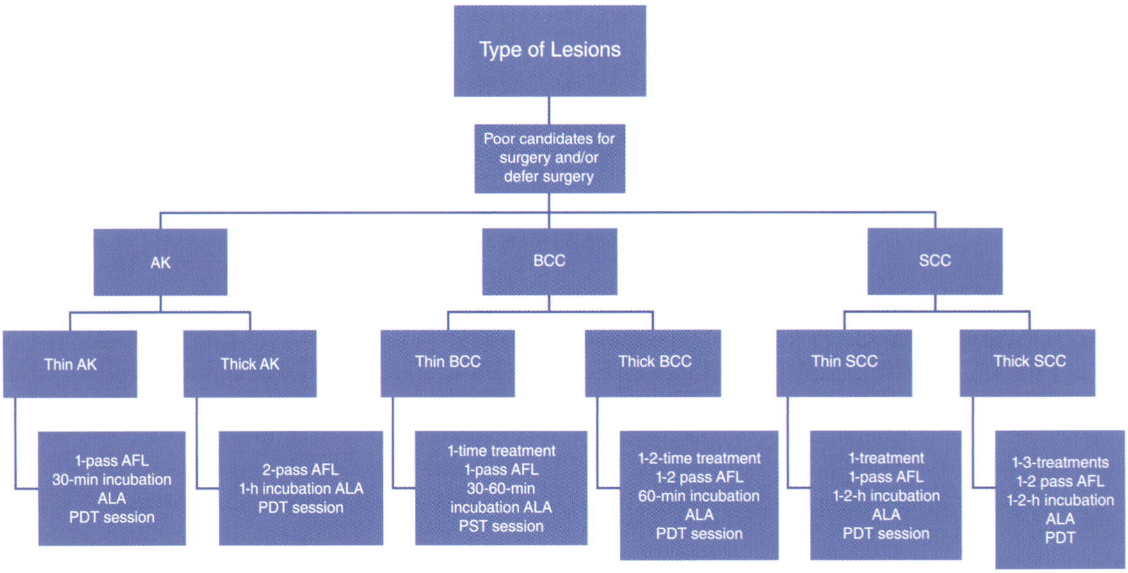

Fig. 5.6 A summary of LAD with PDT in malignant lesions for poor surgical candidates or patients who defer surgical intervention.

PDT-Facilitated Laser Delivery Aesthetic Uses

The aesthetic effects of PDT on photo-aged skin are well documented in the literature. Improvement of lentigines, skin roughness, and fine wrinkles are a few clinical concerns to which patients undergo PDT. Horio demonstrated in 2003 that protoporphyrin IX accumulates within the pilosebaceous unit making sebaceous hyperplasia (SH) a target for PDT.[23] Kim studied eight patients with Fitzpatrick skin type IV and facial SH. Four patients were treated with AFL confined to the site of SH to expose the papillary dermis before applying ALA. Three of the four patients experienced marked 90% improvement in hyperplasia (one patient with moderate 60%–90% improvement) and no lesion

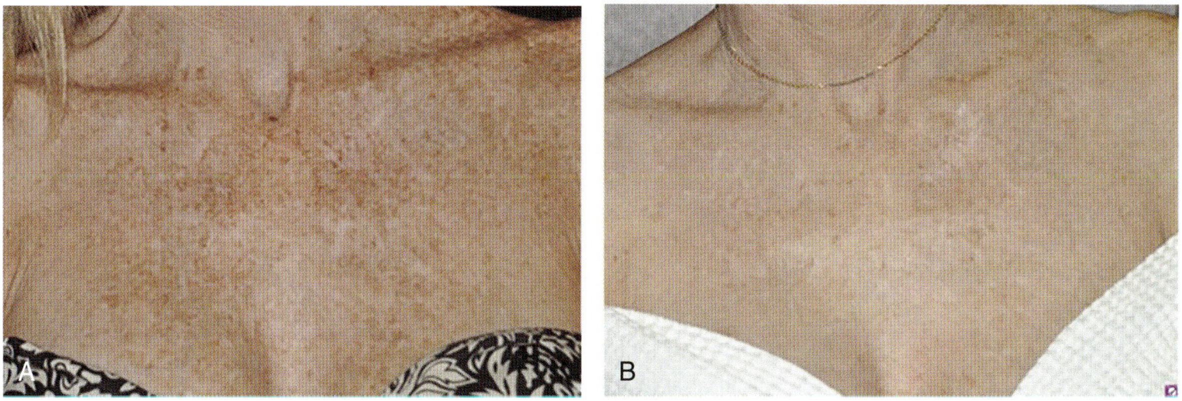

Fig. 5.7 A 54-year-old female with a history of chronic sun exposure before (A) and 3 months after (B) treatment with LAD with PDT on the neck and chest.

recurrence at 4-month follow-up. This was compared to two patients who received 20% ALA to the sebaceous papules and 5 mm surrounding diameter (irradiance of 50 J/cm^2 of 630–650 nm LED) with moderate and mild (30%–60%) improvement. Two patients received ALA only to the SH followed by 100–120 J/cm^2 light with moderate improvement. The number of treatment sessions varied from one to four sessions in the AFL group and one to five sessions in the PDT-only group.[20]

The efficacy of PDT in treatment of infection has gained increasing traction in the literature. Its antimicrobial effects may provide a secondary option for patients wishing to avoid surgical removal of infected epidermal inclusion cysts. Zhang and colleagues treated 39 infected epidermoid cysts on the head, neck, groin, and breast at sizes of 0.5–3.5 cm in diameter and 0.3–3.0 cm in depth. Treatment was initiated with a minimally invasive incision followed by CO_2 laser perforation of the cyst of approximately 2.0–3.0 mm (power of 5 watts, surgical pattern) and content extraction with the use of tangential pressure and a curette. Gauze-soaked 20% ALA solution was incubated inside and outside the wound for 4 h without light followed by light irradiation inside the cavity with a diffuse fiber (power density of 500 mW/cm for 20 min). The surface of the cyst was irradiated with a red LED (power density of 100 mW/cm^2 for 20 min). This procedure, without the initial incision, was repeated three times at weekly intervals. A success rate of 97% was achieved as measured by lack of recurrence at 12 months follow-up, with cyst resolution and patient satisfaction without obvious scar formation (Fig. 5.7).[24]

PDT-Facilitated Laser Delivery: Hamartomas

AFL-PDT may have an advantage in providing an even surface for the treatment of hamartomas. This combination therapy was effective in the setting of facial angiofibromas secondary to tuberous sclerosis. Wang and colleagues utilized CO_2 AFL followed by 10% ALA with 3-h incubation and irradiation with 633 nm red light at 90 mW/cm^2 for 20 min. This was followed by three additional sessions of PDT with ALA at 1-week intervals without further LAD. Resolution without scarring or hypopigmentation was achieved without recurrence at a 6-month follow-up.[25]

PDT-Facilitated Laser Delivery: Scarring

AFL-PDT has been explored in the setting of acne scarring. Moy studied 52 patients with hypertrophic mandibular acne scars. This group compared CO_2-assisted PDT to microneedling-assisted PDT and direct intralesional steroid injections at the scar site with all treatments completed monthly for 3 months. In the microneedling group (16 patients), treatment started with needling resulting in bleeding, followed by PDT with ALA under 3-h occlusion. CO_2 AFL (28 patients) (laser energy: 29 W, dot pitch: 0.8 mm, dot stay: 1.8 ms, dot energy: 52.2 mJ, coverage rate: 31%) was followed by the PDT protocol above. The intralesional steroid group utilized 1 mL of compounded betamethasone with 1.5 mL of normal saline injected to the point of mild blanching. Scars were evaluated based on pigmentation, scar height, vascularity, and pliability. Researchers found a lack of significant difference in clinical efficacy among the three treatment

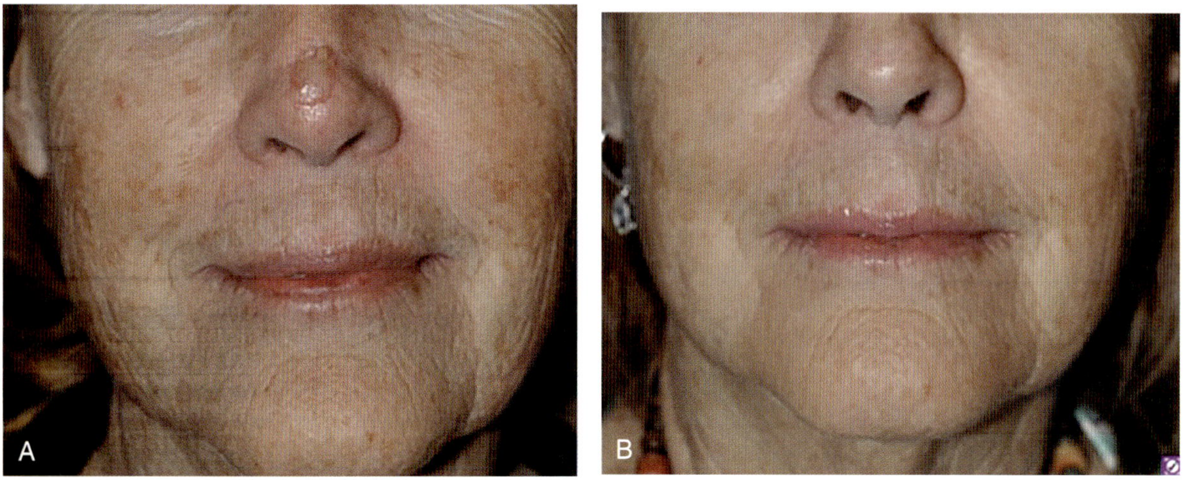

Fig. 5.8 A 60-year-old female with hypertrophic scar of the tip of the nose before (A) and 4 months after 2 (B) treatment sessions with CO_2 AFL and PDT.

groups. However, the microneedling and laser treatment groups demonstrated faster clinical improvement of pigmentation and vascularity as compared to the steroid group alone. The ablation laser group had decreased recurrence compared to the steroid-treated group at 6-month follow-up (Fig. 5.8).

Discussion

Despite the numerous benefits of AFL-PDT, increased pain experienced both during ablative treatment and during subsequent illumination is higher as compared to conventional PDT and may be a limiting factor for patients.[15] Lesions of large size or located on the face or scalp are reported as more painful to treat.[26,27] As in all laser procedures, the training of the laser operator is important. Although UV-derived photodamage, such as AKs, occurs in lighter Fitzpatrick skin types (I and II) with increased frequency, solar damage, and other PDT-treatable conditions can occur in all skin types. Fraction laser ablation, both with CO_2 and ER:YAG, carries a risk of dyspigmentation increasing with the degree of natural pigmentation and necessitating a skilled laser operator to utilize laser-facilitated delivery.[28]

Conclusion

This chapter presented several approaches reported in the literature for the improvement of topical PDT with the use of LAD. Some of the techniques presented are being increasingly used and incorporated into PDT protocols. Laser-assisted drug delivery has continued to evolve and has provided a passage into the skin for penetration of transcutaneous drug delivery. This combination treatment is generally well tolerated and should be considered for patients for efficacious treatment of field cancerization, cosmetic concerns, and those who refuse surgery for superficial cutaneous malignancies or are not surgical candidates. As with other treatment modalities, close follow-up is needed after PDT and laser-facilitated PDT treatment of any cutaneous malignancy.

REFERENCES

1. Nino M, Calabrò G, Santoianni P. Topical delivery of active principles: the field of dermatological research. *Dermatol Online J.* 2010;16(1):4.
2. Yoshioka E, Shankar Chelakkot V, Licursi M, et al. Enhancement of cancer-specific protoporphyrin IX fluorescence by targeting oncogenic Ras/MEK pathway. *Theranostics.* 2018;8(8):2134–2146. doi:10.7150/thno.22641.
3. Lopez RFV, Lange N, Guy R, Bentley MVLB. Photodynamic therapy of skin cancer: controlled drug delivery of 5-ALA and its esters. *Adv Drug Deliv Rev.* 2004;56(1):77–94. doi:10.1016/j.addr.2003.09.002.
4. Forster B, Klein A, Szeimies RM, Maisch T. Penetration enhancement of two topical 5-aminolaevulinic acid formulations for photodynamic therapy by erbium: YAG laser ablation of the stratum corneum: continuous versus fractional ablation. *Exp Dermatol.* 2010;19(9):806–812. doi:10.1111/j.1600-0625.2010.01093.x.
5. Alexiades M. Randomized, controlled trial of fractional carbon dioxide laser resurfacing followed

by ultrashort incubation aminolevulinic acid blue light photodynamic therapy for actinic keratosis. *Dermatol Surg*. 2017;43(8):1053–1064. doi:10.1097/DSS.0000000000001117.

6. Sasaki GH, Travis HM, Tucker B. Fractional CO_2 laser resurfacing of photoaged facial and non-facial skin: histologic and clinical results and side effects. *J Cosmet Laser Ther*. 2009;11(4):190–201. doi:10.3109/14764170903356465.
7. Zhang LW, Fang YP, Fang JY. Enhancement techniques for improving 5-aminolevulinic acid delivery through the skin. *Dermatol Sin*. 2011;29(1):1–7. doi:10.1016/j.dsi.2011.02.002.
8. Haedersdal M, Katsnelson J, Sakamoto FH, et al. Enhanced uptake and photoactivation of topical methyl aminolevulinate after fractional CO_2 laser pretreatment. *Lasers Surg Med*. 2011;43(8):804–813. doi:10.1002/lsm.21096.
9. Blume JE, Oseroff AR. Aminolevulinic acid photodynamic therapy for skin cancers. *Dermatol Clin*. 2007;25(1):5–14. doi:10.1016/j.det.2006.09.005.
10. Kohl E, Karrer S. [New developments in photodynamic therapy]. *Hautarzt*. 2013;64(5):363–369. doi:10.1007/s00105-012-2513-x.
11. Champeau M, Vignoud S, Mortier L, Mordon S. Photodynamic therapy for skin cancer: how to enhance drug penetration? *J Photochem Photobiol B*. 2019;197:111544. doi:10.1016/j.jphotobiol.2019.111544.
12. Alexiades-Armenakas M. Laser-mediated photodynamic therapy. Clin Dermatol. 24(1):16–25. doi:10.1016/j.clindermatol.2005.10.027.
13. Lee WR, Shen SC, Pai MH, Yang HH, Yuan CY, Fang JY. Fractional laser as a tool to enhance the skin permeation of 5-aminolevulinic acid with minimal skin disruption: a comparison with conventional erbium: YAG laser. *J Control Release*. 2010;145(2):124–133. doi:10.1016/j.jconrel.2010.03.017.
14. Huang A, Nguyen JK, Austin E, Mamalis A, Jagdeo J. Updates on treatment approaches for cutaneous field cancerization. 2019;8:122–132. doi:10.1007/s13671-019-00265-2.
15. Togsverd-Bo K, Haak CS, Thaysen-Petersen D, Wulf HC, Anderson RR, Hædesdal M. Intensified photodynamic therapy of actinic keratoses with fractional CO_2 laser: a randomized clinical trial. *Br J Dermato*. 2012;166(6):1262–1269. doi:10.1111/j.1365-2133.2012.10893.x.
16. Wlodek C, Ali FR, Lear JT. Use of photodynamic therapy for treatment of actinic keratoses in organ transplant recipients. *Biomed Res Int*. 2013;2013:349526. doi:10.1155/2013/349526.
17. Lonsdorf AS, Keller A, Hartmann J, Enk AH, Gholam P. Ablative fractional laser-assisted low-irradiance photodynamic therapy for treatment of actinic keratoses in organ transplant recipients: a prospective, randomized, intraindividual controlled trial. *Acta Derm Venereol*. 2022;102:adv00694. doi:10.2340/ACTADV.V102.1057.
18. Woźniak Z, Trzeciakowski W, Chlebicka I, Ziółkowski P. Photodynamic diagnosis and photodynamic therapy in basal cell carcinoma using a novel laser light source. *Photodiagnosis Photodyn Ther*. 2020;31:101883. doi:10.1016/j.pdpdt.2020.101883.
19. Šmucler R, Vlk M. Combination of Er: YAG laser and photodynamic therapy in the treatment of nodular basal cell carcinoma. *Lasers Surg Med*. 2008;40(2):153–158. doi:10.1002/lsm.20606.
20. Kim SK, Do JE, Kang HY, Lee ES, Kim YC. Combination of topical 5-aminolevulinic acid photodynamic therapy with carbon dioxide laser for sebaceous hyperplasia. *J Am Acad Dermatol*. 2007;56(3):523–524. doi:10.1016/j.jaad.2006.10.044.
21. Cai H, Wang YX, Zheng JC, et al. Photodynamic therapy in combination with CO_2 laser for the treatment of Bowen's disease. *Lasers Med Sci*. 2015;30(5):1505–1510. doi:10.1007/s10103-015-1754-1.
22. Marini L, Marini S. Lentigo maligna and intensified ablative fractional laser-assisted PDT: a promising, minimally invasive treatment approach. *J Eur Acad Dermatol Venereol*. 2020;34(3):440–441. doi:10.1111/jdv.16262.
23. Horio T, Horio O, Miyauchi-Hashimoto H, Ohnuki M, Isei T. Photodynamic therapy of sebaceous hyperplasia with topical 5-aminolaevulinic acid and slide projector. *Br J Dermatol*. 2003;148(6):1274–1276. doi:10.1046/J.1365-2133.2003.05360.X.
24. Zhang LC, Hao LM, Tan JX, et al. Efficacy of the combination of minimally invasive CO_2 laser incision with photodynamic therapy for infected epidermoid cysts. *Photodiagnosis Photodyn Ther*. 2020;30:101791. doi:10.1016/j.pdpdt.2020.101791.
25. Wang B, Yao Y, Huang X, Zhang L, Peng D, Zhang G. The combination of photodynamic therapy and ultrapulse carbon dioxide laser for facial angiofibromas in tuberous sclerosis complex: a case report. *Photodiagnosis Photodyn Ther*. 2022;37:102725. doi:10.1016/j.pdpdt.2022.102725.
26. Ericson MB, Wennberg AM, Larkö O. Review of photodynamic therapy in actinic keratosis and basal cell carcinoma. *Ther Clin Risk Manag*. 2008;4(1):1–9.
27. Grapengiesser S, Gudmundsson F, Larkö O, Ericson M, Rosé A, Wennberg AM. Pain caused by photodynamic therapy of skin cancer. *Clinical and Experimental Dermatology* 2002;27(6):493–497.
28. Sriprachya-anunt S, Marchell NL, Fitzpatrick RE, Goldman MP, Rostan EF. Facial resurfacing in patients with Fitzpatrick skin type IV. *Lasers Surg Med*. 2002;30(2):86–92. doi:10.1002/lsm.10012.

6

Photodynamic Therapy Combination Protocols

Jill S. Waibel, Alexander A. Daoud, Rebecca L. Quiñonez, Mary Dick, Emily Sedaghat, Karan Rajalingam

KEY POINTS

- PDT is an effective therapy for treating actinic keratoses, acne vulgaris, and ultraviolet-induced photodamage.
- The choice of light source in PDT is influenced by the photosensitizer's absorption spectrum, light wavelength, and penetration depth.
- Combining PDT with other treatments can enhance efficacy, reduce side effects, and shorten treatment duration.
- Current combination therapies use different light sources alongside PDT to improve outcomes for conditions like actinic keratosis, acne, and photodamage.
- PDT monotherapy is effective, but combination therapies can provide better therapeutic results.
- The use of combination therapies has expanded the applicability of PDT in both medical and cosmetic dermatology.
- This structure reflects a comprehensive overview of PDT, its current uses, and the exploration of combination therapies to improve treatment outcomes.

OBJECTIVES

- To explore and discuss the current combination therapies of light sources in photodynamic therapy (PDT), emphasizing their application for actinic keratosis, acne vulgaris, ultraviolet-induced photodamage, and other cosmetic uses.
- The goal is to expand the understanding and effectiveness of PDT by combining it with other therapeutics to improve treatment outcomes.

INTRODUCTION

Photodynamic therapy (PDT) is an effective field-directed therapy for the treatment of medical conditions, such as actinic keratoses (AKs) and acne vulgaris, and cosmetic use in the treatment of ultraviolet-induced photodamage. The choice of light sources for PDT is determined by two main factors: the absorption spectrum of the photosensitizing agent applied to the skin, and the wavelength and penetration depth of the light itself. While monotherapy with PDT is successful, physicians may elect to combine PDT with other therapeutics to increase treatment efficacy, diminish the risk of treatment side effects, or shorten the duration of treatment for a specific condition. In this chapter, we will discuss several current combination therapies of light sources that have expanded our understanding and use of PDT for actinic keratosis, acne, photodamage, and other cosmetic uses.

What Is ALA?

Previous chapters have expanded on the principle of PDT in which aminolevulinic acid (ALA), a photosensitizing agent, undergoes a photochemical, auto-fluorescent reaction and becomes a prometabolite upon exposure to specific wavelengths of light. Topical ALA is absorbed with greater avidity by the metabolically active keratinocytes in various disease states, where it is then converted intracellularly into the potent photosensitizer protoporphyrin IX (PpIX). When PpIX is exposed to a light source within the absorption spectrum of the selected photosensitizer, it generates reactive oxygen species that lead to apoptosis and autophagy of the target cells. The resultant inflammatory cascade creates a microenvironment rich in proinflammatory cytokines and chemokines that stimulate epidermal healing and turnover, induce fibroblast activation, and thereby promote collagen synthesis and overall dermal remodeling.[1,2]

At present, there are two FDA-approved forms of ALA. ALA HCl in topical solution form contains 20% ALA, as well as an endogenous 5-carbon aminoketone. The solution comes in a two-ampule applicator that is enclosed in a protective cardboard sleeve and cap. The ampules are lightly broken at the time of use and mixed by shaking the contents of the applicator. More recently, a nanoemulsion form of ALA was developed as a gel, favoring easier application and greater stability than the ampule presentation.

Light Source Matters

PpIX has an absorption spectrum with a maximal peak at 410 nm (blue region) and lesser peaks at 509, 544, 584, and 635 nm. Penetration depth increases in direct proportion to wavelength across the visible spectrum. While many studies have detailed the efficacy of single light source PDT for the treatment of various disease states, there is limited data in the literature describing the serial use of multiple light sources for photosensitizer activation. Given the multiple accessory absorption peaks seen with PpIX, use of light sources within these ranges may guarantee that multiple absorption peaks of PpIX are successfully targeted during treatment, theoretically leading to increased prodrug activation and a more effective therapeutic response (Fig. 6.1).

Blue Light Source

Blue light peaks at a wavelength of 405–415 nm. Aside from being used for AKs, blue light PDT is also used for inflammatory acne, as well as other dermatologic conditions. While *Cutibacterium acnes* (formerly *Propionibacterium*) emits its own photosensitizer, thereby making it sensitive to the blue light wavelength spectrum, the use of topically applied photosensitizers allows for the anti-inflammatory benefits of PDT to contribute to its antimicrobial effects.[3] A study conducted by Gilcrest and colleagues produced excellent cosmetic outcomes and decreased texture of scars on two subjects when combining the use of ALA-PDT with 417 nm blue light for treatment of multiple basal cell carcinomas in patients with basal cell nevus (Gorlin) syndrome.[4] The energy settings used were 10 J/cm^2 for two (2) consecutive treatments, one (1) week apart for a total of two (2) courses of PDT with ALA two to four (2–4) months apart.

Smith and colleagues compared the efficacy of broad area PDT using ALA + blue light, ALA + PDL, or topical 5-FU in the treatment of AK of the face and scalp in 36 Caucasian patients with hyperkeratotic lesions in the face and scalp.[5] The subjects were divided into two groups. A total of two treatments were 30 days apart. Patients were further randomized for the topical application of 5-FU to the treatment areas once or twice daily for 4 weeks. The authors found that both 5-FU and blue light PDT groups had 75% or more clearance of AK lesions in comparison to 43% for the PDL-PDT group. Furthermore, the effects of photoaging on all three treatment groups showed improvement in tactile, roughness, and mottled hyperpigmentation. The 5-FU and blue light + PDT group have greater outcomes in skin texture, while 5-FU and PDL-PDT favored pigmentation.[5]

Other studies have compared the safety of blue versus red light therapy for patients with BCC and found that both are equally safe and effective for such conditions.[6]

Intense Pulsed Light (IPL)

The combination treatment of IPL with PDT has been used for actinic keratosis and photoaging, proving to be an effective alternative treatment. One study examined 17 patients treated with ALA-IPL and were evaluated for improvement of telangiectasias, blotchy pigment, fine wrinkles, coarseness of skin, and number of actinic keratosis.[7] A 68% clearance of AKs was noted after one treatment, but with only a minimal change in fine wrinkle appearance.

Another study by Kim and colleagues suggests that IPL is a potentially effective light source for PDT after clearing 50% of AKs in seven patients with a single treatment.[8] Furthermore, Dover and colleagues performed three split-face treatments 3 weeks apart where half of

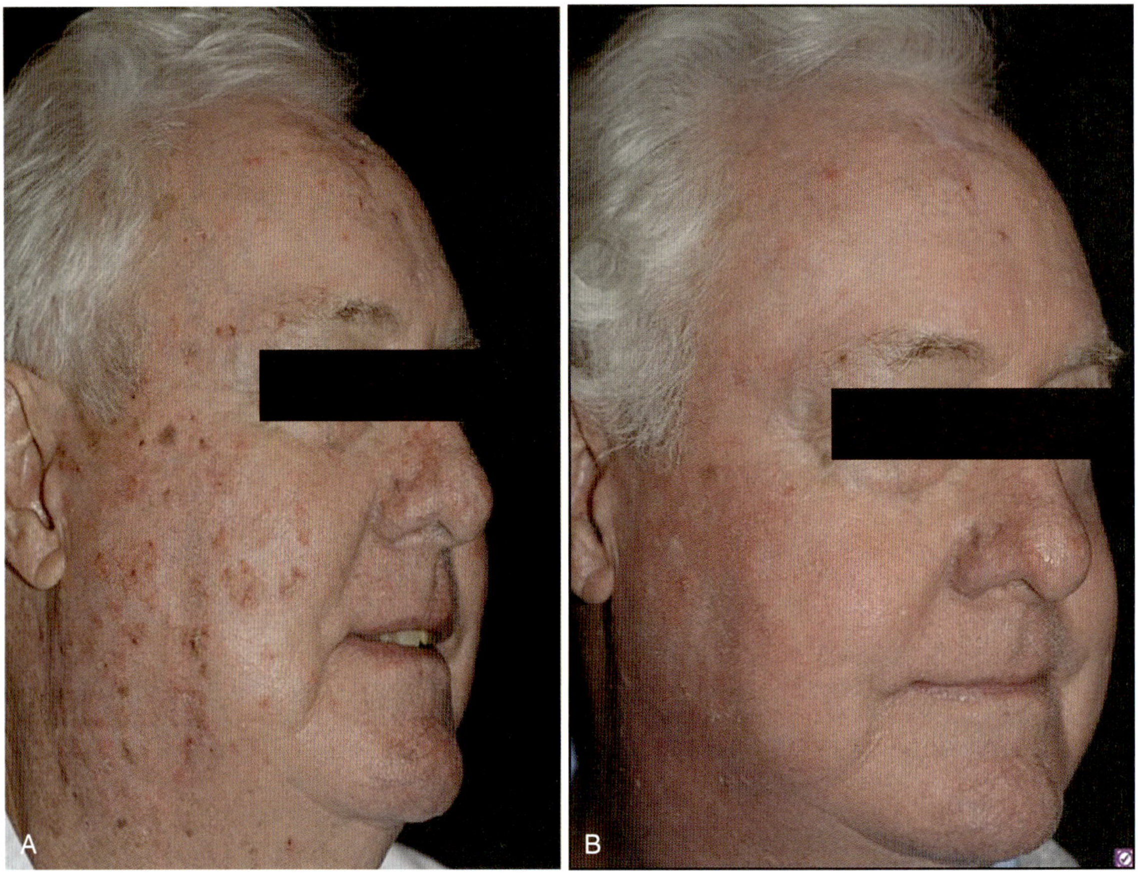

Fig. 6.1 A 68-year-old patient with Fitzpatrick Skin Type II with a history of SCCIS of forehead, BCC of right ear and diffuse AKs on the face, chest and bilateral arms, and rosacea before (A) and after (B) two sessions of IPL/BBL/PDT.

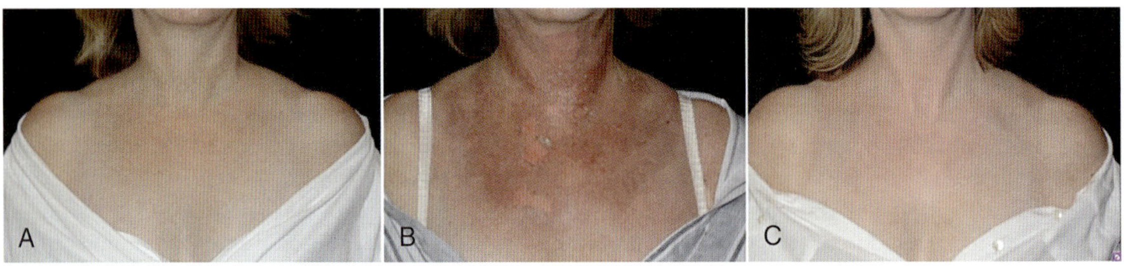

Fig. 6.2 A 54-year-old female with actinic damage of the chest before (A), 1 week post-op (B), and 2 months after (C) PDT treatment.

the face was pretreated with 5-ALA followed by IPL treatment while the other half of the face was treated with IPL alone, with an additional full-face treatment of IPL alone delivered 3 weeks apart. The adjunctive use of 5-ALA with facial photoaging with IPL provided greater improvement in photodamage, pigmentation, and fine lines, and greater patient satisfaction than IPL alone (Fig. 6.2).

Pulsed Dye Laser

The combination of PDT and PDL (PDT-PDL) can be utilized for the treatment of AKs, acne, and lichen sclerosus. Examining the absorption spectrum for protoporphyrin IX, the potential efficacy of this combination is clear: with its lesser absorption peak from 585 to 600 nm, 595 nm pulsed dye laser may result in activation of more PpIX and therefore enhance therapeutic response as compared to blue light monotherapy alone. For the treatment of AKs, Alexiades-Armenakas and Geronemus utilized long-pulse pulsed dye laser (LP-PDL) as an alternative light source to blue light, achieving a mean percentage of 90%–100% clearance of AKs on the head and extremities, respectively, at 8 months. They demonstrated no difference in 3-h incubation under occlusion compared to a 14–18 h incubation time. Additional benefits of LP-PDL include enhanced patient comfort: by virtue of the dynamic cooling of pulsed dye lasers, over treatment comfort may be enhanced. In addition, alterations in spot size grant physicians both greater specificity and control over treatment areas.

Combination Treatment	Authors	Photosensitizer	Incubation Time	Settings
Blue light source				
Blue light	Itkin and Gilchrest[4]	Delta-ALA	1–5 h before treatment	417 ± 5 nm blue light Irradiance 10 mW/cm^2 1000 s (10 J/cm^2) 2–4 months apart
Blue light vs. PDL	Smith et al.[5]	20% ALA	1 h	Two treatments 30 days apart
Blue vs. Red	Maytin et al.[6]	20% ALA	4 h	Blue light 417 nm power density 10 mW/cm^2 1000 s to deliver a fluence of 10 J/cm^2 red light 630 nm power density ~75 mW/cm^2 ~8 min to deliver a fluence of 37 J/cm^2
Intense pulsed dye				
	Avram and Goldman[7] Kim et al.[8]	20% ALA		
Pulsed dye laser				
Long-pulse Pulse dye laser (595 nm Vbeam)	Alexiades-Armenakas and Geron-oemus[9]	20% ALA with	3 h under occlusion	1–4 nonoverlapping pulses with 30-ms delay prior to each pulse Fluence: 4–7.5 J/cm^2 Pulse duration: 10-ms Spot size: 10-mm spot size Cooling: 30-ms cryogen spray
Long-pulse Pulse dye laser (595 nm Vbeam)	Alexiades-Ar-menakas[10]	20% ALA	45 min under occlusion	1 minimally overlapping pass Fluence: 7.0–7.5 J/cm^2 Pulse duration: 10-ms Spot size: 10-mm spot size Cooling: 30-ms with 30-ms delay cryogen spray

Continued

Combination Treatment	Authors	Photosensitizer	Incubation Time	Settings
Long-pulse Pulse dye laser (595 nm Vbeam)	Alexiades-Armenakas	20% ALA	1 h under occlusion	2 minimally overlapping passes Fluence: 7.5 J/cm^2 Pulse duration: 10-ms Spot size: 10-mm spot size Cooling: 30-ms with 30-ms delay cryogen spray

Cutibacterium acnes produces endogenous protoporphyrin. Accordingly, *Cutibacterium* is sensitive to the blue light wavelength spectrum. Photoactivation of this endogenous compound production results in an inherent low-grade bactericidal PDT reaction, decreasing both inflammatory and comedonal acne.[11] *C. Acnes* is further reduced by the application of exogenous photosensitizers, which accumulate within the bacterium themselves. Subsequent treatment with an exogenous light source, be it blue light, red light, pulsed dye laser, IPL, or natural sunlight introduces an additional therapeutic benefit for patients: beyond the antimicrobial effects of photoactivation within bacterium, PDT alters the chemokine/cytokine profile in the local microenvironment toward one of anti-inflammatory cascades. Alexiades-Armenakas had a 100% clearance rate in 14 patients with comedonal, inflammatory, and cystic acne who previously failed classic oral and topical acne therapies after a mean of 2.9 PDT treatments completed with LP-PDL.[10]

Lichen sclerosus, also known as lichen sclerosis atrophicus, is the most common vulvar inflammatory dermatosis with poorly elucidated pathogenesis. It is classically seen in the anogenital region of elderly females but can occur in males, children, and in extragenital locations. Pruritus, pain, and disfigurement due to skin shrinkage can have a profound effect on daily life activities and be refractory to first-line treatments of topical hormones and ultrapotent topical steroids.[12] The treatment of pruritus associated with extragenital lichen sclerosis with LP-PDL-mediated PDT has been published in a case report with success after three treatment sessions.[13]

Light Emitting Diode (LED) and Handheld Devices

PDT light sources include LED portable light sources, handheld devices, and the organic source, the sun. LED handheld devices have gained popularity for the treatment of acne and photoaging.[14] The FDA categorizes these devices as cosmetic products which allows them to be readily available over the counter to consumers. Unlike medical devices used by practitioners in offices, handheld devices do not undergo double-blinded randomized controlled trials to obtain FDA clearance. Cosmetic products are not held to the same standard as medical devices; thus the evidence of efficacy is not well studied.

LED is a medical technology that alters skin biology and manages skin conditions. Jagdeo and colleagues determined that acne, herpes simplex and zoster, and acute wound healing were the three conditions with the highest reported use of LED therapy since 1968.[15] The current practice of dermatology combines systemic and topical therapies with LEDs to provide clinically advantageous results.

Sadick and colleagues compared the effects of red (633 nm) and blue (415 nm) LED on 17 patients who underwent twice-weekly 20-min sessions alternating between both light sources as the only treatment and noted improvement of noninflammatory lesions in 7/11 patients that completed the study.[16]

For the treatment of acne, Kwon assessed a randomized controlled trial of the use of LED for mild-to-moderate acne in 35 patients with combination treatment of 420 nm blue light and 660 nm red light device (OCimple Light Therapy System, MP 200; CERAGEM MEDISYS, Inc., Cheonan, Korea). The regimen consisted of 2.5 min, twice daily for 4 weeks where patients achieved a decrease of inflammatory lesions by 76.8% decrease at their 12-week checkup.

Gold and colleagues tested Silk'n Blue (Home Skinovations, Inc.) twice weekly for 3–5 min per section for the treatment of mild-to-moderate inflammatory acne in 17 patients and noted a 36.4% improvement at 3 months post-treatment.[17] Hellman and Ramirez examined the same device in a prospective uncontrolled trial of

15 patients instructed to use the device daily for 3–5 min per section for 12 weeks and noted a 41.8% reduction of acne lesions at 3 months follow-up.[18] The authors of both studies did not control the use of topical acne treatments.

A split-face study compared the use of the 412 nm Tria blue light device (Tria Beauty; SpectraGenics, Inc.) at two different fluences for mild-to-moderate acne on 32 subjects. Treatment at the higher fluence was associated with significant reductions in lesions from baseline within 1 week of treatment compared to the lower fluence group, which showed reduction at week three.[19,20]

In 2009, Dr. Pearson's AcneApp via Apple App Store, gained popularity after claiming to clear acne. It used an alternating blue (antibacterial) and red (anti-inflammatory) light technology, believed to kill bacteria associated with acne. Although light therapy can help treat acne, the low levels of light from the iPhone device were not sufficient and there was no proof that they worked as advertised.[21]

Organic sunlight. Conventional PDT via external light sources often results in post-treatment photosensitivity, erythema, and varying levels of discomfort/pain. Additionally, the therapeutic depth from the skin is 1–2 mm with blue light and 1–6 mm with red light, limiting its clinical use to the availability of resources.[22] To circumvent these effects, some may elect to pursue daylight or organic PDT. In this treatment fashion, photosensitizer is applied, and the patient is exposed to sunlight for varying lengths of time. As natural sunlight encompasses the absorption peaks of most available photosensitizers, albeit at lower intensity and energy levels than those emitted by mechanical, manmade sources, daylight PDT may offer patients a less expensive, less intense therapeutic option to mechanical light source-driven PDT. Limitations to using daylight PDT include seasonal and weather limitations, variations in sunlight intensity both geographically and chronologically throughout the day, and the inherent risks of unprotected UV exposure.

Wiegell and colleagues compared the efficacy of MAL-PDT with 1½ versus 2½ h of light exposure in a randomized controlled study on 120 patients with AKs.[23] Subjects' lesions were prepared, and then sunscreen was applied to the face and scalp. MAL was applied to the entire treatment areas and were then instructed to expose themselves to daylight according to randomization. The amount of daylight exposure was monitored with a wristwatch dosimeter. The authors concluded that daylight-mediated MAL-PDT is an effective, convenient, and nearly pain-free treatment for patients with multiple thin AKs. Shive and colleagues assessed the safety and efficacy of daylight PDT in treating AKs on the face and scalp using ALA on 30 patients.[24] The authors instructed patients to incubate for 30 min and then were told to seek sun exposure for 2 h in a shaded area. Daylight PDT led to a 78.5% reduction in AK count at 6 months with no significant side effects.

One therapeutic modality that may circumvent both the risks and lack of control associated with daylight PDT is IPL-driven PDT. As a light-based treatment modality, unfiltered IPL exposes patients to a broad range of wavelengths, ranging from 500 to 1400 nm. Accordingly, IPL provides a source that targets all absorption peaks of ALA, thereby increasing prodrug activation and potentially increasing therapeutic efficacy.

In a study of 220 subjects with either photodamage or AKs, individuals were assigned to one of four groups: PDT with IPL as the sole light source, PDT with IPL and blue light as dual light sources, PDT with PDL as the sole light source, or PDT with PDL and blue light as dual light sources.[25] Treatment with IPL and blue light dual-source treatment (both completed in the same session, single treatment setting) resulted in an 84.4% reduction of AKs at 1-month follow-up. In comparison, IPL and PDL monotherapy resulted in 70.8% and 70.5% reductions of AKs, respectively. Interestingly, treatment with PDL and blue light dual therapy offered the lowest reduction rate, 69.3% (Fig. 6.3). As compared to baseline, statistically significant improvements in photoaging were seen in subjects assigned to all four groups.[25]

Topical Treatment In Combination With PDT

Diclofenac. Topical treatment use in combination with PDT has evidence of creating more efficacious outcomes in overall appearance of treatment benefits. The nonsteroidal anti-inflammatory drug, diclofenac, can be used in treating AKs in conjunction with PDT as it inhibits COX-2 of the prostaglandin synthesis pathway resulting in increased production of arachidonic acids.[26] The role of arachidonic acid, a fatty acid, is to stimulate angiogenesis.

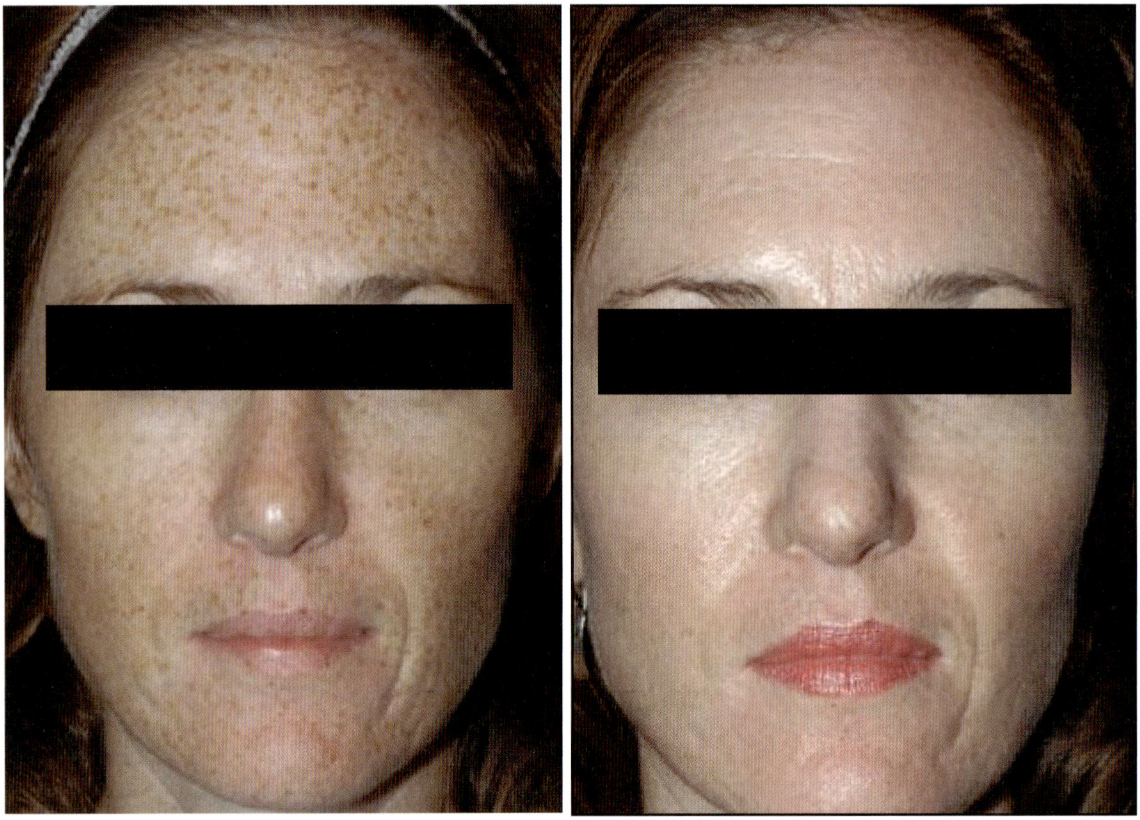

Fig. 6.3 A 42-year-old female with extensive photodamage before (left) and 1 month after (right) treatment with PDL and blue light.

In a study by Van Der Geer and colleagues, administration of diclofenac twice daily for 4 weeks prior to ALA-PDT treatment resulted in improved outcomes, although patients reported pain exacerbation with treatment due to its ability to arouse the peripheral somatosensory system.[26] The application of diclofenac and hyaluronic acid alone, with longer use, has shown benefits as well, thus a longer administration of diclofenac in conjunction with PDT therapy should be attempted, perhaps leading to increased improvement and effectiveness as the short time of 4 weeks did not result in a significant difference in outcome.

Imiquimod. The role of imiquimod is to modify the body's immune response by binding to toll-like receptor (TLR) 7.[27] TLR7 and 8 agonists assist antiviral and antibacterial activity in addition to their cancer-targeting properties, resulting in antitumor effects. The antiviral and antitumor properties of imiquimod come into effect by the stimulation of activating the nuclear factor kappa B (NF-κB) production pathway. NF-κB induces proinflammatory cytokine transcription stimulating the immune response to react to infected or tumorous cells.[28] When applied topically, imiquimod has the potential to create pro-apoptotic actions by binding to death receptors. Its role as a therapeutic agent for AKs has been shown to reduce the risk of further development and cause tumor regression. When combined with PDT, improved AK reduction was seen with twice-a-week application at 3-day intervals. Shaffelburg treated AK patients by first treating them with ALA-PDT at baseline at 1 month, then proceeding to add imiquimod cream at 2 months on one half of the face. Twelve months later, those treated with combination therapy showed improved results compared to those treated with solely ALA-PDT.[29]

In a similar study by Serra and colleagues, patients were placed into three groups—imiquimod alone, PDT alone, and combined therapy. Findings showed improved patient satisfaction with the combined therapy results in comparison to both single therapy groups.[26]

Topical retinoid. Topical retinoid therapy has different uses, but, in treatment of AKs, combined therapy of twice daily tazarotene gel (0.1%) a week prior to PDT showed increased reduction of AK lesions. A study by Galitzer to demonstrate benefits of 10% ALA-PDT and red light illumination in combination with adapalene gel (0.1%) showed improvement of almost 20%.[26]

5-fluorouracil. Pretreatment with 5-fluorouracil therapy twice daily for a week prior to PDT compared to those without pretreatment was shown to be more effective in a study by Niessen and colleagues. After 3 months, combination therapy of 5-FU and PDT had significantly better results in comparison to PDT alone.[30]

Calcitriol and calcipotriol. Calcitriol and calcipotriol are vitamin D analogs that have been used for pretreatment of AKs, although they have been associated with increased reactions in the skin. Initially studied by Galimberti, a 3-month treatment with calcitriol in combination showed 85% response compared to 70% of PDT alone, although some patients expressed erythema with calcitriol application, with daily application as a nuisance. For thicker lesions, these topical vitamin D analogs have shown improved efficacy. In another study by Torezan and colleagues, these findings were confirmed as areas treated with combined therapy compared to areas solely treated with MAL-PDT had improved outcomes.[26]

Concurrent treatment of topical therapy with PDT can show results that are significantly superior. Pretreatment therapy can be more beneficial than isolated PDT.

DISCUSSION

Since the first descriptions of the "photodynamic effect" of various dyes by Raab and von Tappeiner in the early 1900s, PDT has become an indispensable therapeutic modality across a variety of medical specialties.[31] In dermatology, PDT holds a rare place due to its applicability across the breadth of our field. In modern clinical settings, the same PDT setup that treats a pediatric patient with acne vulgaris can be used later that day to treat a superficial nonmelanoma skin cancer in an elderly patient. This same photosensitizer and light source combination may then be enhanced by various laser devices to treat poikiloderma in a young cosmetic patient. PDT's applications are broad, effective, and ever-evolving with the latter especially highlighted by contemporary research focused on modes of enhancing PDT's efficacy through novel combination approaches.

To this effect, a trend appears upon closer inspection of modern PDT research. There is a seeming departure from the 20th century's emphasis on classifying that disease states would respond to PDT. Instead, modern research endeavors hearken back to the era of Raab and von Tappeiner, with the focus returning to the unique physical and chemical properties that maximize PDT's efficacy. Specifically, increasing recognition has been given to the complete absorption spectra of our photosensitizing agents; a phrase referred to by one of the authors of this chapter as "seeking beyond the Soret band." Such investigations have ushered the introduction of nontraditional light sources into the PDT arena, where both monotherapy with these devices, as well as combinations of light sources themselves, demonstrate increased treatment efficacy, decreased adverse effects of treatment, and improved patient outcomes.

PDT's efficacy, as well as the therapeutic benefits seen with as few as one treatment session, warrants its high placement in the dermatologist's treatment algorithm for a variety of conditions. One such example is field precancerization: in the tropical climate of Miami, FL, where several of the authors practice, patient adherence to 2 or 4 weeks of topical chemotherapeutic agents is inconsistent at best. When offered the alternative of a single session of PDT, patient willingness to undergo treatment increases to a significant degree. Coupled with the increasing presence of laser and energy-based devices (such as pulsed dye laser and IPL) in the outpatient setting, clinicians now possess the tools necessary to obtain maximum success for their medical, surgical, pediatric, and cosmetic dermatology patients.

The future of PDT research will likely advance on three fronts: the light source, the photosensitizer, and the conditions treated. As we classify further light sources and devices that may be used in PDT combination treatments, so too will we augment (and improve) our current treatment algorithms. Further development of novel photosensitizers, both in active agents as well as topical vehicles, will also aid this therapeutic effort. Lastly, the classification of other disease states that show response to PDT may not only improve treatment outcomes for various conditions but will afford patients more treatment options and improved autonomy during their care.

CONCLUSION

PDT treatment can be used in practice to treat a myriad of medical and cosmetic dermatological conditions. Clinical efficacy of PDT depends on the major light sources and delivery devices used. Further studies need to be performed to continue assessing the efficacy of combined treatments for other disease states. Herein, we have discussed PDT combination treatment and the future of PDT.

REFERENCES

1. Gollnick SO, Evans SS, Baumann H, et al. Role of cytokines in photodynamic therapy-induced local and systemic inflammation. *Br J Cancer*. 2003;88(11):1772–1779. doi:10.1038/sj.bjc.6600864.
2. Wang P, Han J, Wei M, et al. Remodeling of dermal collagen in photoaged skin using low-dose 5-aminolevulinic acid photodynamic therapy occurs via the transforming growth factor-β pathway. *J Biophotonics*. 2018;11(6):e201700357. doi:10.1002/jbio.201700357.
3. Sakamoto FH, Lopes JD, Anderson RR. Photodynamic therapy for acne vulgaris: a critical review from basics to clinical practice: part I. Acne vulgaris: when and why consider photodynamic therapy? *J Am Acad Dermatol*. 2010;63(2): 183–193; quiz 193–194. doi:10.1016/j.jaad.2009.09.056.
4. Itkin A, Gilchrest BA. delta-Aminolevulinic acid and blue light photodynamic therapy for treatment of multiple basal cell carcinomas in two patients with nevoid basal cell carcinoma syndrome. *Dermatol Surg*. 2004;30(7):1054–1061. doi:10.1111/j.1524-4725.2004.30317.x.
5. Smith S, Piacquadio D, Morhenn V, Atkin D, Fitzpatrick R. Short incubation PDT versus 5-FU in treating actinic keratoses. *J Drugs Dermatol*. 2003;2(6):629–635.
6. Maytin EV, Kaw U, Ilyas M, Mack JA, Hu B. Blue light versus red light for photodynamic therapy of basal cell carcinoma in patients with Gorlin syndrome: a bilaterally controlled comparison study. *Photodiagnosis Photodyn Ther*. 2018;22:7–13. doi:10.1016/j.pdpdt.2018.02.009.
7. Avram DK, Goldman MP. Effectiveness and safety of ALA-IPL in treating actinic keratoses and photodamage. *J Drugs Dermatol*. 3(1 Suppl):S36–S39.
8. Kim HS, Yoo JY, Cho KH, Kwon OS, Moon SE. Topical photodynamic therapy using intense pulsed light for treatment of actinic keratosis: clinical and histopathologic evaluation. *Dermatol Surg*. 2005;31(1):33–36; discussion 36–7. doi:10.1111/j.1524-4725.2005.31003.
9. Alexiades-Armenakas MR, Geronemus RG. Laser-mediated photodynamic therapy of actinic keratoses. *Arch Dermatol*. 2003;139(10):1313–1320. doi:10.1001/archderm.139.10.1313.
10. Alexiades-Armenakas M. Long-pulsed dye laser-mediated photodynamic therapy combined with topical therapy for mild to severe comedonal, inflammatory, or cystic acne. *J Drugs Dermatol*. 2006;5(1):45–55.
11. Touma DJ, Gilchrest BA. Topical photodynamic therapy: a new tool in cosmetic dermatology. *Seminars in Cutaneous Medicine and Surgery*. 2003;22(2).
12. Nair P. Vulvar lichen sclerosus et atrophicus. *J Midlife Health*. 2017;8(2):55–62. doi:10.4103/jmh.JMH_13_17.
13. Alexiades-Armenakas M. Laser-mediated photodynamic therapy of lichen sclerosus. *J Drugs Dermatol*. 2004;3(6):S25–S27.
14. Hession MT, Markova A, Graber EM. A review of hand-held, home-use cosmetic laser and light devices. *Dermatol Surg*. 2015;41(3):307–320. doi:10.1097/DSS.0000000000000283.
15. Jagdeo J, Austin E, Mamalis A, Wong C, Ho D, Siegel DM. Light-emitting diodes in dermatology: a systematic review of randomized controlled trials. *Lasers Surg Med*. 2018;50(6):613–628. doi:10.1002/lsm.22791.
16. Sadick NS. Handheld LED array device in the treatment of acne vulgaris. *J Drugs Dermatol*. 2008;7(4):347–350.
17. Gold MH, Biron JA, Sensing W. Clinical and usability study to determine the safety and efficacy of the Silk'n blue device for the treatment of mild to moderate inflammatory acne vulgaris. *J Cosmet Laser Ther*. 2014;16(3):108–113. doi:10.3109/14764172.2013.854638.
18. Hellman J, Ramirez CA. Evaluation of self-treatment of acne using Silk'n blue phototherapy system. *J Cosmet Dermatol Sci Appl*. 2014;04(03):179–184. doi:10.4236/jcdsa.2014.43025.
19. Wheeland RG, Dhawan S. Evaluation of self-treatment of mild-to-moderate facial acne with a blue light treatment system. *J Drugs Dermatol*. 2011;10(6):596–602.
20. Wheeland RG, Koreck A. Safety and effectiveness of a new blue light device for the self-treatment of mild-to-moderate acne. *J Clin Aesthet Dermatol*. 2012;5(5):25–31.
21. Dolan B. *US regulators remove two acne medical apps*. Mobi Health News. (2011, September 9). https://www.mobihealthnews.com/13123/us-regulators-remove-two-acne-medical-apps/.
22. Nguyen M, Sandhu SS, Sivamani RK. Clinical utility of daylight photodynamic therapy in the treatment of actinic keratosis - a review of the literature. *Clin Cosmet Investig Dermatol*. 2019;12:427–435. doi:10.2147/CCID.S167498.

23. Wiegell SR, Fabricius S, Stender IM, et al. A randomized, multicentre study of directed daylight exposure times of 1½ vs. 2½ h in daylight-mediated photodynamic therapy with methyl aminolaevulinate in patients with multiple thin actinic keratoses of the face and scalp. *Br J Dermatol*. 2011;164(5):1083–1090. doi:10.1111/j.1365-2133.2011.10209.x.
24. Shive ML, Coakley BJ, Bierman DF, et al. Use of 5-aminolevulinic acid and daylight photodynamic therapy for the treatment of actinic keratoses. *Dermatol Surg*. 2019;45(4):529–535. doi:10.1097/DSS.0000000000001771.
25. Abrouk M, Gianatasio C, Li Y, Waibel JS. Prospective study of intense pulsed light versus pulsed dye laser with or without blue light in the activation of PDT for the treatment of actinic keratosis and photodamage. *Lasers Surg Med*. 2022;54(1):66–73. doi:10.1002/lsm.23492.
26. Piaserico S, Mazzetto R, Sartor E, Bortoletti C. Combination-based strategies for the treatment of actinic keratoses with photodynamic therapy: an evidence-based review. *Pharmaceutics*. 2022;14(8):1726. doi:10.3390/pharmaceutics14081726.
27. Bubna AK. Imiquimod - its role in the treatment of cutaneous malignancies. *Indian J Pharmacol*. 2015;47(4):354–359. doi:10.4103/0253-7613.161249.
28. Patinote C, Karroum NB, Moarbess G, et al. Agonist and antagonist ligands of toll-like receptors 7 and 8: ingenious tools for therapeutic purposes. *Eur J Med Chem*. 2020;193:112238. doi:10.1016/j.ejmech.2020.112238.
29. Held L, Eigentler TK, Leiter U, Garbe C, Berneburg MJ. Effective combination of photodynamic therapy and imiquimod 5% cream in the treatment of actinic keratoses: three cases. *Biomed Res Int*. 2013;2013:102698. doi:10.1155/2013/102698.
30. Galimberti GN. Daylight photodynamic therapy versus 5-fluorouracil for the treatment of actinic keratosis: a case series. *Dermatol Ther (Heidelb)*. 2018;8(1):137–141. doi:10.1007/s13555-017-0219-9.
31. Kessel D. Photodynamic therapy: a brief history. *J Clin Med*. 2019;8(10):1581. doi:10.3390/jcm8101581.

7

Photodynamic Therapy for Skin Cancer and Precursor Lesions in Organ Transplant Recipients

Emily Wenande, Rajeev Chavda, Merete Haedersdal

KEY POINTS

- Organ transplant recipients (OTRs) are a high risk population for skin cancer requiring preventative therapy.
- Photodynamic therapy (PDT) is is used to manage skin dysplasia in high-risk populations with documented success.
- PDT management therapy for keratinocyte carcinomas and precursor lesions in OTR population is covered.

OBJECTIVES

- Understand the epidemiology, risk factors and cancer burden in the OTR population.
- Learn the PDT guidelines and protocols in OTR to treat existing lesions and as preventative and ongoing management.

INTRODUCTION

Organ transplant recipients (OTRs) represent a high-risk population for skin cancer due to the chronic immunosuppression necessary for graft survival. In the past decades, the increasing sophistication of organ transplantation has translated to a longer life expectancy for patients receiving transplants.[1] Additionally, the number of transplants being performed is steadily rising, and an older patient population is now eligible for transplantation.[2,3] In parallel with an intensified focus on post-transplant care, including skin cancer screening, the demand for improved therapeutic and preventative strategies for keratinocyte carcinomas (KCs) in the OTR setting is increasing.[4]

While ultraviolet (UV) exposure plays a major role in development of skin cancers similar to the general population, the lifelong immunosuppressive maintenance regimens of OTRs confer added KC risk.[5] Some immunosuppressive agents directly enhance UV radiation's carcinogenic effects,[6] while general immunosuppression results in abnormal anticancer immune surveillance that may be exacerbated by oncogenic viruses, host genetic susceptibility, and tumor genetic/epigenetic factors.[5,6] KCs, including cutaneous squamous cell carcinoma (SCC) and basal cell carcinoma (BCC), as well as precursor skin lesions such as actinic keratoses (AKs) and SCC in situ, are consequently a major source of morbidity in OTRs.[1,7,8] It has been estimated that the risk of SCC is increased between 65 and 250x in OTR patients, while risk of BCC is increased approximately 10-fold.[5,9,10] OTRs also suffer from greater skin cancer mortality, including greater risk of advanced or metastatic disease.[11,12] As a result, skin cancer is a leading cause of cancer-related OTR deaths.[13]

Photodynamic therapy (PDT) has been studied to manage skin dysplasia in high-risk populations with documented success.[14] For OTRs specifically, systematic reviews recently found that PDT represented a promising prevention and treatment approach for AK and SCC.[15,16] In the following chapter, PDT is discussed as a management strategy for KC and precursor lesions in OTR populations. The chapter specifically summarizes disease epidemiology and PDT regimens, in addition to exploring the evidence supporting PDT both as treatment strategy and a primary/secondary preventative approach in this high-risk population.

EPIDEMIOLOGY OF KERATINOCYTE CARCINOMA IN THE ORGAN TRANSPLANT RECIPIENT POPULATION

While elevated KC risk in transplant recipients is well-known, skin cancer epidemiology in OTR populations is variable. In studies from 2010 to 2013, the standardized incidence ratio (SIR, a measure of incidence vs. general population) for KCs showed wide variability, ranging from 4.1 to 357 depending on country and OTR subpopulation.[1] Reported cumulative incidences similarly ranged from 6% to 64.3% (Table 7.1).[1,17–20] Strikingly, a 30-year cohort study of OTR patients in Finland from 1987 to 2016, reported that 53% of post-transplant cancers were KCs.[21] Thus a SIR of 6.5 (95% CI, 6.1–7.1) was reported for BCC, lowest among liver recipients (4.1; 95% CI, 3.2–5.2) and highest in heart recipients (8.5; 95% CI, 6.8–10.5).[21] For SCCs, SIR was particularly elevated at 30.7 (95% CI, 27.8–33.9), highest in lung recipients (52.5; 95% CI, 27.1–91.8).[21] These rates are, however, evolving; most recent evidence now indicates falling relative risks for skin cancer in OTRs compared to background populations, likely due to improvements in immunosuppressive regimens for OTRs and rising skin cancer rates in the general population.[22,23]

Burden of KC in Transplant Patients

Skin cancers are a leading contributor to mortality in OTR patients.[24] Compared with skin cancers in the general population, KC tumors of OTRs are often more aggressive and have a higher likelihood of local recurrence and metastasis even when treated.[25,26] Additionally, OTR patients have a tendency toward multiple lesions, with a 5-year cumulative risk of about 70%.[24] The rate of metastasis of SCC in the OTR population is 8%, substantially higher than the 1% noted in the general population.[27] In addition, metastatic disease has a 3-year mortality rate of up to 46%.[9,27,28] Indeed, Garrett and colleagues note that skin cancer-related mortality among OTRs exceeds mortality in patients with breast or colon cancer.[13,25]

KC Risk Factors in OTRs

Much attention has surrounded the concept of individualized risk analysis as a means to tackle the burden of skin cancer screening in the OTR population.[1] Correspondingly, patient-oriented assessment of risk factors (Fig. 7.1) can guide clinicians in determining which patient stands to benefit most from therapeutic and preventative PDT strategies. Like immunocompetent patients, a history of exposure to UV radiation is a key risk factor for AK and KC development in OTRs.[5] As such, lesions are typically found in sun-exposed skin areas[5,29] and associated risk factors are fair skin type/white race, history of outdoor work, sunburns, cumulative sun exposure, and geographical location.[1] Multiple studies of OTRs furthermore find male sex to be an independent risk factor for skin cancer.[30,31] Transplantation-related factors are also of marked importance for KC risk and specifically include age at transplantation (>50 years), duration since transplantation, transplanted organ type, and type (i.e., azathioprine) and number of immunosuppressive agents included in patients' maintenances regimens.[1] Accordingly, 5%–12% of OTRs develop skin cancer within 5 years after transplantation, rising to 28%–40% within 15 years post transplant.[1] While all types of solid organ transplants are associated with increased skin cancer risk, a higher frequency after thoracic versus nonthoracic organ transplants has been shown.[32] Finally, history of skin cancer and precursor lesions are significant predictors of future skin cancer risk, since OTRs often go on to develop multiple lesions over time.[33,34]

TABLE 7.1 Cumulative Incidence of SCC, BCC and Keratinocyte Carcinoma (KC) Among OTR Recipients

	Study, Location	Years Post Transplant	Kidney	Liver	Heart	Lungs
SCC	Rashtak et al.,[17] USA	5				28%
		10				42%
	Fortina et al.,[18] Italy	5	6%		16%	
		10	17%		33%	
	Haagsma et al.,[19] Netherlands	5		4%		
		10		13%		
		15		28%		
	Ramsay et al.,[20] Australia	<5	16.9%			
		5–10	35.9%			
		10–20	52.4%			
		≥20	75%			
BCC	Rashtak et al.,[17] USA	5				12%
		10				21%
	Ramsay et al.,[20] Australia	<5	21.5%			
		5–10	39.1%			
		10–20	56.2%			
		≥20	64.3%			
KC	Rashtak et al.,[17] USA	5				31%
		10				47%
	Ramsay et al.,[20] Australia	<5	29.1%			
		5–10	52.2%			
		10–20	72.4%			
		≥20	82.1%			

PHOTODYNAMIC THERAPY GUIDELINES IN ORGAN TRANSPLANT RECIPIENTS

Available Guidelines for Use of PDT in OTR

The European Dermatology Forum 2020 guidelines for use of PDT gave a B recommendation for use of PDT in OTR, as supported by high-quality level 1 evidence from systematic review.[35] Specifically, authors recommend that PDT should be used to treat precursor lesions such as AK or Bowen's disease, as well as for KC prevention, particularly when field cancerization is observed (Fig. 7.2).[35] A 2021 international Delphi consensus group acknowledged the need for early and aggressive strategies for SCC in OTRs, noting that small, split-patient studies indicate that PDT outperforms 5-FU and imiquimod as AK treatment in transplant populations.[15,36] Among PDT regimens, a recent European consensus group noted that methyl aminolevulinate (MAL)-PDT remains the best-studied intervention for the treatment of AK in OTRs.[37]

PHOTODYNAMIC THERAPY REGIMENS IN ORGAN TRANSPLANT RECIPIENTS

Mechanism of Action of PDT

PDT is a minimally invasive treatment approach that targets cancer cells while largely sparing surrounding normal

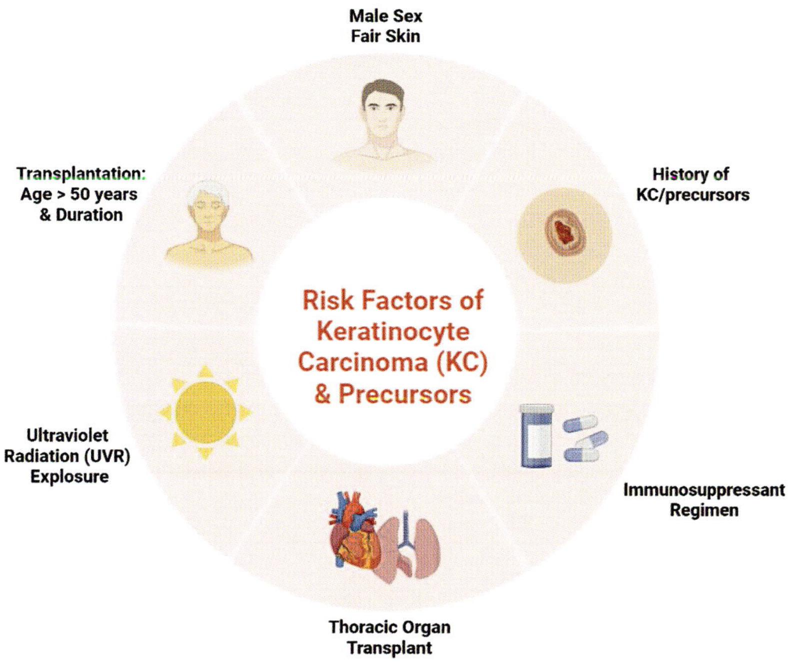

Fig. 7.1 Risk factors for keratinocyte carcinoma (KC) and precursors in organ transplant recipients (OTRs). (Figure created with BioRender.com.)

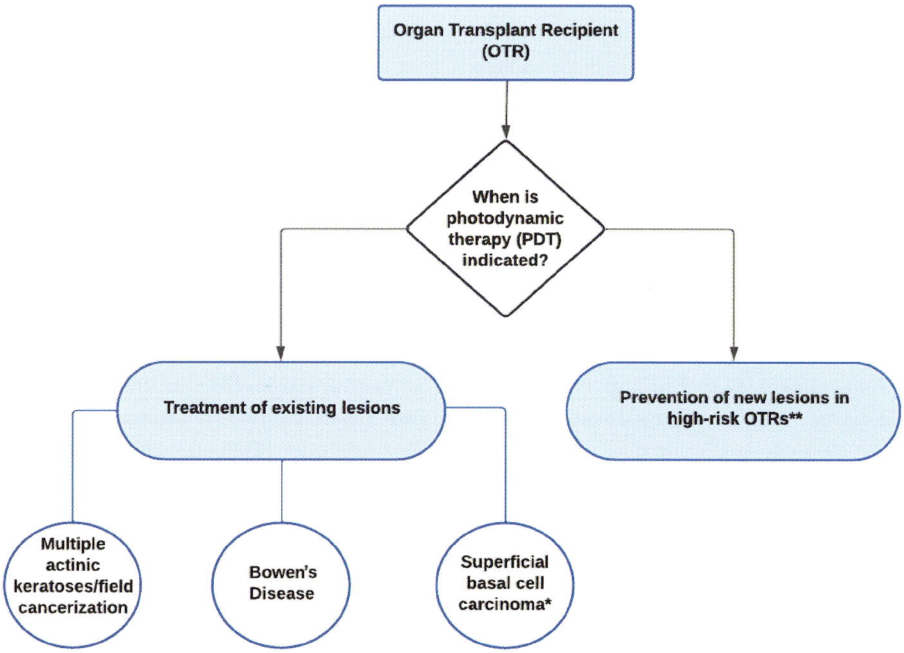

Fig. 7.2 Decision-making flowchart for photodynamic therapy (PDT) in organ transplant recipients (OTRs). For OTR patients, the European Dermatology Forum 2020 guidelines recommend PDT to treat instances of widespread actinic damage with multiple actinic keratoses (AK), known as field cancerization, as well as for Bowen's disease. For basal cell carcinoma (BCC)*, little evidence supports the use of PDT as a treatment for other than low-risk tumors, such as superficial BCCs. Based on current evidence, OTRs with a history of multiple AK or keratinocyte carcinoma** may benefit from PDT as a preventative strategy against new lesions.

tissue.[38] During PDT, a photosensitizing agent is taken up by malignant or premalignant cells.[14] Intracellularly, the agent is converted into the active photosensitizer, protoporphyrin IX (PpIX), through the heme synthesis biochemical pathway.[14] Upon introduction of a light source, PpIX is activated to form reactive oxygen species, killing malignant cells.[14] In addition, the inflammation caused by PDT involves local recruitment of antitumoral immune cells; an aspect that may partly explain lower efficacy of PDT in immunosuppressed patients.[39] On a genetic level, transcriptome studies in OTRs furthermore reveal that PDT corrects abnormal proliferation-related genes, induces extracellular matrix genes, and reverses abnormal expression of cancer-linked genes.[40,41]

PDT Photosensitizing Agents and Enhancement Approaches

PDT regimens typically employ 5-aminolevulinic acid (ALA) 20% or the more lipophilic agent MAL 16%.[14] While the agents are chemically distinct, they are both precursors of PpIX.[42,43] To enhance photosensitizer delivery and increase the efficacy of PDT, various pretreatment methods are employed including simple curettage of hyperkeratotic lesions, physical drug delivery strategies such as microneedling and laser, as well as the use of keratolytic agents like urea or salicylic acid.[5] Ongoing, cyclic regimens of PDT at 4- to 8-week intervals may also be employed to enhance the effect of PDT in OTR patients.[44,45]

PDT Regimens

For conventional PDT, MAL, and ALA have been utilized in combination with red light (633 ± 15 nm) or additionally for ALA-PDT, blue light (417 nm).[46,47] Prior to treatment, 1 mm thick MAL or ALA cream is applied to the affected skin area along with 5 mm margin of surrounding normal tissue.[43,47] After 3 h under semipermeable occlusion, the skin site is illuminated for 9 min.[47] For treatment of existing lesions, two PDT cycles are typically spaced 1–2 weeks apart.[47,48] For lesion prevention, a 6-month interval has been proposed.[49] During the more recently introduced daylight PDT (dPDT), MAL is applied for 30 min without occlusion. After, a 2-h period of exposure to daylight and sun avoidance for the remainder of the 24-h period is performed. MAL-dPDT has been shown to be as effective as conventional red or blue light PDT and is associated with decreased pain and better overall tolerance.[14,50]

PHOTODYNAMIC THERAPY AS TREATMENT FOR EXISTING LESIONS IN ORGAN TRANSPLANT RECIPIENTS

The European Dermatology Forum 2020 guidelines recommend PDT as a treatment for precursor lesions such as AK or Bowen's disease in the OTR population.[35] AKs and their management in OTR context are discussed below.

Actinic Keratoses (AKs)

AKs are epithelial lesions consisting of keratotic macules, papules, or plaques with superficial scaly growth.[51] These lesions are very commonly seen by dermatologists and occur more often in patients of increased age, male sex, fair skin, and with a history of sun exposure.[52] A systematic review found that the estimated transformation risk of an AK lesion ranged between 0.05% and 0.096% per year in immunocompetent patients, or 1% over 10 years.[53,54] Compared to the general population, AKs are more prevalent in OTRs, with a mean occurrence of 38% after 5 years of immunosuppression.[16] Less likely to regress, lesion progression rates seem accelerated in OTRs, where AKs often colocalize into confluent areas of "field cancerization" that give rise to SCC.[55–57] OTR patients with this clinical presentation have a threefold higher risk of SCC than patients with solitary AKs.[55] To reduce the total AK burden and mitigate SCC risks, international guidelines therefore recommend treatment of AK.

AK treatment options are divided into lesion-directed approaches (i.e., cryotherapy, curettage, or ablation) or field-directed approaches that address the broader skin field. Topical field therapies should be considered when widespread actinic damage with multiple AKs, known as field cancerization, is clinically present (Fig. 7.3), and approved field treatments include PDT, 5-fluorouracil (5-FU), imiquimod, diclofenac sodium, and tirbanibulin.[44] In immunocompetent individuals, PDT response rates range between 69% and more than 90% after one and two sessions, respectively.[58–60] For OTRs, a 2019 systematic review found PDT to be an efficacious therapeutic and preventative strategy for AK.[16] In the following, evidence supporting the use of PDT for existing AKs in the OTR population is presented (Table 7.2).

PDT for Existing AKs: Evidence in OTR Populations

Although comparative treatment studies are limited, MAL-PDT currently remains the best-documented

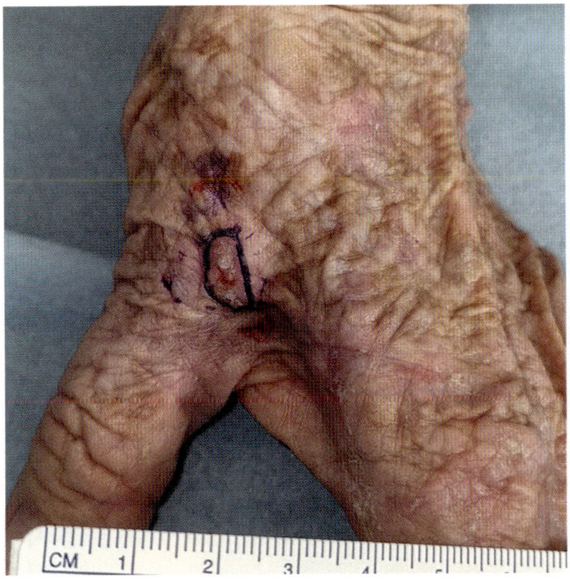

Fig. 7.3 Field cancerization with multiple AKs and a histologically confirmed SCC in situ (encircled in blue) on the dorsal hand of an elderly organ transplant recipient.

treatment of AKs in the OTR setting.[15] Dragieva and colleagues studied 17 OTRs with a total of 129 AKs in a prospective, intra-individually controlled RCT. Patients were treated with MAL or placebo cream followed by visible light (600–730 nm) in two sessions, 1 week apart.[61] At 16 weeks, complete response was noted in 13/17 (76.5%) patients and 90% of individual AK lesions, with three additional individuals demonstrating a partial (>75%) response. No AKs were cleared in the placebo arm.[61] A similar 71% complete response rate was reported by Piaserico and colleagues after two MAL-PDT treatments 2 weeks apart in renal transplant recipients, with facial/scalp AKs demonstrating superior responses (72%) versus acral lesions (40%), attributed to increased hyperkeratosis.[48] Hasson and colleagues administered 1–2 conventional MAL-PDT sessions 12 weeks apart to 16 OTRs with facial/scalp AKs and reported 100% remission at week 24.[62]

Compared to immunocompetent populations, AKs of OTRs seem less responsive to therapy, including PDT. Dragieva and colleagues demonstrated this phenomenon by comparing efficacy of ALA-PDT in OTR patients and immunocompetent controls ($n = 20$ in each group).[75] Following one to two sessions (5-h incubation + visible light illumination), complete response rates at 12 weeks were 68% and 8% in immunocompetent versus immunosuppressed groups, respectively ($P < 0.05$), with comparable cosmetic outcomes. These findings support the theory that PDT efficacy, at least in part, is immunologically mediated.[75]

Intensified PDT regimens are also reported in the OTR literature. Helsing and colleagues compared ablative fractional laser (AFL)-assisted PDT versus AFL alone in 10 patients with multiple AKs on dorsal hands in an intra-individual study.[63] Regions were randomized to receive AFL-assisted PDT or AFL alone.[63] After 16 weeks, complete responses were more common after combination therapy (73%) versus AFL alone (31%, $P = .002$).[63] Additionally, combination therapy was more likely to improve AK lesion grades versus AFL (82% vs. 52%, $P = .008$).[63] Another intra-individual study by Togsverd-Bo and colleagues compared four different MAL-PDT/laser interventions in 16 OTRs, including AFL-assisted dPDT, dPDT, conventional PDT, and AFL alone.[64] At 3 months, complete patient response rates were 74%, 46%, 50%, and 5%, respectively ($P < .001$).[64] As shown in studies of immunocompetent populations, dPDT was associated with less pain compared to conventional PDT ($P < .001$).[64] Rizvi and colleagues also assessed AFL-assisted MAL-dPDT versus dPDT alone in an assessor-blinded, intra-individual study of 12 OTR patients with AKs on the scalp/forehead.[65] After 4 months, complete response was observed in 75.5% of patients after AFL-assisted dPDT versus 64.0% after dPDT. Up to 2 days post therapy, pain was, however, higher in the combination arm ($P < .03$).[65] A systematic review echoed this finding, noting that compared to other topical field strategies, local skin reactions were most severe in OTR patients who were treated with AFL-assisted MAL-dPDT.[15] Finally in 2022, Lonsdorf and colleagues evaluated AFL-assisted, low irradiance PDT versus conventional PDT for facial/scalp AKs.[7] At 3 months, significantly greater lesion response rate was seen after AFL-PDT using low irradiance versus conventional PDT (77.3% vs. 61.8%, $P = .025$).[7]

Compared to other field treatments including 5-FU, imiquimod, and diclofenac, there is some evidence to suggest that MAL-PDT demonstrates superior efficacy for treating AK in the OTR setting.[47,75] Indeed, Heppt and colleagues performed a systematic review of AK treatments in OTRs, reporting that MAL-PDT had the highest rates of complete clearance (ranging from 40% to 76.4%), followed by imiquimod (range 27.5%–62.1%), diclofenac (41%), and 5-FU (11%).[15] Authors noted similar results with regard to lesion-specific clearance.[15] In an open-label, randomized study by Perrett and colleagues, two sessions of conventional MAL-PDT (1 week apart) were compared with 5-FU (twice daily for 3 weeks) in eight

TABLE 7.2 Overview of PDT Studies for Treatment and Prevention of Actinic Keratosis (AK) and Keratinocyte Carcinoma (KC) in Organ Transplant Recipients (OTRs)

Study	Population	Intervention	Comparator	Outcomes	Side Effects	Follow-up
Treatment – AKs and Bowen's Disease						
Dragieva et al.[61] (RCT, Intra-patient)	17 OTR, 13M, 4F (129 AK)	MAL-PDT (blue light) 2 Tx, 1 week apart	Placebo	AK complete remission 16 weeks PDT: 76% Placebo: 0%	Pain: PDT > placebo Erythema + crust: PDT > placebo	4 months
Dragieva et al.[61] (RCT)	20 OTR 18M, 2F, 20 non-OTR controls 14M, 6F (AKs and Bowen's disease)	ALA-PDT (visible light) 1– 2 Tx	Non-OTR patients	Complete response 12 weeks: OTR: 68% Non-OTR: 89%	Pain: Equivalent in both groups Erythema, edema, crusts: Equivalent in both groups	4, 12, and 48 weeks
Piaserico et al.[48] (OL)	15 OTR, gender not reported (245 AK)	MAL-PDT 2 Tx, 2 weeks apart	None	Lesional response: 71% Complete patient response: 64%	Severe pain: 47%	3 months
Hasson et al.[62] (OL)	16 OTR, 12M, 4F	MAL-PDT 1–2 Tx, 12 weeks apart	None	AK complete remission 24 weeks: 100%	Mild erythema: 100% Burning: 12.5% Mild pain: 94%	12 and 24 weeks
Helsing et al.[63] (RCT)	10 OTR, 5M, 5F (680 AK)	Intrapatient AFL-MAL-PDT (red light)	AFL alone	AK complete remission: AFL + PDT: 73% AFL alone: 31%	Pain: MAL-PDT > AFL alone	4 months
Togsverd-Bo et al.[64] (RCT, Intra-patient)	16 OTR, 10M, 6F (542 AK)	3 interventions AFL + dPDT; MAL-dPDT; Conventional MAL-PDT 1 Tx	AFL alone	AK complete remission: AFL-dPDT: 74% dPDT: 46% cPDT: 50% AFL alone: 5%	Pain: cPDT > dPDT Erythema + crust: AFL-dPDT > dPDT or cPDT	3 months
Rivzi et al.[65] (RCT, Intra-patient)	12 OTRs, gender not reported (209 AK)	AFL-MAL-dPTD, 1 Tx	MAL-dPDT 1 Tx	Complete response: AFL-dPDT: 75.5% dPDT: 64%	Pain: AFL-dPDT > dPDT	4 months

TABLE 7.2 **Overview of PDT Studies for Treatment and Prevention of Actinic Keratosis (AK) and Keratinocyte Carcinoma (KC) in Organ Transplant Recipients (OTRs)—cont'd**

Study	Population	Intervention	Comparator	Outcomes	Side Effects	Follow-up
Lonsdorf et al.[7] (RCT, Intra-patient)	18 OTR, 17M, 1F (172 AK)	AFL-low irradiance MAL-PDT (red LED light), 1 Tx	Conventional MAL-PDT (red light) 1 Tx	Complete response: AFL-PDT: 77.3% cPDT: 61.8%	Pain: No difference	3 months
Perrett et al.[47] (OL, Intra-patient)	8 OTR, 6M, 2F (10 Bowen's disease, 8 AK)	MAL-PDT (red light) 2 TX, 1 week apart	5-FU (5%) twice daily for 3 weeks	Complete remission 3 months: PDT: 89% 5-FU: 11%	Pain in first 3 days: PDT > 5-FU Erythema after 3 days: 5-FU > PDT	1, 3, 6 months
Togsverd-Bo et al.[66] (RCT, Intra-patient)	35 OTR, 22M, 13F (572 AK)	MAL-PDT (red light) repeated after 3 months when incomplete response (n = 25)	Imiquimod 3x/ week for 4 weeks, repeated after 2 months when incomplete response (n = 29)	AK complete remission (after 2 sessions Tx): PDT: 78% IMQ: 61%	Pain: PDT > IMQ Cosmesis: PDT = IMQ	3 months
Geusau et al.[41] (RCT, Intra-patient)	9 OTR, 8M, 1F (128 AK)	MAL-PDT (red light) 2 TX 2 weeks apart	Imiquimod 3x/ week for 4 weeks	PDT > IMQ	Side effects similar in both groups	12 weeks
Prevention of New AKs						
Wulf et al.[67] (RCT, Intra-patient)	27 Renal transplant pts, 17M, 10F (129 AK)	MAL-PDT (red light) 1 Tx	No treatment	Time to new lesion PDT: 9.6 months Control: 6.8 months lesion free area PDT: 62% Control: 35%	Burning (70%) Erythema (26%) Stinging (22%)	1 year

Continued

TABLE 7.2 Overview of PDT Studies for Treatment and Prevention of Actinic Keratosis (AK) and Keratinocyte Carcinoma (KC) in Organ Transplant Recipients (OTRs)—cont'd

Study	Population	Intervention	Comparator	Outcomes	Side Effects	Follow-up
De Graaf et al.[68] (RCT, Intra-patient)	40 OTR, 21M, 19F (with keratotic lesions, including AK)	ALA-PDT (blue light 400–450 nm), 2nd Tx at 6 months	No treatment	New keratotic lesions PDT: 206 Control: 383	Burning (38%) Pain (31%)	2 year
Wennburg et al.[69] (RCT, Intra-patient)	81 OTR, 55M, 26F (889 keratotic lesions; 90% AK)	MAL-PDT (red light), 6 monthly Tx	Excluding PDT/5FU/ Imiquimod	New AK at 30 months PDT: 43 AK Control: 80 AK	Pain/erythema/ crusting in 75%	≤2 year
Togsverd-Bo et al.[64] (RCT, Intra-patient)	16 OTR, 10M, 6F (542 AK)	4 quadrants AF Laser + dPDT dPDT (MAL) cPDT (MAL, red light)	AFL alone	New AKs AFL-dPDT: 0 dPDT: 0 cPDT: 1 AFL: 2	Pain: cPDT > dPDT Erythema + crust: AFL-dPDT > dPDT or cPDT	3 months
Bernad et al.[70] (RCT, intra-patient)	21 OTR, 21M, mean AK number at BL: 20.6 in active side and 20 control side	MAL-dPDT, 6 sessions at 2 weekly intervals at BL, 3 months, and 9 months	Lesion-directed cryotherapy at BL, 3 and 9 months	New AK (15 months) dPDT: 3.0 Cryo: 4.8 New KC and AK (21 months) dPDT: 13.7 lesions Cryo: 20.3 lesions	Tolerability: MAL-dPDT > Cryo Adverse events: Cryo < MAL-dPDT	15 and 21 months
Togsverd-Bo et al.[49] (RCT, intra-patient)	25 OTR, 20M, 5F, Clinically normal skin	MAL-PDT (red light), 1 session at BL, then every 6 months for 5 years	No treatment	Cumulative no. AKs PDT: 8 Control: 43 New AKs PDT: 28% Control: 63%	Mild pain and erythema	3 years
Togsverd-Bo et al.[71] (intra-patient)	46 OTR, 33M, 13F	MAL-PDT (red light)	No treatment	Probability of AK-free skin PDT: 72% Control: 50%	Moderate pain, localized erythema	6 years

TABLE 7.2 **Overview of PDT Studies for Treatment and Prevention of Actinic Keratosis (AK) and Keratinocyte Carcinoma (KC) in Organ Transplant Recipients (OTRs)—cont'd**

Study	Population	Intervention	Comparator	Outcomes	Side Effects	Follow-up
Treatment – KCs						
Schleier et al.[72] (OL)	5 OTRs, gender not reported (32 lesions: 22 BCC; 2 SCC; 7 AK; KA)	ALA-PDT (red light), 1–3 sessions based on clinical response	None	Lesion clearance: 75% with 1 Tx 93% with up to 3 Tx (2 SCCs did not clear)	Minor pain	12 weeks
Guleng et al.[73] (OL)	18 OTRs, 12M, 6F (18 BCCs)	MAL-PDT, 2 sessions	None	One recurrence	Not reported	22.5 months
Collier et al.[74] (retrospective review)	23 OTRs, 80 Non-OTRs (322 BCCs)	MAL-PDT (red LED light) 2 sessions, 1 week apart	Non-OTRs	No statistically significant difference in recurrence in OTRs (22.6%) vs. non-OTRs (15.2%)	Pain leading to discontinuation in 2 non-OTR patients	Cases between 2003 and 2013
Prevention – SCCs						
De Graaf et al.[68] (RCT, intra-patient)	40 OTRs, 21M, 19F Skin areas with keratotic lesions	ALA-PDT, 1 or 2 treatments, 6 months apart	Untreated skin	New SCC PDT: 15 Control: 10 (No difference)	Pain and burning sensations (mild to severe) in 80% patients	2 years
Willey et al.[45] (intra-patient)	12 OTRs with history of SCC	Cyclic ALA-PDT (blue light) administered at 4 and 8 week sessions over 2 years	New SCCs in treated areas vs. 1 year period prior to treatment	Reduced SCC incidence 12 months: 79% 24 months: 95%	Mild and transient pain, erythema, desquamation, and crusting	24 months
Bernad et al.[70] (RCT, intra-patient)	21 OTR, 21M	MAL-dPDT, 6 sessions at 2 weekly intervals at BL, 3 months, and 9 months	Lesion-directed cryotherapy at BL, 3 and 9 months	Cumulative new KC and AK (21 months) dPDT: 13.7 lesions Cryo: 20.3 lesions	Tolerability: MAL-dPDT > Cryo Adverse events: Cryo < MAL-dPDT	21 months

AFL, Ablative fractional laser; *AK*, actinic keratosis; *ALA*, aminolaevulinic acid; *cPDT*, conventional PDT; *CR*, complete response; *Cryo*, cryotherapy; *dPDT*, daylight PDT; *F*, female; *5-FU*, 5 fluorouracil; *IMQ*, imiquimod; *KA*, keratoacanthoma; *KC*, keratinocyte carcinoma; *M*, male; *MAL*, methyl aminolevulinate; *OL*, open label; *OTR*, organ transplant recipients; *PDT*, photodynamic therapy.

patients with AKs and SCC in situ.[47] PDT was found to be superior to 5-FU assessed 1, 3, and 6 months post treatment based on complete remission rates per mean area of lesions, and cosmetic results (PDT: 8/9 areas cleared; 5-FU: 1/9 areas ($P = .02$)).[47] Imiquimod has also been compared to PDT regimens for AK. Togsverd-Bo and colleagues compared conventional MAL-PDT with imiquimod (3x weekly for 4 weeks) in 35 transplant patients in 2018.[66] In instances of incomplete response, treatments were repeated at 2 months (imiquimod arm) or 3 months (PDT arm).[66] At 3-month follow-up, PDT had a 78% rate of complete response, compared to 61% with imiquimod ($P < .001$).[66] Geusau and colleagues performed an intra-individual comparison of MAL-PDT (2 cycles, 2 weeks apart) and imiquimod 5% cream (3x weekly for 4 weeks) in 10 OTRs.[41] Although both PDT and imiquimod significantly improved AKs at up to 6 months post treatment, imiquimod showed lower efficacy in comparison to MAL-PDT.[41] Compared to other field therapies, PDT's efficacy may in part be explained by its lower reliance on patient adherence: while other topical AK field therapies may require up to 3x daily application over weeks, PDT can be performed in-office over 1–2 sessions.[24]

Lesion-directed AK therapy was also compared to PDT when Bernad and colleagues assessed MAL-dPDT versus cryotherapy in a randomized split-face trial.[70] dPDT was administered over the course of one year, with two sessions 2 weeks apart, repeated at 3 and 9 months post baseline.[70] AKs on control sides received cryotherapy (2 × 5–10 s freeze-thaw cycles) at baseline, months 3 and 9.[70] At 21 months, dPDT-treated areas had 4.7 lesions compared to 5.8 on areas receiving cryotherapy.[70] dPDT was also associated with fewer new lesions at all evaluations ($P < 0.05$ up to month 15, $P = .06$ at month 21).[70] In addition, the investigators report that patients preferred dPDT over cryotherapy.[70]

In summary, AKs in OTRs demonstrate higher progression rates and greater treatment resistance compared to that of immunocompetent populations. PDT remains the best-studied field-directed approach for AK treatment in OTRs, and available studies suggest that overall, MAL-PDT generally achieves superior clearance rates versus 5-FU, imiquimod, and cryotherapy in this population. Laser-assisted PDT strategies are particularly efficacious for treatment-resistant AK but are associated with intensified side effects. In terms of tolerability, dPDT is better tolerated with similar efficacy compared to conventional PDT and represents a less resource-intensive strategy for treatment of existing AK lesions.[76]

Basal Cell Carcinomas (BCC)

BCC arises from the basal membrane of the epidermis. Although tumors rarely metastasize, BCCs are often accompanied by local invasion, tissue destruction, and occur in multiples, leading to morbidity.[77] Overall, little evidence supports the use of PDT as a treatment for other than low-risk BCC, such as superficial and small nodular tumors. Existing studies on the subject are reviewed in the following section.

PDT for Existing BCCs: Evidence in OTR Populations

Initial case reports of PDT for treatment of BCC tumors in OTRs were encouraging. In 2006, Perrett and colleagues published a case describing successful conventional MAL-PDT in a liver transplant patient with a BCC on the nasal tip. Complete clearance and good cosmetic outcomes were achieved 12 months after two sessions, 1 week apart.[78] A second case report in 2009 described CO_2 laser-assisted PDT in a kidney transplant patient with multiple recurrent BCCs on the trunk. Five tumors were treated with a single session of laser-assisted MAL-PDT with LED illumination, with no recurrences after 3 years.[79] In a case series by Schleier and colleagues, ALA-PDT was used to treat 32 facial tumors (21 clinical BCCs) in five OTRs, leading to complete clearance in 75% after the first session and 93.8% after two to three sessions.[72]

In a larger study of 18 OTRs, Guleng and Helsing reported conventional MAL-PDT for BCCs on the head and trunk (two sessions, 1 week apart). Over a mean of 22.5 months, a single recurrence was reported.[73] A large retrospective case review by Collier and colleagues examining 103 OTRs with 322 PDT-treated BCCs further found no significant difference in BCC recurrence in transplant recipients versus the general population ($P = .18$).[74] Examining peritumoral infiltrates in BCCs from OTRs treated with PDT, Kanitakis and colleagues found significantly lower inflammatory density, suggesting that anticancer immune responses after PDT may be hampered by inherent immunosuppression. This factor, on the other hand, does not seem reflected in the aforementioned clinical outcomes.[39]

PHOTODYNAMIC THERAPY AS A PREVENTATIVE STRATEGY IN ORGAN TRANSPLANT RECIPIENTS

Strategies to prevent skin cancer are critical in the organ transplant population. Patients should be educated and empowered to practice sun avoidance and protection.[24]

Daily sunscreen over 2 years has been shown to reduce the number of both AKs and SCCs in OTR patients.[80] In addition, patients should understand the value of skin vigilance and regular dermatology consultations.[24] When possible, patients should undergo a baseline skin evaluation around the time of transplantation in order to develop a predictive skin cancer risk assessment and devise appropriate management strategies.[24] After transplantation, annual skin cancer screening is recommended for OTRs, with increased frequency for higher-risk individuals. A number of pharmacological approaches have furthermore been devised to reduce development of KC and precursors in OTR populations. Among these, PDT has emerged as a promising preventative strategy.

PDT for AK Prevention: Evidence in OTR Populations

Using PDT to prevent AK lesions before they debut may be a useful means to reduce skin cancer morbidity in the OTR population (Table 7.2). Evidence supporting PDT as a primary prevention strategy against AK is in part provided by Togsverd-Bo and colleagues.[49,71] In 2015, the group investigated 25 kidney transplant patients with clinically normal skin. Areas of the face, forearm, or hand underwent conventional MAL-PDT at 6-month intervals for 5 years, using the contralateral side as the untreated control.[49] Blinded evaluation found that prophylactic PDT significantly delayed the occurrence of AKs versus untreated skin ($P = .020$).[49] After 3 years, the presence of AK was noted in 28% of PDT areas versus 63% of controls, with a lower AK number overall (8 vs. 43 lesions, $P = .005$).[49] Later, Togsverd-Bo and colleagues also showed that a cyclic PDT regimen delayed first onset of AKs in a larger study of OTR patients.[71] Thus in a split-face RCT, 46 renal transplant recipients with no history of AK or KC had conventional MAL-PDT or no treatment at 6-month intervals for 5 years.[71] Six years from baseline, the probability of being AK-free was 72% in PDT-treated skin versus 50% in untreated sites.[71] The number of lesions was significantly lower in PDT-treated skin (32 vs. 76, $P < .01$), as was the median AK number per patient (1.0 vs. 1.8, $P = .030$).[71] Although these findings support the use of PDT as a form of early prophylaxis against AK, authors argue that MAL-PDT should likely be reserved for high-risk patients since 43% of untreated sites did not develop AKs in the 6-year time frame.[71]

Secondary prevention aims to mitigate the impact of a disease that has already debuted. In OTRs with a previous history of AK, the use of PDT as secondary prevention of new AKs has been reported in multiple studies. Wennberg and colleagues conducted a large open-label, randomized intra-individual study in 81 OTRs with 889 skin lesions (90% of which were AKs) examining cyclic conventional MAL-PDT (two sessions, 1 week apart) at baseline, month 3, 9, and 15 versus lesion-specific therapies (83% cryotherapy).[69] At 3 months, MAL-PDT significantly reduced the occurrence of new lesions (AK, SCC, BCC, or warts) (65 vs. 103 control, $P = .01$). At 27 months, a nonsignificant reduction in PDT areas versus control was shown (253 vs. 312, $P = .06$).[69] Also, Wulf and colleagues investigated secondary prevention using conventional MAL-PDT in 27 kidney transplant patients with AKs and other related skin lesions. In an intra-individual study, two contralateral regions were assigned to PDT or no treatment. PDT significantly delayed occurrence of new lesions (defined as AK, SCC, BCC, keratoacanthoma, or wart) versus control (9.6 vs. 6.8 months, $P = .034$). After 12 months, 62% of treated areas remained lesion free versus 35% in control areas, supporting the concept of PDT as a preventative approach.[77]

PDT for Prevention of Squamous Cell Carcinoma (SCC)—Evidence in OTR Populations

Cutaneous SCCs arise from epidermal keratinocytes, often in skin areas where AKs colocalize.[66,81,82] In contrast to immunocompetent populations, SCCs are the most common skin cancers in transplant recipients, outnumbering BCCs by an updated ratio of 3:1.[23] Within 5 years of the first SCC tumor, most OTRs go on to develop multiple additional KCs.[83] Importantly, risk of SCC development increases in cases where multiple AK lesions or field cancerization is present.[55] As an example, one study found that 82% of SCC tumors developed in close proximity to, or even within, AK lesions.[24] The underlying mechanism is thought to be driven by genetically altered stem cells that develop into fields, that in turn mature into areas of precancerous cells.[24] The majority of KC-related morbidity and mortality is consequently linked to AK-laden, field-cancerized skin.[24,84] For this reason, timely management of AK skin is a crucial aspect of SCC prevention in OTRs.

While PDT is not recommended as a therapeutic strategy for SCC, some studies have explored PDT's efficacy as a means to prevent SCC in OTRs with mixed results (Table 7.2). In 2006, de Graaf and colleagues found that a single treatment ALA-PDT with violet light (400–450 nm) failed to prevent new SCCs in OTRs over a 2-year follow-up period.[68] Authors speculated that insufficient follow-up duration, patient selection (patients had a history of ≥1 SCCs and at least 10 hyperkeratotic lesions), superficially penetrating violet light, and omission of curettage pretreatment potentially led to suboptimal results.[68] Contrastingly in 2010, Willey and colleagues reported results of an ALA-PDT regimen in 12 high-risk OTRs with a history of SCC. PDT sessions (1 h incubation; 1000 s blue light 417 nm) were administered at 4- and 8-week intervals over a 2-year period. After 12 months, PDT was found to reduce SCC incidence by 79.0%, rising to 95.0% at 24 months. Thus cyclic rather than single-session PDT may be useful to prevent SCCs in high-risk patients.[45]

PDT-RELATED ADVERSE EVENTS AND TREATMENT RESISTANCE IN ORGAN TRANSPLANT RECIPIENTS

Side effects that endanger organ grafts have not been reported following PDT in OTRs.[24] Rather, typical adverse events with MAL and ALA are mild to moderate, transient in nature, and self-limiting.[43] Pain is the most common and limiting side effect, and may be more prominent in OTRs versus immunocompetent patients.[24] Localized erythema, peeling, or crusting may also occur. In addition, PDT of facial lesions may be more painful compared with other anatomical areas.[14] Options to manage pain in OTRs include transcutaneous electrical nerve stimulation (TENS), cold air fans, cold water spray, and nerve block.[24] As noted previously, dPDT has better general tolerability than conventional blue or red light regimens.[71]

DISCUSSION

OTRs are at a markedly increased risk of developing skin cancer and KCs are a leading contributor to mortality in this population.[24] For OTRs with widespread actinic damage and a history of KC, PDT remains the best-studied treatment option, having the potential to treat existing AK lesions as well as prevent new AK and KC. Compared to other field therapies, PDT is less reliant on patient adherence and may provide superior clearance rates versus other alternatives including 5-FU, imiquimod, and cryotherapy. Particularly for KC, however, the use of PDT has garnered mixed results, and an improved understanding of how to optimize PDT regimens, tailor PDT to specific KC subtypes, and enhance efficacy via combination with other therapies and drug delivery techniques is needed. In the future, a more targeted use of PDT in specific OTR subpopulations (i.e., high-risk individuals and treatment-responsive individuals) is expected, with PDT as primary and secondary KC prevention figuring centrally.[85]

REFERENCES

1. Madeleine MM, Patel NS, Plasmeijer EI, et al. Epidemiology of keratinocyte carcinomas after organ transplantation. *Br J Dermatol.* 2017;177:1208–1216.
2. Watson CJ, Dark JH. Organ transplantation: historical perspective and current practice. *Br J Anaesth.* 2012;108(Suppl 1):i29–i42.
3. Global Observatory on Donation and Transplantation (GODT) data, produced by the WHO-ONT collaboration. 2022. Accessed January 31, 2023. http://www.transplant-observatory.org/.
4. Crow LD, Jambusaria-Pahlajani A, Chung CL, et al. Initial skin cancer screening for solid organ transplant recipients in the United States: Delphi method development of expert consensus guidelines. *Transpl Int.* 2019;32:1268–1276.
5. Basset-Seguin N, Baumann Conzett K, Gerritsen MJ, et al. Photodynamic therapy for actinic keratosis in organ transplant patients. *J Eur Acad Dermatol Venereol.* 2013;27:57–66.
6. Harwood CA, Toland AE, Proby CM, et al. The pathogenesis of cutaneous squamous cell carcinoma in organ transplant recipients. *Br J Dermatol.* 2017;177:1217–1224.
7. Lonsdorf AS, Keller A, Hartmann J, et al. Ablative fractional laser-assisted low-irradiance photodynamic therapy for treatment of actinic keratoses in organ transplant recipients: a prospective, randomized, intraindividual controlled trial. *Acta Derm Venereol.* 2022;102:adv00694.
8. Sinnya S, Zwald FO, Colegio OR. Skin cancer in the crosshairs: highlights from the biennial scientific retreat of international transplant skin cancer collaborative and skin care in organ transplant recipients Europe. *Transplant Direct.* 2015;1:e26.
9. Berg D, Otley CC. Skin cancer in organ transplant recipients: epidemiology, pathogenesis, and management. *J Am Acad Dermatol.* 2002;47:1–17; quiz 8–20.
10. Jensen P, Hansen S, Moller B, et al. Skin cancer in kidney and heart transplant recipients and different long-term immunosuppressive therapy regimens. *J Am Acad Dermatol.* 1999;40:177–186.
11. Euvrard S, Kanitakis J, Claudy A. Skin cancers after organ transplantation. *N Engl J Med.* 2003;348:1681–1691.
12. Jensen AO, Svaerke C, Farkas D, et al. Skin cancer risk among solid organ recipients: a nationwide cohort study in Denmark. *Acta Derm Venereol.* 2010;90:474–479.

13. Garrett GL, Lowenstein SE, Singer JP, et al. Trends of skin cancer mortality after transplantation in the United States: 1987 to 2013. *J Am Acad Dermatol.* 2016;75:106–112.
14. Griffin LL, Lear JT. Photodynamic therapy and non-melanoma skin cancer. *Cancers (Basel).* 2016;8(10):98.
15. Heppt MV, Steeb T, Niesert AC, et al. Local interventions for actinic keratosis in organ transplant recipients: a systematic review. *Br J Dermatol.* 2019;180:43–50.
16. Liew YCC, De Souza NNA, Sultana RG, et al. Photodynamic therapy for the prevention and treatment of actinic keratosis/squamous cell carcinoma in solid organ transplant recipients: a systematic review and meta-analysis. *J Eur Acad Dermatol Venereol.* 2020;34:251–259.
17. Rashtak S, Dierkhising RA, Kremers WK, et al. Incidence and risk factors for skin cancer following lung transplantation. *J Am Acad Dermatol.* 2015;72:92–98.
18. Fortina AB, Caforio AL, Piaserico S, et al. Skin cancer in heart transplant recipients: frequency and risk factor analysis. *J Heart Lung Transplant.* 2000;19:249–255.
19. Haagsma EB, Hagens VE, Schaapveld M, et al. Increased cancer risk after liver transplantation: a population-based study. *J Hepatol.* 2001;34:84–91.
20. Ramsay HM, Fryer AA, Hawley CM, et al. Non-melanoma skin cancer risk in the Queensland renal transplant population. *Br J Dermatol.* 2002;147:950–956.
21. Friman TK, Jaamaa-Holmberg S, Aberg F, et al. Cancer risk and mortality after solid organ transplantation: a population-based 30-year cohort study in Finland. *Int J Cancer.* 2022;150:1779–1791.
22. Menzies S, O'Leary E, Callaghan G, et al. Declining incidence of keratinocyte carcinoma in organ transplant recipients. *Br J Dermatol.* 2019;181:983–991.
23. O'Reilly Zwald F, Brown M. Skin cancer in solid organ transplant recipients: advances in therapy and management: part I. Epidemiology of skin cancer in solid organ transplant recipients. *J Am Acad Dermatol.* 2011;65:253–261.
24. Wlodek C, Ali FR, Lear JT. Use of photodynamic therapy for treatment of actinic keratoses in organ transplant recipients. *Biomed Res Int.* 2013;2013:349526.
25. Blomberg M, He SY, Harwood C, et al. Research gaps in the management and prevention of cutaneous squamous cell carcinoma in organ transplant recipients. *Br J Dermatol.* 2017;177:1225–1233.
26. Zamoiski RD, Yanik E, Gibson TM, et al. Risk of second malignancies in solid organ transplant recipients who develop keratinocyte cancers. *Cancer Res.* 2017;77:4196–4203.
27. Karia PS, Han J, Schmults CD. Cutaneous squamous cell carcinoma: estimated incidence of disease, nodal metastasis, and deaths from disease in the United States, 2012. *J Am Acad Dermatol.* 2013;68:957–966.
28. Silberstein E, Sofrin E, Bogdanov-Berezovsky A, et al. Lymph node metastasis in cutaneous head and neck squamous cell carcinoma. *Dermatol Surg.* 2015;41:1126–1129.
29. Ulrich C, Kanitakis J, Stockfleth E, et al. Skin cancer in organ transplant recipients–where do we stand today? *Am J Transplant.* 2008;8:2192–2198.
30. Cheng JY, Li FY, Ko CJ, et al. Cutaneous squamous cell carcinomas in solid organ transplant recipients compared with immunocompetent patients. *JAMA Dermatol.* 2018;154:60–66.
31. Garrett GL, Blanc PD, Boscardin J, et al. Incidence of and risk factors for skin cancer in organ transplant recipients in the United States. *JAMA Dermatol.* 2017;153:296–303.
32. Wheless L, Anand N, Hanlon A, Chren MM. Differences in skin cancer rates by transplanted organ type and patient age after organ transplant in white patients. *JAMA Dermatol.* 2022;158(11):1287–1292.
33. Hao X, Lai W, Xia X, et al. Skin cancer outcomes and risk factors in renal transplant recipients: analysis of organ procurement and transplantation network data from 2000 to 2021. *Front Oncol.* 2022;12:1017498.
34. Wenande E, Togsverd-Bo K, Hastrup A, Lei U, Philipsen PA, Haedersdal M. Skin cancer development is strongly associated with actinic keratosis in solid organ transplant recipients: a Danish cohort study. *Dermatology.* 2023;239(3):393–402.
35. Morton CA, Szeimies RM, Basset-Seguin N, et al. European dermatology forum guidelines on topical photodynamic therapy 2019 part 2: emerging indications - field cancerization, photorejuvenation and inflammatory/infective dermatoses. *J Eur Acad Dermatol Venereol.* 2020;34:17–29.
36. Massey PR, Schmults CD, Li SJ, et al. Consensus-based recommendations on the prevention of squamous cell carcinoma in solid organ transplant recipients: a Delphi consensus statement. *JAMA Dermatol.* 2021;157:1219–1226.
37. Moscarella E, Di Brizzi EV, Casari A, et al. Italian expert consensus paper on the management of patients with actinic keratoses. *Dermatol Ther.* 2020;33:e13992.
38. Mishchenko T, Balalaeva I, Gorokhova A, et al. Which cell death modality wins the contest for photodynamic therapy of cancer? *Cell Death Dis.* 2022;13:455.
39. Kanitakis J, Alhaj-Ibrahim L, Euvrard S, et al. Basal cell carcinomas developing in solid organ transplant recipients. Clinicopathologic study of 176 cases. *Arch Dermatol.* 2003;139:1133–1137.
40. Joly F, Deret S, Gamboa B, et al. Photodynamic therapy corrects abnormal cancer-associated gene expression observed in actinic keratosis lesions and induces a remodeling effect in photodamaged skin. *J Dermatol Sci.* 2018;S0923-1811(17):30775–30782.

41. Geusau A, Tzaneva S, Petzelbauer P, et al. Peptidase inhibitor 3 and chemokine ligand 27 may serve as biomarkers for actinic keratoses in organ transplant recipients. *Eur J Dermatol.* 2019;29:259–267.
42. Lee PK, Kloser A. Current methods for photodynamic therapy in the US: comparison of MAL/PDT and ALA/PDT. *J Drugs Dermatol.* 2013;12:925–930.
43. Ko DY, Kim KH, Song KH. Comparative study of photodynamic therapy with topical methyl aminolevulinate versus 5-aminolevulinic acid for facial actinic keratosis with long-term follow-up. *Ann Dermatol.* 2014;26:321–331.
44. Wilken R, Carucci J, Stevenson ML. Skin cancers and lung transplant. *Semin Respir Crit Care Med.* 2021;42:483–496.
45. Willey A, Mehta S, Lee PK. Reduction in the incidence of squamous cell carcinoma in solid organ transplant recipients treated with cyclic photodynamic therapy. *Dermatol Surg.* 2010;36:652–658.
46. Mikolajewska P, Iani V, Juzeniene A, et al. Topical aminolaevulinic acid- and aminolaevulinic acid methyl ester-based photodynamic therapy with red and violet light: influence of wavelength on pain and erythema. *Br J Dermatol.* 2009;161:1173–1179.
47. Perrett CM, McGregor JM, Warwick J, et al. Treatment of post-transplant premalignant skin disease: a randomized intrapatient comparative study of 5-fluorouracil cream and topical photodynamic therapy. *Br J Dermatol.* 2007;156:320–328.
48. Piaserico S, Belloni Fortina A, Rigotti P, et al. Topical photodynamic therapy of actinic keratosis in renal transplant recipients. *Transplant Proc.* 2007;39:1847–1850.
49. Togsverd-Bo K, Omland SH, Wulf HC, et al. Primary prevention of skin dysplasia in renal transplant recipients with photodynamic therapy: a randomized controlled trial. *Am J Transplant.* 2015;15:2986–2990.
50. Wiegell SR, Wulf HC, Szeimies RM, et al. Daylight photodynamic therapy for actinic keratosis: an international consensus: international society for photodynamic therapy in dermatology. *J Eur Acad Dermatol Venereol.* 2012;26:673–679.
51. Ezzedine K, Painchault C, Brignone M. Systematic literature review and network meta-analysis of the efficacy and acceptability of interventions in actinic keratoses. *Acta Derm Venereol.* 2021;101:adv00358.
52. Traianou A, Ulrich M, Apalla Z, et al. Risk factors for actinic keratosis in eight European centres: a case-control study. *Br J Dermatol.* 2012;167(Suppl 2):36–42.
53. Werner RN, Sammain A, Erdmann R, et al. The natural history of actinic keratosis: a systematic review. *Br J Dermatol.* 2013;169:502–518.
54. Dodds A, Chia A, Shumack S. Actinic keratosis: rationale and management. *Dermatol Ther (Heidelb).* 2014;4:11–31.
55. Wallingford SC, Russell SA, Vail A, et al. Actinic keratoses, actinic field change and associations with squamous cell carcinoma in renal transplant recipients in Manchester, UK. *Acta Derm Venereol.* 2015;95:830–834.
56. Steeb T, Wessely A, Petzold A, et al. Long-term recurrence rates of actinic keratosis: a systematic review and pooled analysis of randomized controlled trials. *J Am Acad Dermatol.* 2022;86:1116–1119.
57. Basset-Seguin N, Ibbotson SH, Emtestam L, et al. Topical methyl aminolaevulinate photodynamic therapy versus cryotherapy for superficial basal cell carcinoma: a 5 year randomized trial. *Eur J Dermatol.* 2008;18:547–553.
58. Szeimies RM, Karrer S, Radakovic-Fijan S, et al. Photodynamic therapy using topical methyl 5-aminolevulinate compared with cryotherapy for actinic keratosis: a prospective, randomized study. *J Am Acad Dermatol.* 2002;47:258–262.
59. Freeman M, Vinciullo C, Francis D, et al. A comparison of photodynamic therapy using topical methyl aminolevulinate (Metvix) with single cycle cryotherapy in patients with actinic keratosis: a prospective, randomized study. *J Dermatolog Treat.* 2003;14:99–106.
60. Morton CA, Brown SB, Collins S, et al. Guidelines for topical photodynamic therapy: report of a workshop of the British Photodermatology Group. *Br J Dermatol.* 2002;146:552–567.
61. Dragieva G, Prinz BM, Hafner J, et al. A randomized controlled clinical trial of topical photodynamic therapy with methyl aminolaevulinate in the treatment of actinic keratoses in transplant recipients. *Br J Dermatol.* 2004;151:196–200.
62. Hasson A, Navarrete-Dechent C, Nicklas C, et al. Topical photodynamic therapy with methylaminolevulinate for the treatment of actinic keratosis and reduction of photodamage in organ transplant recipients: a case-series of 16 patients. *Indian J Dermatol Venereol Leprol.* 2012;78:448–453.
63. Helsing P, Togsverd-Bo K, Veierod MB, et al. Intensified fractional CO2 laser-assisted photodynamic therapy vs. laser alone for organ transplant recipients with multiple actinic keratoses and wart-like lesions: a randomized half-side comparative trial on dorsal hands. *Br J Dermatol.* 2013;169:1087–1092.
64. Togsverd-Bo K, Lei U, Erlendsson AM, et al. Combination of ablative fractional laser and daylight-mediated photodynamic therapy for actinic keratosis in organ transplant recipients - a randomized controlled trial. *Br J Dermatol.* 2015;172:467–474.
65. Rizvi SM, Veierod MB, Mork G, et al. Ablative fractional laser-assisted daylight photodynamic therapy for actinic keratoses of the scalp and forehead in organ

transplant recipients: a pilot study. *Acta Derm Venereol.* 2019;99:1047–1048.

66. Togsverd-Bo K, Halldin C, Sandberg C, et al. Photodynamic therapy is more effective than imiquimod for actinic keratosis in organ transplant recipients: a randomized intraindividual controlled trial. *Br J Dermatol.* 2018;178:903–909.
67. Wulf HC, Pavel S, Stender I, et al. Topical photodynamic therapy for prevention of new skin lesions in renal transplant recipients. *Acta Derm Venereol.* 2006;86:25–28.
68. de Graaf YG, Kennedy C, Wolterbeek R, et al. Photodynamic therapy does not prevent cutaneous squamous-cell carcinoma in organ-transplant recipients: results of a randomized-controlled trial. *J Invest Dermatol.* 2006;126:569–574.
69. Wennberg AM, Stenquist B, Stockfleth E, et al. Photodynamic therapy with methyl aminolevulinate for prevention of new skin lesions in transplant recipients: a randomized study. *Transplantation.* 2008;86:423–429.
70. Bernad I, Aguado L, Nunez-Cordoba JM, et al. Daylight photodynamic therapy for prevention of new actinic keratosis and keratinocyte carcinomas in organ transplants. A cryotherapy-controlled randomized clinical trial. *J Eur Acad Dermatol Venereol.* 2020;34(7):1464–1470.
71. Togsverd-Bo K, Sandberg C, Helsing P, et al. Cyclic photodynamic therapy delays first onset of actinic keratoses in renal transplant recipients: a 5-year randomized controlled trial with 12-month follow-up. *J Eur Acad Dermatol Venereol.* 2022;36(11):e946–e948.
72. Schleier P, Hyckel P, Berndt A, et al. Photodynamic therapy of virus-associated epithelial tumours of the face in organ transplant recipients. *J Cancer Res Clin Oncol.* 2004;130:279–284.
73. Guleng GE, Helsing P. Photodynamic therapy for basal cell carcinomas in organ-transplant recipients. *Clin Exp Dermatol.* 2012;37:367–369.
74. Collier NJ, Ali FR, Lear JT. Efficacy of photodynamic therapy for treatment of basal cell carcinoma in organ transplant recipients. *Lasers Med Sci.* 2015;30:1407–1409.
75. Dragieva G, Hafner J, Dummer R, et al. Topical photodynamic therapy in the treatment of actinic keratoses and Bowen's disease in transplant recipients. *Transplantation.* 2004;77:115–121.
76. O'Reilly Zwald F, Brown M. Skin cancer in solid organ transplant recipients: advances in therapy and management: part II. Management of skin cancer in solid organ transplant recipients. *J Am Acad Dermatol.* 2011;65:263–279.
77. Khan NH, Mir M, Qian L, et al. Skin cancer biology and barriers to treatment: recent applications of polymeric micro/nanostructures. *J Adv Res.* 2022;36:223–247.
78. Perrett CM, Tan SK, Cerio R, et al. Treatment of basal cell carcinoma with topical methylaminolaevulinate photodynamic therapy in an organ-transplant recipient. *Clin Exp Dermatol.* 2006;31:146–147.
79. Shokrollahi K, Marsden NJ, Whitaker IS, et al. Basal cell carcinoma treated successfully with combined CO2 laser and photodynamic therapy in a renal transplant patient: a case report. *Cases J.* 2009;2:7920.
80. Ulrich C, Jurgensen JS, Degen A, et al. Prevention of non-melanoma skin cancer in organ transplant patients by regular use of a sunscreen: a 24 months, prospective, case-control study. *Br J Dermatol.* 2009;161(Suppl 3):78–84.
81. Stoff B, Salisbury C, Parker D, et al. Dermatopathology of skin cancer in solid organ transplant recipients. *Transplant Rev (Orlando).* 2010;24:172–189.
82. Lindelof B, Dal H, Wolk K, et al. Cutaneous squamous cell carcinoma in organ transplant recipients: a study of the Swedish cohort with regard to tumor site. *Arch Dermatol.* 2005;141:447–451.
83. Ulrich C, Arnold R, Frei U, et al. Skin changes following organ transplantation: an interdisciplinary challenge. *Dtsch Arztebl Int.* 2014;111:188–194.
84. Philipp-Dormston WG, Sanclemente G, Torezan L, et al. Daylight photodynamic therapy with MAL cream for large-scale photodamaged skin based on the concept of "actinic field damage": Recommendations of an international expert group. *J Eur Acad Dermatol Venereol.* 2016;30:8–15.
85. Collier NJ, Rhodes LE. Photodynamic therapy for basal cell carcinoma: the clinical context for future research priorities. *Molecules.* 2020;25(22):5398.

8

Photodynamic Therapy for Actinic Keratoses and Non-Melanoma Skin Cancers in Solid Organ Transplant Recipients

Paul J. Shim, Gyorgy Paragh, Nathalie C. Zeitouni

KEY POINTS

- Solid organ transplant recipients (SOTRs) represent an important high-risk group with increased incidence and morbidity of actinic keratosis and non-melanoma skin cancers.
- The high burden of premalignant and malignant skin disease often requires field-directed rather than lesion-directed therapy.
- Photodynamic therapy (PDT) is a field-directed treatment modality involving a topical or systemic photosensitizer and a light source to target and destroy precancers and cancers in SOTR.

OBJECTIVE

- To review the use of photodynamic therapy for actinic keratoses and non-melanoma skin cancers in solid organ transplant recipients.

INTRODUCTION

Solid Organ Transplant Recipients

Within the past few decades, the number of solid organ transplant recipients (SOTRs) in the United States (US) has significant grown, from roughly 13,000 transplants performed in 1988 to 47,000 today in 2024.[1,2] These patients are at increased risk of developing malignancies due to the long-term immunosuppressive medications required for graft survival. Skin cancer accounts for 50% of all post-transplant malignancies, and the incidence of SOTRs is increasing.[3] Squamous cell carcinoma (SCC) (Fig. 8.1.) is the most common skin cancer in SOTRs with 65–250 times increased risk, depending on the duration of time post transplant, compared to the immunocompetent general population.[4] Basal cell carcinoma (BCC) (Fig. 8.2) is the second most common skin cancer in SOTRs, with 10–16 times increased risk compared to the general population.[4] Additionally, SOTRs have an increased risk of locally advanced and metastatic skin cancers. The mortality risk of SCC in SOTRs is 10–50 times greater than that of the general population.[5] The increased incidence and aggressiveness of skin cancers in this population demand increased surveillance, intervention, and prevention.

Specific risk factors for skin cancers in SOTRs have been identified (Table 8.1). These include Fitzpatrick skin type I–III, cumulative sun exposure, pretransplant skin cancer, age at transplant of 50 years or older, male sex,

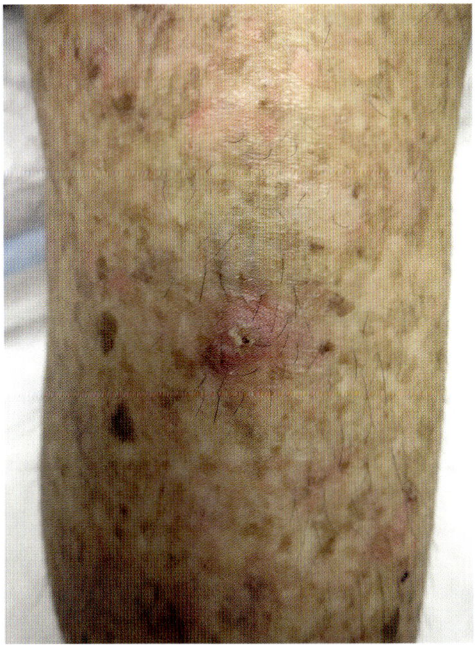

Fig. 8.1 Squamous cell carcinoma in a SOTR.

time elapsed since transplant, and duration of immunosuppressant use.[3] Specific immunosuppressants have also been associated with varying risks of skin cancer. Azathioprine, calcineurin inhibitors, and voriconazole have been shown to have an increased risk of SCCs, while mycophenolic acid has been associated with an increased risk of BCCs.[6,7] Interestingly, mammalian targets of rapamycin (mTOR) inhibitors such as sirolimus may reduce the risk of skin malignancies.[8] Furthermore, the type of transplanted organ may also modify skin cancer risk. Heart and lung transplant recipients were reported to have an increased risk of SCC, while liver transplant recipients had a decreased risk.[4,9] However, patient age may be a confounding factor, and in a cohort study of 5129 SOTRs, the type of organ transplanted did not affect the time to development of second or third skin cancers.[4,10] Ultimately, these risk factors should be used to risk stratify SOTRs to guide clinical decision making.

While surgery is the gold standard for the treatment of NMSCs, additional management options are necessary for SOTRs who can develop multiple lesions over wide

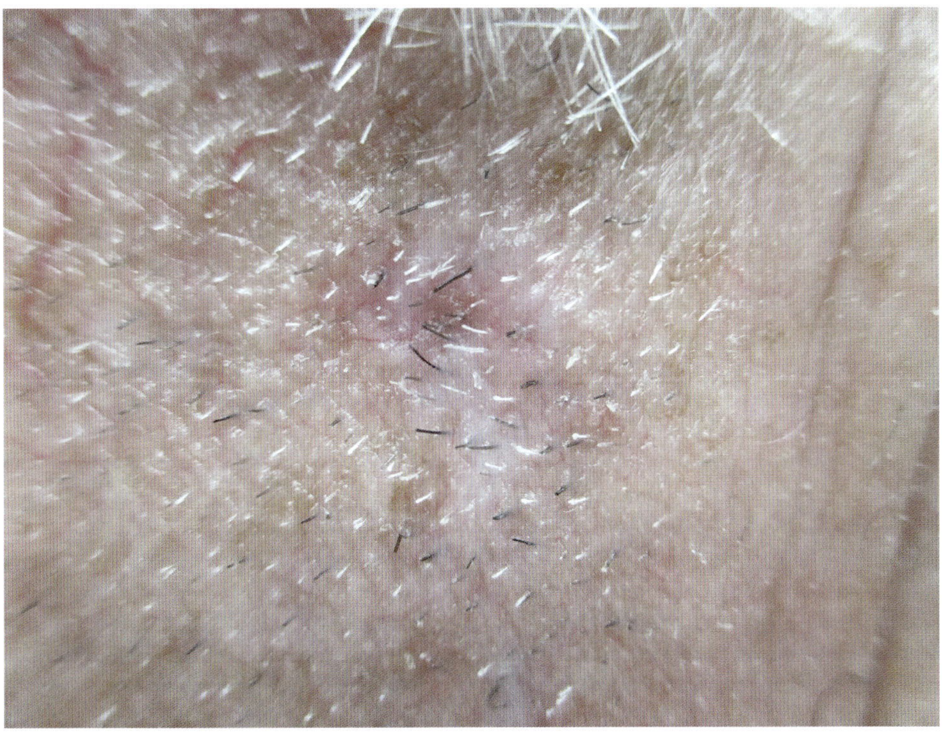

Fig. 8.2 Basal cell carcinoma in a SOTR.

TABLE 8.1 Incidence and Risk Factors for Skin Cancers in SOTRs

NMSC	
– Cumulative sun exposure[5] – Pretransplant skin cancer[5] – Age at transplant 50 or older[5] – Male sex[5] – Time elapsed since transplant[5] – Fitzpatrick skin type I–III[11] – Increased number, dosage, and duration of use of immunosuppressants[19]	
Squamous Cell Carcinoma	**Basal Cell Carcinoma**
– 65–250 x increased risk[5] – Heart and lung transplants[5,12] – Azathioprine[15] – Calcineurin inhibitors[5] – Voriconazole[19]	– 10–16 x increased risk[5] – Liver transplant[5] – Mycophenolic acid[15]

areas as well as tumor recurrence. The high burden of premalignant and malignant skin disease often requires field-directed rather than lesion-directed therapy. Photodynamic therapy (PDT) is a field-directed treatment modality involving a topical or systemic photosensitizer and a light source to target and destroy precancers and cancers. This chapter will cover the role of PDT for actinic keratoses (AKs) and NMSCs in the SOTR population.

Photodynamic Therapy

PDT is a procedure involving the topical or systemic administration of a photosensitizer with affinity to precancerous cells or tumor cells. Tumor cells either directly accumulate the photosensitizer or convert it to protoporphyrin IX (PpIX) via the heme synthesis pathway. After an incubation period, subsequent photodynamic activation by a light source generates reactive oxygen species resulting in direct cytotoxic effects on tumor cells, damage to tumor vasculature, induction of an inflammatory response, apoptosis, and necrosis.[11] There are a variety of photosensitizers, including topical aminolevulinic acid (ALA), methyl-aminolevulinic acid (MAL), and systemic porfimer sodium, as well as different light sources including blue light, red light, white light, and daylight. Currently, PDT is approved by the Food and Drug Administration (FDA) in the US for the treatment of AKs.[12]

PDT offers several advantages in the treatment of AKs and NMSCs in SOTRs. These include the ability to treat large areas of field cancerization, excellent safety profile, potential for repeated use, preservation of function and cosmesis, absence of surgical fatigue, and ability to be used in patients taking immunosuppressive medications. In this chapter, we will review the current literature and offer recommendations for the safe and effective use of PDT in SOTRs for the treatment of AKs and superficial NMSCs.

CURRENT APPLICATIONS

Current Protocols

There are a variety of PDT protocols for the treatment of AKs and NMSC that have been developed and approved by various regulatory agencies worldwide. In the US, ALA HCl in the form of the Levulan Kerastick with a label incubation time of 14–18 h (although in practice 1–3 h) for the scalp or face, and 3 h for the upper extremities with occlusion with the BLU-U (10 J/cm^2, 1000 s) blue light device has been FDA-approved for the treatment of mild-to-moderate AKs.[12] ALA HCl has been similarly approved in Australia since 2014.[13] More recently, ALA 10% nanoemulsion gel in the form of Ameluz with an incubation time of 3 h under occlusion with the BF-RhodoLED lamp (37 J/cm^2, 10 min) has been approved for both lesion-directed and field-directed treatment mild-to-moderate AKs of the face and scalp.[12] In Europe, Ameluz and BF-RhodoLED lamp is also approved by the European Medicines Agency for treatment of AKs of the face or scalp as well as BCCs with a protocol of 3 h incubation under occlusion followed by a red-light source (37 J/cm^2).[14] Furthermore, the use of MAL 16.8% cream with red-light PDT has been approved for non-hyperkeratotic AKs of the face and scalp, superficial or nodular BCCs, and SCC in situ (*SCCis*) in several European countries, New Zealand, Australia, and select South American countries including Brazil.[15–17] It has also been approved in combination with daylight PDT (dPDT) for AKs. In the US, MAL 16.8% cream is no longer commercially available, despite being previously approved in 2008. Of note, these protocols are indicated for the general immunocompetent population and there are currently no separately approved protocols for SOTRs.

The available approved clinical protocols often need more practical utility. The incubation times are unreasonable or rigid, and surface areas of treatment are restrictive for most patients with field disease. Therefore most clinicians perform PDT using their off-label protocols to better address the needs of unique patient populations. This is especially the case for clinicians treating SOTRs with PDT for extensive areas of field damage requiring a much larger treatment area than currently approved protocols suggest. Besides the treatment area, other variables optimized by providers include methods of pre-PDT debridement, photosensitizer incubation time, illumination methods, frequency of treatments, and post-care protocols.

Current Guidelines

Given the high incidence and distribution of AKs and NMSCs in SOTRs compared to the general population, guidelines have been established by expert societies or panels to provide clinicians with a framework on how to manage care for SOTRs. The first practice guidelines were recommended by the International Society for Photodynamic Therapy in Dermatology and the British Photodermatology Group and the British Association of Dermatologists in 2007 and 2008, respectively. However, their recommendations were weak, simply suggesting that PDT may be a possible treatment for the prevention of NMSCs in SOTRs.[18,19] As more clinical data emerged supporting the utility of PDT in SOTRs, the same group strengthened their recommendations in 2018, stating that field PDT can be used prophylactically to reduce the emergence of new NMSCs in SOTRs.[20] Similar statements were made by the PDT subgroup of the European Dermatology Forum guidelines committee in 2013 and 2015.[21,22] Most recently in 2021, an expert panel of dermatologists with greater than 5 years of experience treating SOTRs released consensus-based recommendations for the prevention of SCC in SOTRs.[23] They recommended field therapy, which includes PDT, when AKs were grouped in one anatomical area unless the AKs were thick in which they recommended both field therapy and cryotherapy. Hence, the most up-to-date recommendations promote the use of PDT as a field-directed therapy for treatment as well as prevention of AKs and NMSCs.

CLINICAL DATA

PDT in SOTRs Compared to Immunocompetent Patients

PDT has been demonstrated to be effective in both immunocompetent patients and in SOTRs. In the first trial comparing the use of PDT in SOTRs versus immunocompetent patients, Dragieva and colleagues used red-light ALA-PDT to treat AKs or Bowen's disease in 20 SOTRs and 20 immunocompetent patients.[24] While both groups demonstrated similar complete response (CR) rates at 4 weeks after their last PDT treatment, SOTRs had decreased clearance rates at 12 and 48 weeks after the last PDT treatment as well as an increased risk of recurrence. The authors hypothesized that lesions in SOTRs demonstrated more prominent hyperkeratosis, higher proportion on sites with poorer response rates, and an altered immune response. On the contrary, Lim and colleagues recently performed a retrospective chart review of 281 immunocompetent patients and 33 SOTRs with AKs, BCCs, and SCCis treated with red-light MAL-PDT.[25] The authors found no statistically significant difference between clearance rates at 12 weeks (74% vs. 76%, respectively) and 12 months (80% vs. 73%, respectively). Similarly, a large case series review by Collier and colleagues of 322 BCCs in 23 SOTRs and 80 immunocompetent patients treated with red-light MAL-PDT found no significant differences in recurrence rates or time to recurrence between transplant and non-transplant patients.[26] Importantly, none of these studies demonstrated any significant adverse effect of PDT in SOTRs. Together, these results indicate that PDT is similar in safety and efficacy in SOTRs and immunocompetent patients. However, the likelihood of long-term lesion recurrence after PDT treatment in SOTRs remains uncertain.

PDT to Treat Actinic Keratoses and Squamous Cell Carcinoma in Situ

AKs are UV-induced premalignant scaly lesions that are precursors to SCCs, the most common skin cancer in SOTRs. The incidence of AKs is greater in SOTRs compared to the general population with a mean occurrence of 38% within 5 years of a solid organ transplant.[27] While some AKs in the immunocompetent population may self-resolve even without treatment, the spontaneous regression rate of AKs in SOTRs is 0%.[28] Additionally, the progression of AKs to SCCs is accelerated in SOTRs.[29] In patients with superficial disease without metastasis with frequent recurrence or high lesion incidence, PDT can be integrated into the overall management of these patients. Therefore we will evaluate studies in which PDT was used in the management of AKs and SCCis.

The studies performed by Dragieva and colleagues and Lim and colleagues described earlier in this chapter suggest that PDT is effective in treating AKs and SCCis in SOTRs.[24,25] Dragieva and colleagues performed another trial utilizing red-light MAL-PDT to treat 17 SOTRs with 129 AKs and achieved a CR in 13 patients, a partial response in three, and no response in one patient when measured at 16 weeks after PDT.[30] An even better response was reported by Hasson and colleagues, in which 15 SOTRs treated with red-light MAL-PDT achieved 100% CR at 12 and 24 weeks after PDT.[31] A systematic review and meta-analysis by Liew and colleagues of PDT for the treatment of AKs and SCCis in SOTRs analyzed 86 patients from five RTCs capturing 1931 AKs and 10 SCCis and determined that the PDT group had decreased lesional areas of 77% and a decreased number of lesions of 50%, compared to the control groups.[32] While the results were promising, the authors found great heterogeneity in the five included studies, particularly with the PDT protocols, including the frequency of treatment. Nevertheless, PDT is shown to be effective. In our chapter, we will describe the current literature regarding PDT for AKs and SCCis categorized into co-treatment with other modalities, direct comparisons to other existing treatments, as well as disease prevention.

Combination Therapy for Actinic Keratoses and Squamous Cell Carcinoma in Situ

The effects of PDT can be potentiated by pretreating lesions with mechanical debridement using a variety of tools including ablative fractional lasers (AFL), microneedling, and physical debridement (Table 8.2). These techniques decrease hyperkeratosis and increase photosensitizer and light penetration, which can make PDT more effective.[33] One of the most well-studied combination treatments is AFL pretreatment. In a study by Togsverd-Bo and colleagues, 16 SOTRs with 542 AKs had their affected areas divided into four

TABLE 8.2 Summary of PDT Combination Treatments and Protocols for AKs in SOTRs

Combination Treatment	Study	Protocol	Results
Ablative Fractional Laser + daylight PDT	Togsverd-Bo et al.[34]	Ablative fractional Er:YAG laser pretreatment → MAL (2.5 h incubation without occlusion) → 120 min of daylight exposure	CR of 74% in AKs at 3 months compared to dPDT (46%) or AFL (5%) alone
	Rizvi et al.[35]	Lutronic CO_2 laser pretreatment → MAL (30 min incubation) → 120 min of daylight exposure	CR of 76% in AKs at 4 months compared to PDT alone (64%)
Ablative Fractional Laser + conventional PDT	Helsing et al.[36]	Lutronic CO_2 laser pretreatment → MAL (3 h incubation under occlusion) → 632 nm red-light PDT (37 J/cm^2 light dose)	CR of 73% in AKs at 4 months compared to PDT alone (31%)
	Londsdorf et al.[37]	Ablative fractional Er:YAG laser pretreatment → MAL (3 h incubation) → 635 nm red-light PDT (37 J/cm^2 light dose, intensity at 30%)	CR of 77.3% in AKs at 3 months and no pain compared to PDT alone (61.8%)
Microneedling + conventional PDT	Bencini et al.[39]	Microneedling pretreatment → MAL (3 h incubation) → PDT(90 J/cm^2)	CR of 100% at 4 months and CR of 83% at 9 months
Topical 5-FU + conventional PDT	Jambusaria-Pahlajani et al.[40]	Lesional curettage → 5-FU cream twice daily for 5 days → ALA 20% → blue light PDT (10 J/cm^2) light dose	CR of 100% in AKs at 1 and 6 months

treatment fields.[34] This included MAL incubation followed by either AFL + dPDT, dPDT alone, red-light PDT, or AFL alone. CR was highest in the AFL + dPDT treatment field at 74% compared to either PDT alone (50%), dPDT (46%), or AFL alone (5%). Pain was found to be greatest in the red-light PDT field and was absent in all other fields. Rizvi and colleagues found similar results in a study of 12 SOTRs with 209 AKs in treatment areas divided between either MAL incubation followed by AFL-dPDT or dPDT alone.[35] The addition of AFL to PDT significantly potentiated the effects of PDT, increasing the CR from 64% to 76%. Helsing and colleagues likewise performed a similar study but used red-light PDT.[36] In ten SOTRs with 680 AKs with treatment areas of either AFL-red-light PDT or AFL alone, the combination group demonstrated a significantly higher CR of 73% compared to the AFL alone group of 31%. Furthermore, lesions that had not completely resolved improved to lower-grade lesions. To avoid the increased pain associated with red-light PDT, Lonsdorf and colleagues developed a protocol of using low-irradiance red-light PDT (18.5 mW/cm^2) in combination with AFL compared to conventional PDT (61.67 mW/cm^2) alone.[37] They found that the combination treatment with AFL and low-irradiance PDT achieved significantly higher CR of 77.3% compared to 61.8% of the conventional PDT alone at 3 months post treatment without affecting pain or cosmetic outcomes. Lastly, a review of laser-assisted PDT for AKs by Steeb and colleagues recommended laser-assisted PDT for the treatment of AKs in SOTRs given the higher clearance rate of combination therapy as well as no significant difference in pain.[38] AFL may be synergistic with PDT using all light sources, and thus AFL pretreatment can be considered to improve PDT outcomes in SOTRs.

Besides AFL, other physical pretreatments can also be used before PDT. In recent years microneedling has been gaining traction as a low-cost physical intervention. A study by Bencini and colleagues including 12 SOTRs with 59 AKs resistant to classical PDT demonstrated that all lesions treated with microneedling followed by PDT achieved CR at 4 months with only two of 12 patients relapsing at 9 months.[39] Although physical debridement is the most common lesional pretreatment, its effects are difficult to quantify given the different techniques (e.g., curettage and sandpaper abrasion) and great inter-individual differences in the aggressiveness of the procedures.

Besides physical measures, chemical pretreatment is another way to enhance PDT efficacy. A clinical trial by Maytin and colleagues evaluated the rate of AK clearance in four SOTRs who had treatment fields of either 5-FU pretreatment with MAL red-light PDT or with PDT alone. 5-FU was topically applied for 6 days prior to the PDT session in the pretreatment field. The authors discovered that the clearance rate of AKs in the pretreatment field was nearly double that of the PDT-alone treatment field in both SOTRs and the immunocompetent population at 3 months. Even at 6 and 9 months post treatment, the pretreatment fields continued to have significantly improved clearance rates. A similar study was performed by Jambusaria-Pahlajani and colleagues in which four SOTRs were treated with lesional curettage, topical 5-FU twice daily for 5 days, and then MAL-red-light PDT.[40] All patients achieved CR at 1 and 6 months follow-up, suggesting 5-FU topical pretreatment of the field can also augment PDT efficacy in SOTRs.

Comparison of PDT to Other Treatments for Actinic Keratoses

When used as monotherapy, PDT was shown to be equivalent to, if not more effective than, other treatment modalities for AKs in SOTRs. A study conducted by Togsverd-Bo and colleagues treated 35 SOTRs with 572 AKs in two distinct areas with either MAL-red-light PDT or imiquimod cream.[41] At 3-month follow-up, the PDT-treated areas had significantly higher rates of CR (78% vs. 61%) preexisting AKs, and fewer emergent new AKs (0.7 vs. 1.5 new AKs) compared to the imiquimod-treated sites. A similar study by Perrett and colleagues evaluated the differences between two treatments of MAL-red-light PDT versus topical 5-FU cream in eight OTRs with 18 AKs.[42] At 1, 3, and 6 months after treatment, eight of nine PDT-treated AKs achieved CR compared to only one of nine lesions treated with 5-FU. In both previously described studies, the only drawback was increased pain post treatment, but patients still preferred PDT over topical creams. These studies were further validated by a review of 8 RTCs for local interventions for AKs in SOTRs by Heppt and colleagues in which they found that MAL-PDT has the highest CR (40%–76.4%) compared to imiquimod (27.5%–62.1%), diclofenac (41%), or 5-FU (11%).[43] PDT is effective even in AKs resistant to conventional treatments. Piaserico and colleagues performed a study in which 15 SOTRs with 245 AKs unresponsive to 5-FU, CO_2 laser, curettage, and electrosurgery were treated with two sessions of lesional shaving followed by MAL and red-light PDT.[29] At 3-month follow-up, 64% of the lesions achieved CR. Hence, current data indicates that PDT in SOTRs demonstrates equal or superior effects compared to other treatment modalities for AKs and may be an effective salvage therapy for treatment-resistant lesions. However, given recent well-designed larger studies in evaluating AK treatments in non-immunosuppressed patients, larger studies in SOTRs are necessary to confirm the previously established superiority of PDT.[44,45]

Preventive PDT for Actinic Keratoses and Squamous Cell Carcinoma in Situ

Given the increased incidence and recurrence of AKs and SCCs in SOTRs, prevention is key to reduce overall morbidity in this high-risk population. Current chemoprevention strategies include the use of nicotinamide and oral retinoid therapy in addition to sun protection.[46] In addition to systemic chemoprevention, PDT may be used as it offers well-tolerated, field-directed treatment with minimal side effects.

The first trial exploring the use of PDT for the prevention of AKs in SOTRs was conducted by Wulf and colleagues.[47] In this study, 27 SOTRs had a treatment area of debridement followed by one session of MAL-red-light PDT as well as a no-treatment area. The treatment area had a prolonged mean time-to-occurrence of a single AK of 9.6 months compared to 6.8 months in the untreated areas. At 12 months, 62% of treated areas were lesion-free compared to only 35% of untreated areas. A similar trial was conducted by de Graaf and colleagues in which 40 SOTRs were randomized to either one or two treatments of ALA-violet light PDT or no treatment in different areas.[48] However, no significant difference in new SCCs was found between the treatment and control areas at 1 and 2 years after treatment. The authors postulated that the lack of difference between the treated and untreated areas could be because the existing lesions were not eliminated before the initiation of PDT. Consequently, it is possible that both regular sessions of PDT as well as lesional pretreatment and adequate light sources are necessary for adequate prophylaxis. To determine the effects of regular preventive PDT, Wennberg and colleagues performed a trial in which 81 SOTRs with AKs were treated with either debridement followed by red-light MAL-PDT or lesion-directed cryotherapy at baseline, 3, 9, and 15 months.[49] The authors found that while there was a significant difference in the reduction of new AKs at 3 months, there was no significant difference at 8 or 27 months after the last PDT session. Another similar trial by Bernad and colleagues of 24 SOTRs evaluated the preventive effects of MAL-dPDT at baseline, 3 months, and 9 months compared to lesion-directed cryotherapy and, like the previous trial, a reduction in new lesions was seen when patients were receiving regular PDT, but after patients discontinued regular PDT sessions, no reduction was seen.[50] The loss of preventive effect at the later stages of these trials when the patients were not receiving PDT treatments suggests that PDT must be delivered regularly to prevent AKs. This hypothesis was explored by Togsverd and colleagues in a long-term trial of SOTRs receiving MAL-red-light PDT at 6-month intervals for 5 years on only half of their clinically normal skin.[51,52] Preliminary data at 3-years follow-up comprising 25 SOTRs reported that AKs were found in 28% of treated areas compared to 63% of untreated areas.[51] Subsequent data from 44 SOTRs found that at 6-years follow-up, there was a significant decrease in average AKs per patient (1.0 vs. 1.8) as well as an increased probability of AK-free skin (72% vs. 50%) in PDT-treated skin compared to the untreated skin.[52] When the frequency of PDT is increased, CR may further improve. This was demonstrated by Lindberg and colleagues, who treated seven SOTRs with quarterly ALA-blue light PDT on the face and scalp and reported a 3-year average reduction in NMSC of 83.9% and a number needed to treat of 1.75 to prevent an NMSC.[53] Additionally, a study by Willey and colleagues composed of 12 SOTRs treated with ALA-blue light PDT every 4–8 weeks for 2 years with existing lesions being curetted demonstrated similar results.[54] There was a median reduction in new SCCs of 79% and 95% at 12 and 24 months, respectively, compared to the number of new SCCs developed the year before PDT started. There is currently a clinical trial conducted by Zeitouni and colleagues investigating the long-term safety and efficacy of cyclic ALA-blue light PDT for the prevention of AKs and NMSCs in SOTRs.[55] A meta-analysis by Liew and colleagues including three of the previously described studies analyzed 234 patients and reported PDT-treated patients had lower incidence of future AKs and NMSCs, with a pooled risk difference of 0.14.[32] Current data suggests that SOTRs at high risk of AKs should have all existing lesions adequately treated and then they may benefit from regular preventive PDT.

PDT to Treat Basal Cell Carcinomas

BCCs in SOTRs are more frequently superficial and are more likely to be extracephalic compared to immunocompetent individuals.[56,57] This presents greater difficulty with treatment as extracephalic lesions have been shown to be less likely to respond to PDT.[58] However, the current clinical data regarding the utility of PDT for BCC treatment in SOTRs is promising. A case report by Perrett and colleagues demonstrated that MAL-red-light PDT was effective in treating a nodular BCC on the nose of a liver OTR with no recurrence at 12 months.[59] Additionally, Guleng and colleagues treated 18 SOTRs with nodular and superficial BCCs on the head and trunk with two sessions of MAL-red-light PDT and achieved CR in 17 of 18 patients.[60] Notably, there was only a single recurrence during a follow-up period of a combined 407 months across all patients. In a larger case series review by Collier and colleagues of 23 SOTRS and 80 non-transplant patients with 322 BCCs, two sessions of MAL-red-light PDT led to CR in 77.4% of SOTRs.[26] Furthermore, there were no significant differences in recurrence rates or time to recurrence between the SOTRs and non-transplant patients, indicating that MAL-PDT may work equally well in both populations. Of note, the subtype of BCC was not available in this study. Similar results have also been observed using ALA, in which a study by Schleier and colleagues used red-light PDT in five SOTRs with 21 mostly superficial BCCs (1 patient was also found to have invasive BCCs) and achieved CR of 75% after one treatment and 94% after two treatments, with only a single refractory tumor after three sessions.[61] Consequently, there is evidence that both MAL- and ALA-PDT with red light can effectively treat both superficial and nodular BCCs in SOTRs with a low risk of recurrence.

Adverse Effects of PDT

PDT is generally well-tolerated by most patients. Contraindications to PDT include patients with a past history of hyperphotosensitivity, those with porphyria, and those with allergies to components of the photosensitizers (e.g., soybean, peanut, and almond oil).[62] The predominant adverse effect of PDT is pain often described as "stinging," "sharp," or "burning" during the irradiation process of the procedure, followed by erythema and edema of the targeted skin as part of the phototoxic reaction.[63] These effects can persist for several hours to days after treatment and can interfere with both the desire to perform PDT and the completion of planned treatment. Although pain is variable among patients, factors associated with increased pain include larger treatment areas, facial lesions, and skin phenotype.[64–66] In a review, Wlodek and colleagues suggested that SOTRs may experience more pronounced pain during PDT than immunocompetent patients owing to the increased size and number of their lesions.[67] This was evaluated by Dragieva and colleagues in a study of 20 SOTRs and 20 immunocompetent patients who received ALA-red-light PDT to treat AKs and SCCis.[24] Patients were asked to grade the pain experienced during treatment numerically, and the authors found no significant difference between groups. Consequently, techniques of pain reduction explored in the general population are likely also applicable in SOTRs.

A recent review by Ang and colleagues concerning pain in PDT categorized pain-relieving techniques as either external interventions or modification of PDT parameters, including photosensitizer, incubation time, light source, and light intensity.[68] The authors found that nerve blocks, inhalational anesthesia, and subcutaneous infiltration anesthesia have significant pain-reducing effects, although they may be impractical in the clinical setting.[69–71] Cooling methods, including cold air analgesia, have effects on pain reduction, although to a much lower extent than the previously described invasive analgesic methods.[72] Concerning the modification of PDT parameters, ALA-PDT tends to be more painful than MAL, although some studies have conflicting data.[65,73–75] In addition, dPDT, which results in continuous activation of smaller amounts of PpIX, has been shown to cause significantly less pain than conventional PDT, which quickly activates larger amounts of PpIX.[76] Other less painful light sources include artificial prolonged white light illumination.[77,78] Additionally, modifying the timing of light administration has been shown to alleviate pain. Kaw and colleagues found that immediately starting blue light after ALA application compared to starting 1 h after ALA incubation had identical lesion clearance but significantly less pain.[79] Lastly, modifying the amount of irradiation has also been shown to reduce pain. Zeitouni and colleagues developed a two-step protocol utilizing an initial low irradiance by laser at 40 or 50 mW/cm^2 or LED at 35 mW/cm^2 followed by an irradiance at 70 mW/cm^2 for a total light dose of 75 J/cm^2 which resulted in low pain while maintaining high CR for the treatment of AKs and BCCs.[80,81]

There have been few trials investigating PDT techniques to reduce pain specifically in SOTRs. Lonsdorf and colleagues discovered that using AFL pretreatment with low-irradiance red-light PDT (18.5 mW/cm^2) achieved superior CR response for AKs in SOTRs without causing pain, compared to conventional red-light PDT (61.67 mW/cm^2) alone.[37] Additionally, Lonsdorf and colleagues found that SOTRs overwhelmingly prefer dPDT compared to red or blue light, without any differences in CR for AKs.[34] When PDT was compared to other treatments in SOTRs, PDT was found to be preferred over other treatments, including 5-FU or imiquimod, as patients preferred shorter intense pain compared to prolonged milder pain.[41,42] Overall, techniques for pain management in immunocompetent patients likely have similar effects in SOTRs. These techniques can help improve patient satisfaction and compliance in patients who otherwise cannot tolerate PDT.

DISCUSSION

Our chapter explores the various roles of PDT in the management of AKs and NMSCs in SOTRs. We reviewed the comprehensive data on the safety and efficacy of PDT in SOTRs, with similar short-term effects to those seen in immunocompetent patients. PDT is particularly useful in this patient population, who often experience significant surgical fatigue. Expert guidelines also recommend PDT as a field-directed therapy for treating and possibly preventing AKs and NMSCs in SOTRs. PDT offers good flexibility with the ability to adjust protocols according to the patient's needs and can be efficiently combined with other therapies to further potentiate its efficacy. While the main limiting adverse effect is treatment-related pain, various protocols have been developed to address the issue and ongoing studies are investigating newer strategies to mitigate pain. Additionally, post-PDT care should be emphasized to decrease patient discomfort and additional adverse effects. When topical photosensitizers are used, post-PDT care should include the use of bland emollients as well as avoidance of sun or sources of intense visible light for 48 h with close follow-up 2–4 weeks after the procedure.[33] Along with regular skin exams and patient education concerning sun protection, PDT is an invaluable tool for dermatologic management of SOTRs.[82,83]

An important avenue for the future of PDT delivery in SOTRs is noninvasive in vivo imaging to determine treatment site selection, monitor treatment efficacy, and screen for residual or recurrent tumors. The implementation of such a technique would allow for decreased diagnostic biopsies and optimize PDT treatments with regard to treatment locations. In immunocompetent patients, imaging techniques including multispectral fluorescence imaging, reflectance confocal microscopy (RCM), and optical coherence tomography have been studied and used to evaluate PDT effectiveness as well as detect recurrences after PDT to guide future therapy.[84–88] In SOTRs however, only a single study exists, which evaluates the use of noninvasive imaging to monitor response to PDT. In this study, Astner and colleagues evaluated five SOTRs' AKs with both reflectance and fluorescence confocal microscopy, which confirmed actinic disease.[89] After treatment with ALA-red-light PDT, RCM was used to monitor treatment response which demonstrated a gradual change from diseased to normal RCM characteristics and architecture. Additionally, RCM was able to detect subclinical disease when performed in areas surrounding affected skin sites. Therefore RCM has great potential to optimize PDT in SOTRs and must be further investigated.

CONCLUSION

PDT is an effective and safe treatment modality for AKs, SCCis, and nonaggressive BCCs in SOTRs, who face exceptionally high skin cancer risk and require field-directed therapy. It has the most evidence compared to other non-surgical treatments in SOTRs and has documented advantages compared to other field treatment modalities. Additionally, it can be used with other treatment modalities to further enhance efficacy. In SOTRs with a high disease burden, PDT may play a role in prevention of future AKs and NMSCs. While pain may be a limiting factor to patient compliance, various protocols and techniques exist to reduce pain and improve overall patient satisfaction. Although there is a vast body of literature concerning the use of PDT in SOTRs for AKs and NMSC, there is substantial heterogeneity concerning protocols, including the definition of controls and the timing of follow-up. To further validate the use of PDT in SOTRs, larger randomized controlled trials with standardized protocols should be performed to establish the best practices for preventing and treating AKs and NMSC.

REFERENCES

1. OPTN Metrics. Accessed Nov 5 2024. https://insights.unos.org/OPTN-metrics/.
2. Organ Procurement and Transplantation Network. National data. United States Department of Health and Human Services. 2022. Accessed October 1, 2022. https://optn.transplant.hrsa.gov/data/view-data-reports/national-data/.
3. Garrett GL, Blanc PD, Boscardin J. Incidence of and risk factors for skin cancer in organ transplant recipients in the United States. *JAMA Dermatol.* 2017;153(3):296–303.
4. O'Reilly ZF, Brown M. Skin cancer in solid organ transplant recipients: advances in therapy and management: part I. Epidemiology of skin cancer in solid organ transplant recipients. *J Am Acad Dermatol.* 2011;65(2):253–261.
5. Howard MD, Su JC, Chong AH. Skin cancer following solid organ transplantation: a review of risk factors and models of care. *Am J Clin Dermatol.* 2018;19(4):585–597.
6. Coghill AE, Johnson LG, Berg D, et al. Immunosuppressive medications and squamous cell skin carcinoma: nested case-control study within the skin cancer after organ transplant (SCOT) cohort. *Am J Transplant.* 2016;16(2):565–573.
7. Singer JP, Boker A, Metchnikoff C, et al. High cumulative dose exposure to voriconazole is associated with cutaneous squamous cell carcinoma in lung transplant recipients. *J Heart Lung Transplant.* 2012;31(7):694–699.
8. Knoll GA, Kokolo MB, Mallick R, et al. Effect of sirolimus on malignancy and survival after kidney transplantation: systematic review and meta-analysis of individual patient data. *BMJ.* 2014;349:g6679.
9. Perera GK, Child FJ, Heaton N, O'Grady J, Higgins EM. Skin lesions in adult liver transplant recipients: a study of 100 consecutive patients. *Br J Dermatol.* 2006;154(5):868–872.
10. Wheless L, Anand N, Hanlon A, Chren MM. Differences in skin cancer rates by Transplanted organ type and patient age after organ transplant in white patients. *JAMA Dermatol.* 2022;158(11):1287–1292.
11. Agostinis P, Berg K, Cengel KA, et al. Photodynamic therapy of cancer: an update. *CA Cancer J Clin.* 2011;61(4):250–281.
12. FDA/CEDR Resources Page. Food and Drug Administration website. Accessed September 7, 2022 https://www.accessdata.fda.gov/drugsatfda_docs/label/2018/020965s016lbl.pdf.
13. Australian Public Assessment Report for Aminolevulinic Acid HCl. Australian Government Department of Health. 2014. Accessed October 1, 2022. https://www.tga.gov.au/sites/default/files/auspar-aminolevulinic-acid-140303.pdf.
14. EMA Medicines Page. European Medicines Agency website. Accessed September 7, 2022. https://www.ema.europa.eu/en/documents/product-information/ameluz-epar-product-information_en.pdf.
15. EMC Page. Electronic Medicines Compendium website. Accessed September 7, 2022. https://www.medicines.org.uk/emc/product/6777/smpc#gref.
16. Wan MT, Lin JY. Current evidence and applications of photodynamic therapy in dermatology. *Clin Cosmet Investig Dermatol.* 2014;7:145–163.
17. Issa MCA, Boechat M, Fassini AC. Photodynamic therapy in Brazil: 10 years of history. *Surg Cosmet Dermatol.* 2016;8(4 Supl. 1):S16–S22.
18. Braathen LR, Szeimies RM, Basset-Seguin N, et al. Guidelines on the use of photodynamic therapy for nonmelanoma skin cancer: an international consensus. International Society for Photodynamic Therapy in Dermatology, 2005. *J Am Acad Dermatol.* 2007;56(1):125–143.
19. Morton CA, McKenna KE, Rhodes LE. Guidelines for topical photodynamic therapy: update. *Br J Dermatol.* 2008;159(6):1245–1266.
20. Wong TH, Morton CA, Collier N. British Association of Dermatologists and British Photodermatology Group guidelines for topical photodynamic therapy 2018. *Br J Dermatol.* 2019;180(4):730–739.
21. Morton C, Szeimies RM, Sidoroff A, et al. European Dermatology Forum Guidelines on topical photodynamic therapy. *Eur J Dermatol.* 2015;25(4):296–311.
22. Morton CA, Szeimies RM, Sidoroff A, Braathen LR. European guidelines for topical photodynamic therapy part 2: emerging indications–field cancerization, photorejuvenation and inflammatory/infective dermatoses. *J Eur Acad Dermatol Venereol.* 2013;27(6):672–679.
23. Massey PR, Schmults CD, Li SJ, et al. Consensus-based recommendations on the prevention of squamous cell carcinoma in solid organ transplant recipients: a Delphi consensus statement. *JAMA Dermatol.* 2021;157(10):1219–1226.
24. Dragieva G, Hafner J, Dummer R, et al. Topical photodynamic therapy in the treatment of actinic keratoses and Bowen's disease in transplant recipients. *Transplantation.* 2004;77(1):115–121.
25. Lim CM, Grillo M, Harrison P, Nguyen AM, Gordon L. Photodynamic therapy: a real-world analysis of outcomes of photodynamic therapy in an Australian tertiary dermatology clinic. *Australas J Dermatol.* 2019;60(4):339–340.

26. Collier NJ, Ali FR, Lear JT. Efficacy of photodynamic therapy for treatment of basal cell carcinoma in organ transplant recipients. *Lasers Med Sci.* 2015;30(4):1407–1409.
27. Dréno B, Mansat E, Legoux B, Litoux P. Skin cancers in transplant patients. *Adv Nephrol Necker Hosp.* 1997;27:377–389.
28. Steeb T, Petzold A, Hornung A, et al. Spontaneous regression rates of actinic keratosis: a systematic review and pooled analysis of randomized controlled trials. *Sci Rep.* 2022;12(1):5884.
29. Piaserico S, Belloni Fortina A, Rigotti P, et al. Topical photodynamic therapy of actinic keratosis in renal transplant recipients. *Transplant Proc.* 2007;39(6):1847–1850.
30. Dragieva G, Prinz BM, Hafner J, et al. A randomized controlled clinical trial of topical photodynamic therapy with methyl aminolaevulinate in the treatment of actinic keratoses in transplant recipients. *Br J Dermatol.* 2004;151(1):196–200.
31. Hasson A, Navarrete-Dechent C, Nicklas C, de la Cruz C. Topical photodynamic therapy with methylaminolevulinate for the treatment of actinic keratosis and reduction of photodamage in organ transplant recipients: a case-series of 16 patients. *Indian J Dermatol Venereol Leprol.* 2012;78(4):448–453.
32. Liew YCC, De Souza NNA, Sultana RG, Oh CC. Photodynamic therapy for the prevention and treatment of actinic keratosis/squamous cell carcinoma in solid organ transplant recipients: a systematic review and meta-analysis. *J Eur Acad Dermatol Venereol.* 2020;34(2):251–259.
33. Zeitouni NC, Bhatia N, Ceilley RI, et al. Photodynamic therapy with 5-aminolevulinic acid 10% gel and red light for the treatment of actinic keratosis, nonmelanoma skin cancers, and acne: current evidence and best practices. *J Clin Aesthet Dermatol.* 2021;14(10):E53–E65.
34. Togsverd-Bo K, Lei U, Erlendsson AM, et al. Combination of ablative fractional laser and daylight-mediated photodynamic therapy for actinic keratosis in organ transplant recipients – a randomized controlled trial. *Br J Dermatol.* 2015;172(2):467–474.
35. Rizvi SM, Veierød MB, Mørk G, Helsing P, Gjersvik P. Ablative fractional laser-assisted daylight photodynamic therapy for actinic keratoses of the scalp and forehead in organ transplant recipients: a pilot study. *Acta Derm Venereol.* 2019;99(11):1047–1048.
36. Helsing P, Togsverd-Bo K, Veierød MB, Mørk G, Haedersdal M. Intensified fractional CO_2 laser-assisted photodynamic therapy vs. laser alone for organ transplant recipients with multiple actinic keratoses and wart-like lesions: a randomized half-side comparative trial on dorsal hands. *Br J Dermatol.* 2013;169(5):1087–1092.
37. Lonsdorf AS, Keller A, Hartmann J, Enk AH, Gholam P. Ablative fractional laser-assisted low-irradiance photodynamic therapy for treatment of actinic keratoses in organ transplant recipients: a prospective, randomized, intraindividual controlled trial. *Acta Derm Venereol.* 2022;102:adv00694.
38. Steeb T, Schlager JG, Kohl C, et al. Laser-assisted photodynamic therapy for actinic keratosis: a systematic review and meta-analysis. *J Am Acad Dermatol.* 2019;80(4):947–956.
39. Bencini PL, Galimberti MG, Pellacani G, Longo C. Application of photodynamic therapy combined with pre-illumination microneedling in the treatment of actinic keratosis in organ transplant recipients. *Br J Dermatol.* 2012;167(5):1193–1194.
40. Jambusaria-Pahlajani A, Ortman S, Schmults CD, Liang C. Sequential curettage, 5-fluorouracil, and photodynamic therapy for field cancerization of the scalp and face in solid organ transplant recipients. *Dermatol Surg.* 2016;42(Suppl 1):S66–S72.
41. Togsverd-Bo K, Halldin C, Sandberg C, et al. Photodynamic therapy is more effective than imiquimod for actinic keratosis in organ transplant recipients: a randomized intraindividual controlled trial. *Br J Dermatol.* 2018;178(4):903–909.
42. Perrett CM, McGregor JM, Warwick J, et al. Treatment of post-transplant premalignant skin disease: a randomized intrapatient comparative study of 5-fluorouracil cream and topical photodynamic therapy. *Br J Dermatol.* 2007;156(2):320–328.
43. Heppt MV, Steeb T, Niesert AC, et al. Local interventions for actinic keratosis in organ transplant recipients: a systematic review. *Br J Dermatol.* 2019;180(1):43–50.
44. Steeb T, Wessely A, Harlaß M, et al. A systematic review and meta-analysis of interventions for actinic keratosis from post-marketing surveillance trials. *J Clin Med.* 2020;9(7):2253.
45. Jansen MHE, Kessels J, Nelemans PJ, et al. Randomized trial of four treatment approaches for actinic keratosis. *N Engl J Med.* 2019;380(10):935–946.
46. Chen K, Craig JC, Shumack S. Oral retinoids for the prevention of skin cancers in solid organ transplant recipients: a systematic review of randomized controlled trials. *Br J Dermatol.* 2005;152(3):518–523.
47. Wulf HC, Pavel S, Stender I, Bakker-Wensveen CA. Topical photodynamic therapy for prevention of new skin lesions in renal transplant recipients. *Acta Derm Venereol.* 2006;86(1):25–28.
48. de Graaf YG, Kennedy C, Wolterbeek R, et al. Photodynamic therapy does not prevent cutaneous squamous-cell carcinoma in organ-transplant recipients:

results of a randomized-controlled trial. *J Invest Dermatol*. 2006;126(3):569–574.
49. Wennberg AM, Stenquist B, Stockfleth E, et al. Photodynamic therapy with methyl aminolevulinate for prevention of new skin lesions in transplant recipients: a randomized study. *Transplantation*. 2008;86(3):423–429.
50. Bernad I, Aguado L, Núñez-Córdoba JM, Redondo P. Daylight photodynamic therapy for prevention of new actinic keratosis and keratinocyte carcinomas in organ transplants. a cryotherapy-controlled randomized clinical trial. *J Eur Acad Dermatol Venereol*. 2020;34(7):1464–1470.
51. Togsverd-Bo K, Omland SH, Wulf HC, Sørensen SS, Haedersdal M. Primary prevention of skin dysplasia in renal transplant recipients with photodynamic therapy: a randomized controlled trial. *Am J Transplant*. 2015;15(11):2986–2990.
52. Togsverd-Bo K, Sandberg C, Helsing P, et al. Cyclic photodynamic therapy delays first onset of actinic keratoses in renal transplant recipients: a 5-year randomized controlled trial with 12-month follow-up. *J Eur Acad Dermatol Venereol*. 2022;36(11):e946–e948.
53. Lindberg MR, Kent RA, DeSimone JA. Quarterly photodynamic therapy for prevention of nonmelanoma skin cancer in organ transplant recipients: an observational prospective cohort study. *J Am Acad Dermatol*. 2023;88(2):463–465.
54. Willey A, Mehta S, Lee PK. Reduction in the incidence of squamous cell carcinoma in solid organ transplant recipients treated with cyclic photodynamic therapy. *Dermatol Surg*. 2010;36(5):652–658.
55. Zeitouni NC. Cyclic PDT for the prevention of AK & NMSC in solid organ transplant recipients. Identifier NCT03110159. 2024. https://www.clinicaltrials.gov/ct2/show/NCT03110159.
56. Kanitakis J, Alhaj-Ibrahim L, Euvrard S, Claudy A. Basal cell carcinomas developing in solid organ transplant recipients: clinicopathologic study of 176 cases. *Arch Dermatol*. 2003;139(9):1133–1137.
57. Bastiaens MT, Hoefnagel JJ, Bruijn JA, et al. Differences in age, site distribution, and sex between nodular and superficial basal cell carcinoma indicate different types of tumors. *J Invest Dermatol*. 1998;110(6):880–884.
58. Fantini F, Greco A, Del Giovane C, et al. Photodynamic therapy for basal cell carcinoma: clinical and pathological determinants of response. *J Eur Acad Dermatol Venereol*. 2011;25(8):896–901.
59. Perrett CM, Tan SK, Cerio R, et al. Treatment of basal cell carcinoma with topical methylaminolaevulinate photodynamic therapy in an organ-transplant recipient. *Clin Exp Dermatol*. 2006;31(1):146–147.
60. Guleng GE, Helsing P. Photodynamic therapy for basal cell carcinomas in organ-transplant recipients. *Clin Exp Dermatol*. 2012;37(4):367–369.
61. Schleier P, Hyckel P, Berndt A. Photodynamic therapy of virus-associated epithelial tumours of the face in organ transplant recipients. *J Cancer Res Clin Oncol*. 2004;130(5):279–284.
62. Matsumoto Y, Akita Y. Safety guidelines for PDT of cutaneous lesions. *Laser Ther*. 2012;21(2):124–128.
63. Ibbotson SH. Adverse effects of topical photodynamic therapy. *Photodermatol Photoimmunol Photomed*. 2011;27(3):116–130.
64. Grapengiesser S, Ericson M, Gudmundsson F. Pain caused by photodynamic therapy of skin cancer. *Clin Exp Dermatol*. 2002;27(6):493–497.
65. Gholam P, Denk K, Sehr T, Enk A, Hartmann M, et al. Factors influencing pain intensity during topical photodynamic therapy of complete cosmetic units for actinic keratoses. *J Am Acad Dermatol*. 2010;63(2):213–218.
66. Arits AH, van de Weert MM, Nelemans PJ, Kelleners-Smeets NW. Pain during topical photodynamic therapy: uncomfortable and unpredictable. *J Eur Acad Dermatol Venereol*. 2010;24(12):1452–1457.
67. Wlodek C, Ali FR, Lear JT. Use of photodynamic therapy for treatment of actinic keratoses in organ transplant recipients. *Biomed Res Int*. 2013;2013:349526.
68. Ang JM, Riaz IB, Kamal MU, Paragh G, Zeitouni NC. Photodynamic therapy and pain: a systematic review. *Photodiagnosis Photodyn Ther*. 2017;19:308–344.
69. Klein A, Karrer S, Horner C, et al. Comparing cold-air analgesia, systemically administered analgesia and scalp nerve blocks for pain management during photodynamic therapy for actinic keratosis of the scalp presenting as field cancerization: a randomized controlled trial. *Br J Dermatol*. 2015;173(1):192–200.
70. Fink C, Uhlmann L, Enk A, Gholam P. Pain management in photodynamic therapy using a nitrous oxide/oxygen mixture: a prospective, within-patient, controlled clinical trial. *J Eur Acad Dermatol Venereol*. 2017;31(1):70–74.
71. Borelli C, Herzinger T, Merk K. Effect of subcutaneous infiltration anesthesia on pain in photodynamic therapy: a controlled open pilot trial. *Dermatol Surg*. 2007;33(3):314–318.
72. Stangeland KZ, Kroon S. Cold air analgesia as pain reduction during photodynamic therapy of actinic keratoses. *J Eur Acad Dermatol Venereol*. 2012;26(7):849–854.
73. Ibbotson SH, Valentine R, Hearn R. Is the pain of topical photodynamic therapy with methyl aminolevulinate any different from that with 5-aminolaevulinic

acid? *Photodermatol Photoimmunol Photomed.* 2012;28(5):272–273.

74. Dirschka T, Radny P, Dominicus R. Photodynamic therapy with BF-200 ALA for the treatment of actinic keratosis: results of a multicentre, randomized, observer-blind phase III study in comparison with a registered methyl-5-aminolaevulinate cream and placebo. *Br J Dermatol.* 2012;166(1):137–146.
75. Neittaanmäki-Perttu N, Karppinen TT, Grönroos M, Tani TT, Snellman E. Daylight photodynamic therapy for actinic keratoses: a randomized double-blinded nonsponsored prospective study comparing 5-aminolaevulinic acid nanoemulsion (BF-200) with methyl-5-aminolaevulinate. *Br J Dermatol.* 2014;171(5):1172–1180.
76. Wiegell SR, Haedersdal M, Philipsen PA, et al. Continuous activation of PpIX by daylight is as effective as and less painful than conventional photodynamic therapy for actinic keratoses; a randomized, controlled, single-blinded study. *Br J Dermatol.* 2008;158(4):740–746.
77. Maire C, Vignion-Dewalle AS, Cartier H, Mordon S. Artificial white light photodynamic therapy for actinic keratosis: a study of 38 patients in private office practice. *J Eur Acad Dermatol Venereol.* 2020;34(4): e165–e167.
78. Mordon S, Vignion-Dewalle AS, Abi-Rached H, et al. The conventional protocol vs. a protocol including illumination with a fabric-based biophotonic device (the Phosistos protocol) in photodynamic therapy for actinic keratosis: a randomized, controlled, noninferiority clinical study. *Br J Dermatol.* 2020;182(1):76–84.
79. Kaw U, Ilyas M, Bullock T, et al. A regimen to minimize pain during blue light photodynamic therapy of actinic keratoses: bilaterally controlled, randomized trial of simultaneous versus conventional illumination. *J Am Acad Dermatol.* 2020;82(4):862–868.
80. Zeitouni NC, Sunar U, Rohrbach DJ, et al. A prospective study of pain control by a 2-step irradiance schedule during topical photodynamic therapy of nonmelanoma skin cancer. *Dermatol Surg.* 2014;40(12):1390–1394.
81. Paragh G, Zeitouni NC, et al. Two-step irradiance treatment can achieve excellent pain control during red light 5-aminolevulinic acid photodynamic therapy for actinic keratoses. *Photomed Laser Surg.* 2018;36(3):174–176.
82. Crow LD, Jambusaria-Pahlajani A, Chung CL, et al. Initial skin cancer screening for solid organ transplant recipients in the United States: Delphi method development of expert consensus guidelines. *Transpl Int.* 2019;32(12):1268–1276.
83. Ulrich C, Jürgensen JS, Degen A, et al. Prevention of non-melanoma skin cancer in organ transplant patients by regular use of a sunscreen: a 24 months, prospective, case-control study. *Br J Dermatol.* 2009;161(Suppl 3):78–84.
84. Hewett J, Nadeau V, Ferguson J, et al. The application of a compact multispectral imaging system with integrated excitation source to in vivo monitoring of fluorescence during topical photodynamic therapy of superficial skin cancers. *Photochem Photobiol.* 2001;73(3):278–282.
85. Teoh YL, Kuan LY, Chong WS, et al. The role of reflectance confocal microscopy in the diagnosis and management of squamous cell carcinoma in situ treated with photodynamic therapy. *Int J Dermatol.* 2019;58(12):1382–1387.
86. Venturini M, Sala R, Gonzàlez S, Calzavara-Pinton PG. Reflectance confocal microscopy allows in vivo real-time noninvasive assessment of the outcome of methyl aminolaevulinate photodynamic therapy of basal cell carcinoma. *Br J Dermatol.* 2013;168(1):99–105.
87. Curiel-Lewandrowski C, Myrdal CN, Saboda K, et al. In vivo reflectance confocal microscopy as a response monitoring tool for actinic keratoses undergoing cryotherapy and photodynamic therapy. *Cancers (Basel).* 2021;13(21):5488.
88. Themstrup L, Banzhaf CA, Mogensen M, Jemec GB, et al. Optical coherence tomography imaging of non-melanoma skin cancer undergoing photodynamic therapy reveals subclinical residual lesions. *Photodiagnosis Photodyn Ther.* 2014;11(1):7–12.
89. Astner S, Swindells K, González S, Stockfleth E, Lademann J, et al. Confocal microscopy: innovative diagnostic tools for monitoring of noninvasive therapy in cutaneous malignancies. *Drug Discov Today Dis Mech.* 2008;5(1):e81–e91.

PART III

PDT for Neoplasia/ Skin Cancer

9

Photodynamic Therapy for Non-High-Risk Invasive Cutaneous Squamous Cell Carcinoma

Ron R. Allison

KEY POINTS

- Cutaneous squamous cell carcinoma (cSCC) is common
- cSCC should always be diagnosed by histology
- cSCC that is invasive should be evaluated for high risk of spread
- cSCC that is invasive and not at high risk for spread can be cured by various local treatments including, in select cases, photodynamic therapy (PDT)
- cSCC that is invasive is best treated by definitive surgery or radiation therapy
- cSCC that is invasive should not routinely be treated by PDT due to high failure rates

OBJECTIVES

- To differentiate between non-high-risk vs high-risk invasive cutaneous squamous cell cancer.
- To understand the different treatment options available for non-high-risk cutaneous squamous cell cancer.
- To understand the limited and off label role for photodynamic therapy in non-high-risk cutaneous squamous cell cancer.
- To understand the underutilized roll of fluorescence in detecting and monitoring non-high-risk cutaneous squamous cell cancer.

INTRODUCTION

As the skin is our largest organ, critical to homeostasis and a first line of defense against disease it should come as no surprise that it is a common location for cancer development and even metastasis.[1] In our environment, mutagenic and carcinogenic toxins are rampant, as is ionizing radiation from sunlight and cosmic sources, all potentially leading to skin cancer initiation and growth.[2] While the body has repair and elimination mechanisms to mitigate these risks, tumor progression remains common. Each cell type of the skin may be affected by a histologically identifiable lesion that generally progresses from in situ to invasive cancer. When these growths are identified and successfully eliminated in the noninvasive stage, the risk for tumor morbidity and mortality is virtually eliminated.[3] In contrast, invasive skin cancer, particularly those that are deeply penetrating or with lymphatic spread can be fatal.[4] It is largely for this reason, that skin cancer, particularly in situ and early invasive squamous cell cancer of the skin has had great effort made for early diagnosis and therapy.

Squamous epithelium forms the outer keratinizing layer of the skin, so lesions and changes originating here are often visible and generally brought to medical attention, most commonly in relatively early stages of development. In situ tumors are also termed Bowen's disease and may be solitary or more likely multifocal in origin.[5] These early lesions present with irregular appearance, may be nonhealing, bleed, have altered coloration and pigmentations, and may itch. As this may also describe a variety of benign skin diseases, clinical suspicion for malignancy needs to be high. The treatment of in situ disease is a focus of the preceding chapter. As lesions progress, they may form a spreading, nonhealing solitary mass, which histologically may invade beyond the epidermis but not yet spread to the lymphatic channels. Here again, local control of the tumor can be curative and is the focus of this chapter. Higher-grade squamous cell skin tumors may grow rapidly and invade deeply to include lymphatic spread.[6] Neglected tumors, particularly those hidden by hair on the scalp may also grow to impressive size and depth. In these latter instances, a high degree of clinical suspicion is needed to ensure that these tumors have not yet metastasized, requiring treatment beyond the primary tumor bed to control disease spread. Treatment of these high-risk patients is the focus of the next chapter.

Histologically confirmed invasive squamous cell cancers can be treated through many different techniques to include various surgical procedures, radiation therapy, systemic and targeted therapy, and potentially photodynamic therapy (PDT). The optimal intervention or combination of interventions is clinically determined on a case-by-case basis as will be seen in this chapter.

SCOPE OF ISSUE

Worldwide, squamous cell skin cancer is diagnosed in several million people annually, fortunately, most commonly in the noninvasive stage.[7] Excessive unprotected sun exposure, environmental toxins, immunosuppression for organ transplantation, and secondary to chronic disease have caused a dramatic increase in incidence and prevalence.[8] Historically, cSCC was a disease of older individuals but now due to intentional exposure to UV radiation (from sun and tanning beds) individuals in their 20s may present with these tumors.[9] Generally, lesions develop in sun-exposed skin such as the scalp, neck, and back of hands. Those with light skin (Fitzpatrick type I/II), outdoor work schedules, and geographic locations associated with intense sunlight are at higher risk for cancer development.[10] Albinism and *Xeroderma pigmentosum* create extremely high risk for cSCC development, even before the teenage years.[11]

PATHOPHYSIOLOGY

cSCC tumors begin with damage to the epidermal keratinocyte, ultimately resulting in uncontrolled progression to invasive and metastatic cancer.[5] The initiating factors can be manifold but ultraviolet radiation from sunlight exposure is considered a common starting point.[12] Often, UV damage can be repaired, or the damaged cell eliminated by apoptotic mechanisms preventing cancer progression.[13] Similarly, other injuries such as thermal burns leading to scar may be an initiator. Various viruses including human papillomavirus (HPV) have been implicated.[14] The immune system plays a role in eliminating these tumors as immunosuppressed individuals either through age, chronic disease, or transplant are at extremely high risk of cSCC lesion development and spread.[15]

CLINICAL PRESENTATION

While most commonly a disease of the Caucasian elderly with a history of excess sun exposure, cSCC tumors can also affect the young, those with pigmented skin, and particularly those with genetically susceptible and immunosuppressive states.[16] Therefore a high level of clinical suspicion is always required to allow for rapid and accurate diagnosis. In most case presentations, early forms of cSCC are to be found. These are termed actinic keratosis (AK) and are considered premalignant lesions by most, and by some, in situ cancers. They are irregular in shape, often raised, and erythematous. Generally, lesions are very slowly progressing in size and have been noted by the patient for months or even years. Actinic cheilitis (AC) is a noninvasive precancerous lesion originating on the sun-exposed lip.[17] It may appear at first small and eroded, and evolve into a large and ulcerative plaque. Of note a substantial number of individuals with AC may have an associated invasive cSCC of the lip, therefore diagnostic caution is critical. Keratoacanthoma is considered a cSCC, and may appear not on the lip vermilion border but is also noted in areas of hair follicles.

This lesion has low metastatic potential and is generally treated locally for cure. Bowen's disease is considered true cSCC in situ. Bowen's disease presents as a well-demarcated erythematous hyperkeratotic plaque but may also appear as a poorly demarcated flesh-colored lesion. Erythroplasia of Queyrat is carcinoma in situ of the penis and appears ruddy and velvety. HPV-associated squamous cell cancer is often associated with a mucosal surface such as the lips, vulva, penis, and perianal regions. These tumors are often confused with warts. True invasive cSCC tumors may arise de novo or as a progression of AK.[18] They generally appear as an ulcerated nonhealing lesion though they can appear as small plaques or nodules. It is important to note that invasive tumors may extend far beyond what is visible or palpable. Rarely a solitary lymph node may be palpable which must be evaluated for metastasis.[19] In neglected or aggressive cases, the primary tumor can be large and associated with multiple nodal metastasis.[20] Systemic spread is also a possibility in these advanced cases. In particular, cSCC tumors associated with burn (Marjolin tumor) are at very high risk for nodal and regional tumor spread.[21]

DIAGNOSIS

As many skin lesions may be benign, histologic confirmation of cSCC is always required prior to any oncologic therapy.[3] Often needle or incisional biopsy will be diagnostic. In select, small, and well-demarcated tumors excisional biopsy with appropriate margin may be diagnostic and therapeutic. Optical methods such as photodiagnosis may assist in diagnosis and eventually eliminate the need for histology, but until clinically validated, tissue histology is of great importance.[3] Pretreatment, a clear photograph of the lesion with tumor measurements should be mandatory. A good description including any suspicion of spread is helpful, particularly for the follow-up exam. The final pathological report should include data that assists in staging, prognostic classification, and treatment. This should always include lesion size, depth, level of dermal invasion (Clark's level), status of margins, differentiation, perineural invasion, lymphatic invasion, and vascular invasion. Having this information is critical to allow for optimal intervention and the clinician should demand all this be present in the final pathology report.[22]

Several pathological variants of cSCC are recognized and may be included by the pathologist in their comments. Most importantly these include:

1. **Verrucous:** Well-differentiated and slow-growing with low metastatic potential.[23] This is a cauliflower-like mass. When located on the penis, scrotum, or perianal anatomy this is termed Buschke-Lowenstein Verrucous SCC. When located on the plantar foot it is referred to as carcinoma cuniculatum.
2. **Desmoplastic:** This is generally a high-grade tumor often with perineural and vascular infiltration. These lesions have high local recurrence rates and high metastatic potential.[24]
3. **Spindle cell:** While bizarre in appearance and sometimes mistaken for melanoma, these lesions are generally nonaggressive. The exception may be spindle cell tumors arising in previously radiated areas where local control is often difficult.[25]
4. **Acantholytic:** Extensive pseudo glandular structures are seen on histologic evaluation. These tumors can be highly locally aggressive and develop metastatic disease.[26]

WORKUP

In addition to an examination and a detailed report on the primary tumor, a complete skin exam should always be undertaken to assess the possibility of other lesions.[27] Head and neck cSCC may spread to the many lymph nodes found in this anatomy. Therefore careful nodal palpation should always be done. Special attention to the parotid, preauricular, postauricular, neck, and supraclavicular region is required. Lesions of the nose and lip should always have submental node assessment.

Lesions on the arm and upper body spread to epitrochlear and axillary nodes. Lesions of the lower body and trunk should have the groin nodes highlighted during the exam.

A small percentage of patients will be found to have clinically enlarged nodes.[28] While most often these will be benign or reactive, radiologic workup and biopsy procedures for one or more of the suspicious nodes may be needed. Sentinel node biopsy may be an optimal option.[29] Ultrasound may assist in the detection of these abnormal nodes and ultrasound guidance may also assist in the needle biopsy of suspicious nodes to rule metastatic disease in or out.

A cohort of patients with biopsy-proven cSCC are felt to have "high-risk" lesions that may spread locally or systemically.[27] High-risk patients have one or more of the following characteristics: tumor >2 cm, poorly differentiated, invasion >6 mm, located on ear or lip, located on soul of foot, arising in scar/burn, spindle, acantholytic, perineural invasion, vascular invasion, nodal invasion, incomplete excision, recurrent tumor after treatment, immunosuppressed. Patients with multiple "high-risk" factors appear to develop nodal and metastatic disease at even higher rates. Select studies show only a 30% 5-year survival rate in patients with lymph node involvement.[30] Positive margins on re-excision appear to be a strong, independent risk factor.[31] So too is perineural invasion, which if found on primary tumor histology offers a 35% risk of associated nodal metastasis.[31] It should be noted that small (<0.1 mm caliber) nerve infiltration has a lower, but still definite, risk of finding metastatic disease. Immunosuppression of any kind is among the highest risk factors for development of metastasis. On long-term follow-up, immunosuppression patients may be associated with a tenfold increased risk for development of metastatic disease.[28] These patients require specialized care and frequent follow-up.[32] All high-risk patients should undergo further staging workup to make sure disease has not spread.

CT scans can assist in detection of bone infiltration, disease extent, and nodal abnormalities. CT scans easily detect enlarged nodes greater than 1 cm. In select series, CT scans have changed the clinical stage for cutaneous squamous cell of more than 50% of patients.[33] MRI scans are excellent to evaluate perineural invasion and for those select patients with head and neck SCC presenting with new onset of cranial nerve findings.[34] PET/CT may be employed when systemic spread is felt to be at hand, particularly for extensive tumors and those that are recurrent.[35] Judicious use of imaging may also assist those patients opting for surveillance.

TREATMENT DECISIONS FOR INVASIVE SCC OF SKIN

Treatment for invasive SCC starts with clear communication between the medical provider and patient. Outcomes and morbidity must be clearly defined and documented in a medical-legal informed consent document. Not all therapies are locally available and patients may need to travel to achieve their desired intervention. A variety of studies, mainly small and retrospective, also with very select patients, have attempted to show superiority or inferiority of many different interventions. However, upon critical analysis, these publications generally show some bias and their outcomes for the population or procedure reported upon cannot be readily extrapolated to the general patient population.[36–42]

Treatment for invasive SCC can generally be divided between surgical excision (which may include knife or laser) and nonsurgical ablation which is generally radiation therapy.[36,37] In some aggressive cases, chemotherapy, targeted therapy, and immunotherapy will be chosen; in select aggressive cases several treatment types may be required for tumor control.[38]

In each patient consideration of cosmetic outcome and functional outcome are also critical, particularly in clinically obvious regions such as the face. Further, treatment that allows for continuing normal or near-normal organ function is favored particularly for treatment around the eyes, lips, ears, and nose.

When treating standard-risk squamous cell tumors intervention is focused on the primary lesion. High-risk lesions should include not only consideration of treatment of the primary but also evaluation for nodal disease and for the possibility, while rare, of systemic disease being present.[37]

TREATMENT APPLICATIONS AND OPTIONS FOR NON-HIGH-RISK INVASIVE CSCC

The following are the standard possible treatment options generally available with an overview of outcome and morbidity for standard-risk squamous cell cancers of the skin. This is summarized in Table 9.1.

Primary Site Surgery

Surgical excision remains a treatment of choice as it can offer histologic evaluation, local control, and satisfactory cosmesis.[39] Surgery can be performed on both in situ and invasive lesions and is particularly beneficial when it is unclear if the lesion is invasive or not. Resection margins are critical to long-term tumor control and outcome.[40]

Standard-risk patients require a 5 mm margin while high-risk patients need at least 1 cm margin. Neither is always possible. In cases with suspected SCC and multiple AK or in situ lesions, surgery can be employed to remove those lesions felt to be invasive, followed by

TABLE 9.1 Treatment Applications and Options for Non-High-Risk Invasive Sq Cell Ca of the Skin

Treatment	Eligible Patients	Local Control	Morbidity
Mohs or Mohs-like surgery	• All surgical candidates	>98%	• Pain • Scar • Function loss • Bleeding • Infection
Surgery with wide margins	• All patients where ≥5 mm surgical margin can be achieved	>95%	• Pain • Scar • Function loss • Bleeding • Infection
Radiation therapy	• All patients • Nonsurgical candidates • Cosmetically critical • Positive margins post-op	>95%	• Acute inflammation • Alopecia • Fibrosis
PDT with systemic photosensitizer	• Off label • Nonsurgical candidates	>90%	• Pain during PDT • Wound healing • Photosensitivity
PDT with topical photosensitizer	• Off label • Not acceptable as stand-alone treatment	>50%	• Pain during PDT

regional treatment for noninvasive lesions with PDT, Cryosurgery, curettage, electrocoagulation, Imiquimod cream, 5- fluorouracil, etc. As these later treatments are unable to routinely offer histology, surgery will provide the needed information to achieve optimal management.

Surgical techniques vary but the goal in curative cases is always complete excision of the tumor. When complete excision is achieved local tumor control rates at 5-year follow-up is 95% or more.[41] While cosmesis and maintaining function, particularly for the face, is critical, the priority in terms of tumor control is clear resection margins. To achieve clear resection margins may also require cosmetic surgical repair and in some cases, cosmesis/function may be impacted. Thus it behooves the physician/surgeon to be clear about this to the patient and in the consent form.

Two forms of surgical excision are generally considered suitable for invasive SCC.[42] Cold knife excision can be an outpatient procedure where the lesion is clinically resected and sent for post-op pathological evaluation. It has the advantage of being widely available, does not require specialized equipment, and is cost effective. In contrast, a Mohs or Mohs-like surgery requires specialized tools and training.[43,44] This is micrographic surgery which is time-consuming but allows for pathological evaluation in near real-time. This provides for a high degree of certainty in defining all tumor margins, including depth of invasion. Consequently, Mohs techniques allow for extremely high confidence in achieving clear resection margins. The optimal patient for Mohs surgery is a point of some controversy, particularly as this is a relatively expensive procedure and may often require cosmetic repair due to the surgical defect.[45] It should certainly be considered the standard for high-risk patients. This includes lesions of the scalp, face, lips, hand, and nail; tumors with high grade; tumors >2 cm and recurrent tumors. Several select studies show that local control rates may improve with Mohs surgery over conventional surgery.[46] A survival benefit may also be seen in select cases.[47]

Radiation Therapy

Radiation is an established modality in the treatment of cSCC with control rates equivalent to surgery.[48] It can be employed as a primary treatment or as adjunct therapy.[49] This therapy is pain free, outpatient, and widely available.

Radiation can be delivered through brachytherapy (up close) or via teletherapy (from a distance). Currently, a linear accelerator (for teletherapy) delivers x-rays or electrons generated by electricity. Historically, superficial 250 kV x-rays were employed which do not penetrate skin deeply, and recently these devices have again become commercially available. Gamma rays, generated by radioactive decay of a brachytherapy radioactive source may also be used, but require significant precautions due to government regulations of radioactive sources. An innovative electronic brachytherapy device using electricity to generate superficial x-rays is also currently widely available.[49]

In all cases, the clinical goal is to sterilize the tumor and minimally damage surrounding normal tissue.[50] As per surgical technique, this requires clinical expertise and optimal use of quality equipment. Total dose of radiation (measured in Gray), field size of treatment, and fractionation of radiation for daily therapy can vary widely depending on the clinical situation. As a rule of thumb brachytherapy is delivered once per day, two or three times a week for 2 weeks. Though, with the electronic brachytherapy device this may be daily therapy for 5 weeks. External beam therapy is also delivered daily five times weekly for 2–5 weeks. Therapy is painless and is noninvasive. Each treatment session is generally less than 10 min for both brachytherapy and teletherapy. The number of fractions delivered, total dose, lesion size, and anatomic location are critical to tumor control and cosmesis.

Increasing fractionation has a biologically based ability to diminish side effects and enhance cosmesis. It is clinically proven that a greater number of smaller fractions of radiation delivered will minimize skin and subcutaneous structure damage. However, increased fractionation adds cost and inconvenience to the patient and staff. Higher total doses of radiation generally can increase tumor control but also definitively increase morbidity. Larger tumors are often more difficult to control in part due to disease volume but also in part due to uncertainty in tumor extent. Anatomic location is also critical as the irregular anatomy of the ear, nose, and lip may lead to inhomogeneous doses of radiation delivered. This could lead to underdosing of tumors and overdosing of normal tissue.

For select non-high-risk patients, XRT can be used as definitive therapy, but does not provide for histologic confirmation of outcome, therefore close follow-up will be required.[51,52] Rarely XRT can be used as definitive treatment for high-risk patients should they not be able to undergo surgery or refuse definitive surgery. In these cases, tumor debulking, if possible, is suggested. An important role for XRT is consolidative following incomplete resection.[53] XRT may offer benefits in terms of local/regional disease control to patients with perineural invasion and those thought to be at risk for lymphatic metastasis. Patients with local reoccurrence of tumor can also benefit from re-excision followed by consolidative XRT.[28]

Certain patients may be considered poor candidates for XRT.[54] These include the young who may develop a second malignancy from radiation, immunosuppressed, Xeroderma Pigmentosum, and scleroderma patients. Tumors abutting cartilage such as at the nose and ear should be approached with caution as these regions can heal poorly. In these cases, increasing the number of radiation fractions helps cosmesis dramatically. Re-irradiating a previously treated region is also quite risky. Verrucous carcinoma may be considered a potential contraindication though this is not backed up by clinical documentation.

Photodynamic Therapy (PDT)

This is a light-based treatment that offers excellent cosmesis and high levels of local control for AK and in situ cSCC tumors.[55] Invasive SCC responds less well and should not be considered for PDT as the primary treatment modality, particularly by topical PDT. Regulatory approval varies by country and topical PDT is not approved for invasive SCC in the United States. In PDT, an inert photosensitizer (PS) agent is either topically or intravenously applied and allowed time to accumulate in the target.[56] Then, light of the appropriate wavelength and intensity (fluence) is directed to the target which activates the PS. This activation creates a well-described photochemical reaction, termed the photodynamic reaction (PDR), which is ablative through creation of highly toxic singlet oxygen.[57,58]

When light energy is introduced to the PS, an alternative pathway may be activated that is of great interest in dermatology. Instead of activating to create the cytotoxic PDR, the PS may be coaxed to intentionally release this light energy as fluorescence.[59] Fluorescence can serve as a tool to demarcate the extent of the tumor allowing the surgeon guidance as to margins of disease extent. This is the basis of the rapidly expanding field of fluorescence-guided resection (FGR), which has shown clinical benefit in improving tumor control and minimizing normal tissue resection.[60] Please see Fig. 9.1A and B. Further, the loss of fluorescence can indicate

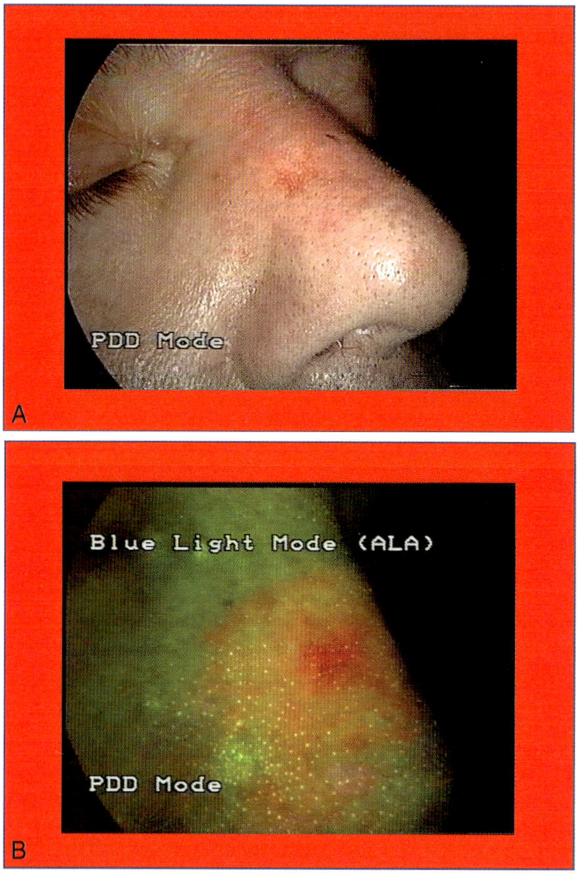

Fig. 9.1 (A, B) Fluorescent outline of lesion following ALA application.

tumor ablation. A developing aspect of fluorescence is to use this as a diagnostic tool which may one day augment or replace histological biopsy.[61] Potentially, the fluorescent activity of topical PS may be its greatest use for invasive squamous cell cancer of the skin as it would permit highly accurate fluorescent-based surgery.

Most commonly for dermatological treatment, the PS is applied directly to the skin lesion (topical PDT). The currently available topical photosensitizers (PSs) are aminolaevulinic acid (ALA) or methylated ALA. Both versions of ALA are a pro-drug, which is enzymatically converted to Protoporphyrin IX (PpIX), a potent PS. Blue light (400 nm region) can activate PpIX to create a highly effective PDR that can control many lesions including AK. Both topical ALA and blue light penetrate tissue to perhaps 1–2 mm, therefore treatment is superficial. Deeper penetrating red light (630 nm range) may

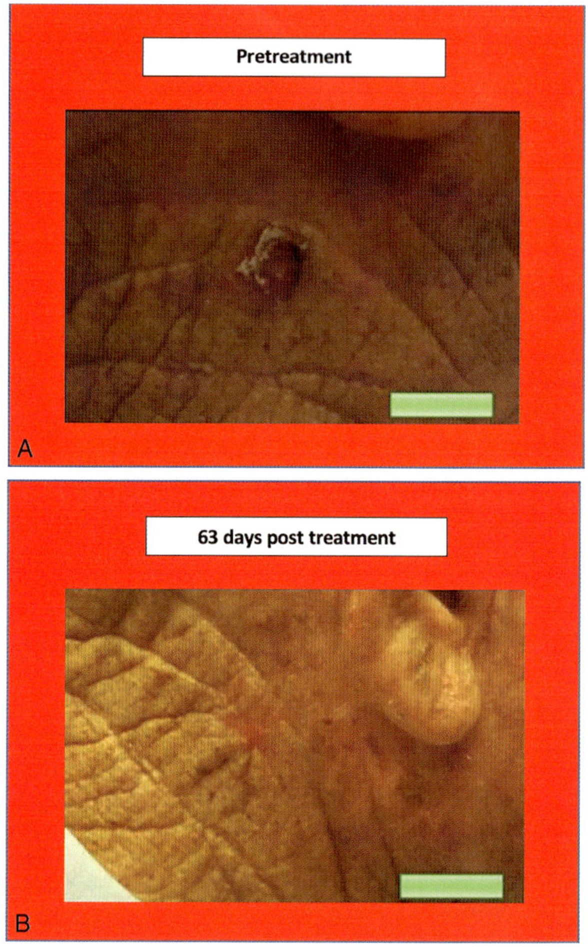

Fig. 9.2 PDT with intravenous Photofrin (off label) successfully treating a recurrent squamous cell cancer that failed surgery and radiation. (A) Pretreatment. (B) Excellent cancer control and cosmetic outcome at 63 days.

also activate PpIX and illuminate effectively to 0.5–1 cm, but again topical ALA or MAL may itself not penetrate beyond 2 mm.[62] Mechanical means to improve tissue penetration are common, still, lesions beyond 2 mm will not likely be successfully treated by topical PDT alone.[63] Some clinicians will debulk the lesion and then offer PDT to try to work around this depth limitation.[64]

Alternatively, intravenous PS is available, for example, Photofrin in the US, which can deeply penetrate tumors.[65] One can then ablate tumor to 1 cm (depth of red light) but this is off-label therapy and unfortunately rarely applied.[42] Still, IV PS for PDT can offer superb tumor control and cosmesis for invasive cSCC (see Fig. 9.2A and 9.2B). The standard dose of Photofrin is 2 mg/kg but cutaneous lesions appear to respond well to 1 mg/kg. In a select group of patients, PDT with intravenous PS could be an optimal option particularly when cosmetic outcome is critical, as PDT often allows for functional and cosmetic preservation. In a small report on invasive skin cancers arising in the head and neck region, Schweitzer found high control rates for recurrent tumors often treated in combination with surgery.[66] Similarly good results were reported by Jerjes employing Foscan, another systemic PS, for T1 (less than 1 cm) primary squamous cell cancers, showing high complete response rates with preservation of cosmesis and function.[67]

While topical PDT has a large and excellent literature showing high levels of clinical control with superior cosmesis for superficial lesions such as AK, it must be emphasized that the use of topical PDT for invasive tumors is both off label and cannot currently be recommended as a primary treatment.[42] For SCC of low risk, small size, and a minimal depth of invasion (microinvasion), multiple PDT sessions (often after debulking) may offer high clinical response but again suffer from a high failure rate.[68] This modality also suffers from lack of histologic confirmation of response which can be critical when dealing with invasive tumors. Recently Choi reported on the combination of ablative fractional laser treatment in combination with MAL-PDT for microinvasive SCC limited to the papillary dermis. The combination allowed for an 88% control rate at 24 months as compared to a nearly 40% failure rate with MAL alone.[69] Similarly, the control rate for fractional laser ablation in combination with MAL-PDT for AC achieved 92% local control at 12 months versus 50% with MAL alone, showing the potential for this combination treatment in microinvasive and other select clinical situations, but further and larger clinical trials are needed.[70] Conceptually, topical PDT may help achieve clear margins when employed following surgery. This might allow for a more limited surgery and still maintain organ function and tumor control but requires clinical trial investigation.

Currently, topical PDT is not indicated in invasive cSCC management due to high local failure rates and the possibility that this high failure rate will allow for tumor progression and possibly spread. European interdisciplinary guidelines do not include PDT for this group of patients. In a large systemic review and pooled analysis, invasive cSCC treated by PDT had an average 26% failure rate (range: 12.3–43.7), far higher than other treatment modalities.[71] A more recent systemic review and meta-analysis again showed poor outcomes with topical PDT in invasive cSCC with only a 51% control rate for squamous cell tumors.[72]

Cryosurgery

Cryosurgery has a track record for treatment of superficial disease but caution is urged if this is considered for invasive cSCC.[73,74] For select, small, well-defined, and low-grade tumors, cryotherapy has had success on the extremities.[75] Cryosurgery should not be considered for lesions with indefinite margins or lesions with depth of 3 mm or more. When used, multiple freeze-thaw cycles are suggested. For lesions of 5 mm or more, its use is not considered standard of care as some of these larger lesions will contain more deeply invasive cancer that may progress due to partial treatment.

Curettage and Electrodessication

This technique is also widely available with an excellent track record for noninvasive and in situ disease.[76] It has shown success in minimally invasive cSCC.[77] For lesions of 5 mm or more, its use is not considered standard of care as the deeper, possibly invasive regions of these tumors may silently grow due to partial treatment with curettage.[78]

Topical Agents

These include Imiquimod, which is not currently recommended, as nonresponding patients can develop progressing invasive SCC at short-term follow-up.[79,80] Topical 5-FU can potentially clear cSCC but a high percent age of patients develop progressive invasive disease at short-term follow-up.[79] Cosmetic results were inferior too as compared to other minimally invasive treatments.

Systemic and Targeted Therapy

These are generally employed for unresectable, recurrent, and progressing tumors that have failed primary therapy.[81] Cetuximab epidermal growth factor receptor (EGFR) inhibitor, has shown responses in squamous cell tumors and could be considered in these cases.[82] Most report disease stabilization in 40% of patients, though again this was short lived.[83] Select cSCC can respond to immunotherapy as some have altered PD 1 (programmed death) receptors.[84] For those patients found to have, on testing, a 1% or higher tumor proportion score, PD-1 inhibition therapy is an option. In these select cases, objective response of 40% or more can be expected with 20% achieving complete response, with response generally lasting 6–12 months.[85] In real-world outcomes, response may be lower and morbidity higher than reported in pivotal clinical trials.[86] Chemotherapy may also be attempted, but immunotherapy is currently preferred due to less toxicity and equivalent outcomes.[28] In a retrospective review, advanced squamous cell cancers of the skin may respond to cis-platin-containing regimens, where 44% partial response was reported for a median progression-free survival of 5.5 months. Patients treated with taxanes had poorer responses than those treated with platin-containing regimens.[87] Agents to improve response rates are needed and future trials should address the use of novel targeted and new chemotherapy combinations in cSCC.

FOLLOW-UP

Patients diagnosed with invasive and advanced cSCC may have a 50% risk of developing new lesions within 5 years.[42] Therefore follow-up is crucial. In several studies, most recurrences occurred within 2 years.[88] Low-risk patients rendered no evidence of disease (NED), should therefore be followed at least two or three times a year for the first- and second-year post therapy, then at least every 6 months until year five and annually thereafter. It is suggested that higher-risk patients rendered NED by treatment be examined at least every 3 months or more often for 2 years. Any suspicious findings or changes in cutaneous/nodal exam should be rapidly evaluated in detail for this cohort. These higher-risk patients should also be carefully examined at least three times a year for follow-up years three, four, and five. At that point, depending on risk factors, a minimal follow-up of every 6 months for life is recommended.

FUTURE DIRECTIONS

Mohs and radiation therapy offer very high rates of tumor control, but these may still be improved upon by the addition of optical techniques such as optical coherence tomography which could increase both tumor localization and also prevent noninvolved regions from being treated.[89] This might also result in diminished treatment-related morbidity as treatment fields might be limited in volume and more normal tissue spared. Radiation therapy for skin cancer also recently has included image guidance through ultrasound for target localization and follow-up, achieving improved outcomes.[90,91]

Topical PDT will not become a significant option for cSCC until improved topically applied PSs that have the ability to treat beyond several millimeters become available. Nanotechnology may assist with this.[92] In contrast, systemic PDT with intravenous PS does treat to the required depth and may be an option for these patients, but additional clinical trials and support for this are required. It is unfortunate that systemic PDT is not as readily accessible to patients, as PDT could serve this select population well, particularly those patients in many parts of the world where state-of-the-art surgery and radiation are not routinely available.

One underutilized aspect of PDT that could readily improve outcomes is utilization of the fluorescence of currently available PS to demarcate tumors and preserve surrounding normal tissues.[93] FGR have proven worth in other surgeries with the ability to enhance tumor removal while simultaneously respecting preservation of normal tissue. FGR for squamous cell cancer of the skin is an indication waiting to happen.

REFERENCES

1. Linares MA, Zakaria A, Nizran P. Skin cancer. *Prim Care.* 2015;42:645–659.
2. Narayanan DL, Saladi RN, Fox JL. Ultraviolet radiation and skin cancer. *Int J Dermatol.* 2010;49:978–986.
3. Dorrell DN, Strowd LC. Skin cancer detection technology. *Dermatol Clin.* 2019;37:527–536.
4. Corchado-Cobos R, García-Sancha N, González-Sarmiento R, Pérez-Losada J, Cañueto J. Cutaneous squamous cell carcinoma: from biology to therapy. *Int J Mol Sci.* 2020;21:2956. doi:10.3390/ijms21082956.
5. Fania L, Didona D, Di Pietro FR, et al. Cutaneous squamous cell carcinoma: from pathophysiology to novel therapeutic approaches. *Biomedicines.* 2021;9:171. doi:10.3390/biomedicines9020171.
6. Rabinowits G, Migden MR, Schlesinger TE, et al. Evidence-based consensus recommendations for the evolving treatment of patients with high-risk and advanced cutaneous squamous cell carcinoma. *JID Innov.* 2021;1:100045.
7. Khandelwal AR, Echanique KA, St John M, Nathan CA. Cutaneous cancer biology. *Otolaryngol Clin North Am.* 2021;54:259–269.
8. In GK, Thomas JS. Silk AW. Cutaneous malignancies of the head and neck. *Hematol Oncol Clin North Am.* 2021;35:991–1008.

9. Dessinioti C, Pitoulias M, Stratigos AJ. Epidemiology of advanced cutaneous squamous cell carcinoma. *J Eur Acad Dermatol Venereol.* 2022;36:39–50.
10. Madani S, Marwaha S, Dusendang JR, et al. Ten-year follow-up of persons with sun-damaged skin associated with subsequent development of cutaneous squamous cell carcinoma. *JAMA Dermatol.* 2021;157:559–565.
11. Baykal C, Atcı T, Yılmaz Z, Büyükbabani N. Skin tumors in xeroderma pigmentosum: evaluation of a large series and a literature review. *J Cutan Pathol.* 2021;48:884–895.
12. Chang D, Shain AH. The landscape of driver mutations in cutaneous squamous cell carcinoma. *NPJ Genom Med.* 2021;6:61 -021.
13. Vechtomova YL, Telegina TA, Buglak AA, Kritsky MS. UV radiation in DNA damage and repair involving DNA-photolyases and cryptochromes. *Biomedicines.* 2021;9:1564. doi:10.3390/biomedicines9111564.
14. Becerril S, Corchado-Cobos R, García-Sancha N, et al. Viruses and skin cancer. *Int J Mol Sci.* 2021;22:5399. doi:10.3390/ijms22105399.
15. Stenz NA, Stampf S, Arnold AW, et al. Skin cancer development in solid organ transplant recipients in Switzerland (Swiss Transplant Cohort Study). *Dermatology.* 2021;237:970–980.
16. Leiter U, Keim U, Garbe C. Epidemiology of skin cancer: update 2019. *Adv Exp Med Biol.* 2020;1268:123–139.
17. Trager MH, Farmer K, Ulrich C, et al. Actinic cheilitis: a systematic review of treatment options. *J Eur Acad Dermatol Venereol.* 2021;35:815–823.
18. Stratigos AJ, Garbe C, Dessinioti C, et al. European interdisciplinary guideline on invasive squamous cell carcinoma of the skin: Part 1. Epidemiology, diagnostics and prevention. *Eur J Cancer.* 2020;128:60–82.
19. Saito Y, Fujikawa H, Takatsuka S, Abe R, Takenouchi T. Risk factors for lymph node metastasis in cutaneous squamous cell carcinoma: a long-term retrospective study of Japanese patients. *Int J Clin Oncol.* 2021;26:606–612.
20. Yan F, Tillman BN, Nijhawan RI, et al. High-risk cutaneous squamous cell carcinoma of the head and neck: a clinical review. *Ann Surg Oncol.* 2021;28:9009–9030.
21. Kanth AM, Heiman AJ, Nair L, et al. Current trends in management of Marjolin's ulcer: a systematic review. *J Burn Care Res.* 2021;42:144–151.
22. Stratigos A, Garbe C, Lebbe C, et al. Diagnosis and treatment of invasive squamous cell carcinoma of the skin: European consensus-based interdisciplinary guideline. *Eur J Cancer.* 2015;51:1989–2007.
23. Fawaz B, Vieira C, Decker A, Lawrence N. Surgical treatment of verrucous carcinoma: a review. *J Dermatolog Treat.* 2022;33:1811–1815.
24. Parekh V, Seykora JT. Cutaneous squamous cell carcinoma. *Clin Lab Med.* 2017;37:503–525.
25. Choi JH, Ro JY. Cutaneous spindle cell neoplasms: pattern-based diagnostic approach. *Arch Pathol Lab Med.* 2018;142:958–972.
26. Sajin M, Hodorogea Prisăcaru A, Luchian MC, et al. Acantholytic squamous cell carcinoma: pathological study of nine cases with review of literature. *Rom J Morphol Embryol.* 2014;55:279–283.
27. Que SKT, Zwald FO, Schmults CD. Cutaneous squamous cell carcinoma: management of advanced and high-stage tumors. *J Am Acad Dermatol.* 2018;78:249–261.
28. Maubec E. Update of the management of cutaneous squamous-cell carcinoma. *Acta Derm Venereol.* 2020; 100(11):309–317.
29. Kofler L, Kofler K, Schulz C, Breuninger H, Häfner HM. Sentinel lymph node biopsy for high-thickness cutaneous squamous cell carcinoma. *Arch Dermatol Res.* 2021;313:119–126.
30. Burton KA, Ashack KA, Khachemoune A. Cutaneous squamous cell carcinoma: a review of high-risk and metastatic disease. *Am J Clin Dermatol.* 2016;17:491–508.
31. Stewart TJ, Saunders A. Risk factors for positive margins after wide local excision of cutaneous squamous cell carcinoma. *J Dermatolog Treat.* 2018;29:706–708.
32. Mittal A, Colegio OR. Skin cancers in organ transplant recipients. *Am J Transplant.* 2017;17:2509–2530.
33. Prehn RB, Pasic TR, Harari PM, Brown WD, Ford CN. Influence of computed tomography on pretherapeutic tumor staging in head and neck cancer patients. *Otolaryngol Head Neck Surg.* 1998;119:628–633.
34. Pérez García MP, Mateu Puchades A, Sanmartín Jiménez O. Perineural invasion in cutaneous squamous cell carcinoma. *Actas Dermosifiliogr (Engl Ed).* 2019;110:426–433.
35. Belkin DA, Wysong A. Radiographic imaging for skin cancer. *Semin Cutan Med Surg.* 2016;35:42–48.
36. Keohane SG, Botting J, Budny PG, et al. British Association of Dermatologists guidelines for the management of people with cutaneous squamous cell carcinoma 2020. *Br J Dermatol.* 2021;184:401–414.
37. García-Foncillas J, Tejera-Vaquerizo A, Sanmartín O, et al. Update on management recommendations for advanced cutaneous squamous cell carcinoma. *Cancers (Basel).* 2022;14:629. doi:10.3390/cancers14030629.
38. Stanganelli I, Spagnolo F, Argenziano G, et al. The multidisciplinary management of cutaneous squamous cell carcinoma: a comprehensive review and clinical recommendations by a panel of experts. *Cancers (Basel).* 2022;14:377. doi:10.3390/cancers14020377.
39. Waldman A, Schmults C. Cutaneous squamous cell carcinoma. *Hematol Oncol Clin North Am.* 2019;33:1–12.
40. Dessinioti C, Stratigos AJ. Overview of guideline recommendations for the management of high-risk and

advanced cutaneous squamous cell carcinoma. *J Eur Acad Dermatol Venereol*. 2022;36(Suppl 1):11–18.
41. Dessinioti C, Stratigos AJ. Recent advances in the diagnosis and management of high-risk cutaneous squamous cell carcinoma. *Cancers (Basel)*. 2022;14:3556. doi:10.3390/cancers14143556.
42. Work Group, Invited Reviewers, JYS Kim. Guidelines of care for the management of cutaneous squamous cell carcinoma. *J Am Acad Dermatol.*. 2018;78:560–578.
43. Hunt WTN, Earp E, Brown AC, Veitch D, Wernham AGH. A review of Mohs micrographic surgery for skin cancer. Part 3: squamous cell carcinoma. *Clin Exp Dermatol*. 2022;47(10):1765–1773.
44. Bittner GC, Cerci FB, Kubo EM, Tolkachjov SN. Mohs micrographic surgery: a review of indications, technique, outcomes, and considerations. *An Bras Dermatol*. 2021;96:263–277.
45. Tokede O, Jadotte YT, Nkemjika S, et al. Effectiveness of Mohs micrographic surgery for nonmelanoma skin cancer: a systematic review protocol. *JBI Database System Rev Implement Rep*. 2017;15:666–675.
46. van Lee CB, Roorda BM, Wakkee M, et al. Recurrence rates of cutaneous squamous cell carcinoma of the head and neck after Mohs micrographic surgery vs. standard excision: a retrospective cohort study. *Br J Dermatol*. 2019;181:338–343.
47. Matsumoto A, Li JN, Matsumoto M, Pineider J, Nijhawan RI, Srivastava D. Factors predicting outcomes of patients with high-risk squamous cell carcinoma treated with Mohs micrographic surgery. *J Am Acad Dermatol*. 2021;85:588–595.
48. Cheraghi N, Cognetta A, Goldberg D. Radiation therapy in dermatology: non-melanoma skin cancer. *J Drugs Dermatol*. 2017;16:464–469.
49. Pashazadeh A, Boese A, Friebe M. Radiation therapy techniques in the treatment of skin cancer: an overview of the current status and outlook. *J Dermatolog Treat*. 2019;30:831–839.
50. Fitzgerald TJ, Jodoin MB, Tillman G, et al. Radiation therapy toxicity to the skin. *Dermatol Clin*. 2008; 26:161–172.ix.
51. Roth W, Beer RE, Iyengar V, Bender T, Raymond I. Long-term efficacy and safety of superficial radiation therapy in subjects with nonmelanoma skin cancer: a retrospective registry study. *J Drugs Dermatol*. 2020;19:163–168.
52. Yu L, Oh C, Shea CR. The treatment of non-melanoma skin cancer with image-guided superficial radiation therapy: an analysis of 2917 invasive and in situ keratinocytic carcinoma lesions. *Oncol Ther*. 2021;9:153–166.
53. Likhacheva A, Awan M, Barker CA, et al. Definitive and postoperative radiation therapy for basal and squamous cell cancers of the skin: executive summary of an American Society for Radiation Oncology clinical practice guideline. *Pract Radiat Oncol*. 2020;10:8–20.
54. Shore RE. Radiation-induced skin cancer in humans. *Med Pediatr Oncol*. 2001;36:549–554.
55. Allison RR, Moghissi K. Photodynamic therapy (PDT): PDT mechanisms. *Clin Endosc*. 2013;46:24–29.
56. Allison RR, Sibata CH. Photodynamic therapy: mechanism of action and role in the treatment of skin disease. *G Ital Dermatol Venereol*. 2010;145:491–507.
57. Allison RR, Moghissi K. Oncologic photodynamic therapy: clinical strategies that modulate mechanisms of action. *Photodiagnosis Photodyn Ther*. 2013;10:331–341.
58. Allison RR. Photodynamic therapy: oncologic horizons. *Future Oncol*. 2014;10:123–124.
59. Kostron H. Photodynamic diagnosis and therapy and the brain. *Methods Mol Biol*. 2010;635:261–280.
60. Allison RR. Fluorescence guided resection (FGR): a primer for oncology. *Photodiagnosis Photodyn Ther*. 2016;13:73–80.
61. Allison RR, Bagnato VS, Cuenca R, Downie GH, Sibata CH. The future of photodynamic therapy in oncology. *Future Oncol*. 2006;2:53–71.
62. Allison RR, Downie GH, Cuenca R, Hu XH, Childs CJ. Sibata CH. Photosensitizers in clinical PDT. *Photodiagnosis Photodyn Ther*. 2004;1:27–42.
63. Dreyfuss I, Kamath P, Frech F, Hernandez L, Nouri K. Squamous cell carcinoma: 2021 updated review of treatment. *Dermatol Ther*. 2022;35:e15308.
64. Kus KJB, Ruiz ES. Non-surgical treatments for keratinocyte carcinomas. *Adv Ther*. 2021;38:5635–5648.
65. Allison RR, Sibata CH. Oncologic photodynamic therapy photosensitizers: a clinical review. *Photodiagnosis Photodyn Ther*. 2010;7:61–75.
66. Schweitzer VG. Photodynamic therapy for treatment of head and neck cancer. *Otolaryngol Head Neck Surg*. 1990;102:225–232.
67. Jerjes W, Yousif AA, Hamdoon Z, Hopper C. Non-metastatic cutaneous squamous cell carcinoma treated with photodynamic therapy using intravenous mTHPC. *Photodiagnosis Photodyn Ther*. 2019;28:172–176.
68. Allison RR, Sibata CH, Downie GH, Cuenca RE. A clinical review of PDT for cutaneous malignancies. *Photodiagnosis Photodyn Ther*. 2006;3:214–226.
69. Choi SH, Kim KH, Song KH. Effect of Methyl aminolevulinate photodynamic therapy with and without ablative fractional laser treatment in patients with microinvasive squamous cell carcinoma: a randomized clinical trial. *JAMA Dermatol*. 2017;153:289–295.
70. Choi SH, Kim KH, Song KH. Efficacy of ablative fractional laser-assisted photodynamic therapy for the treatment of actinic cheilitis: 12-month follow-up results of a prospective, randomized, comparative trial. *Br J Dermatol*. 2015;173:184–191.
71. Lansbury L, Bath-Hextall F, Perkins W, Stanton W, Leonardi-Bee J. Interventions for non-metastatic squamous

cell carcinoma of the skin: systematic review and pooled analysis of observational studies. *BMJ*. 2013;347:f6153.
72. Yongpisarn T, Rigo R, Minkis K. Durable clearance rate of photodynamic therapy for bowen disease and cutaneous squamous cell carcinoma: a systematic review and meta-analysis. *Dermatol Surg*. 2022;48:395–400.
73. Clebak KT, Mendez-Miller M, Croad J. Cutaneous cryosurgery for common skin conditions. *Am Fam Physician*. 2020;101:399–406.
74. Sapijaszko M, Zloty D, Bourcier M, et al. Non-melanoma skin cancer in Canada chapter 5: management of squamous cell carcinoma. *J Cutan Med Surg*. 2015;19:249–259.
75. Collins A, Savas J, Doerfler L. Nonsurgical treatments for nonmelanoma skin cancer. *Dermatol Clin*. 2019;37:435–441.
76. Ondo AL, Kerner JD, Kerner JV, Ondo IP, Trainor P, Shanler SD. Treatment of cutaneous squamous cell carcinoma in situ with curettage followed by topical imiquimod 5% cream. *Dermatol Surg*. 2021;47:609–612.
77. Fournier S, Laroche A, Leblanc M, et al. Prospective clinical trial comparing curettage and cryosurgery to curettage and electrodesiccation in the management of minimally invasive basal and squamous cell carcinomas. *J Cutan Med Surg*. 2020;24:596–600.
78. Chuang GS, Lu LK, Cummins DL, et al. Incidence of invasive squamous cell carcinomas in biopsy-proven squamous cell carcinomas in situ sent for Mohs micrographic surgery. *Dermatol Surg*. 2012;38:1456–1460.
79. Cheng B, Veerabagu S, Miller CJ, et al. A comparison of invasive squamous cell carcinoma greater than 1 year after treatment with 5-fluorouracil, imiquimod, or photodynamic therapy with aminolevulinic acid. *J Am Acad Dermatol*. 2022;87:592–596.
80. Ahmady S, Jansen MHE, Nelemans PJ, et al. Risk of invasive cutaneous squamous cell carcinoma after different treatments for actinic keratosis: a secondary analysis of a randomized clinical trial. *JAMA Dermatol*. 2022;158:634–640.
81. Savoia P, Cremona O, Fava P. New perspectives in the pharmacological treatment of non-melanoma skin cancer. *Curr Drug Targets*. 2016;17:353–374.
82. Chen A, Ali N, Boasberg P, Ho AS. Clinical remission of cutaneous squamous cell carcinoma of the auricle with cetuximab and nivolumab. *J Clin Med*. 2018;7:10. doi:10.3390/jcm7010010.
83. O'Bryan K, Sherman W, Niedt GW, et al. An evolving paradigm for the workup and management of high-risk cutaneous squamous cell carcinoma. *J Am Acad Dermatol*. 2013;69:595–602 e1.
84. Stravodimou A, Tzelepi V, Balasis S, et al. PD-L1 expression, T-lymphocyte subpopulations and Langerhans cells in cutaneous squamous cell carcinoma and precursor lesions. *Anticancer Res*. 2021;41:3439–3448.
85. In GK, Vaidya P, Filkins A, et al. PD-1 inhibition therapy for advanced cutaneous squamous cell carcinoma: a retrospective analysis from the University of Southern California. *J Cancer Res Clin Oncol*. 2021;147:1803–1811.
86. Amaral T, Osewold M, Presser D, Meiwes A, Garbe C, Leiter U. Advanced cutaneous squamous cell carcinoma: real world data of patient profiles and treatment patterns. *J Eur Acad Dermatol Venereol*. 2019;33(Suppl 8):44–51.
87. Jarkowski AI, Hare R, Loud P, et al. Systemic therapy in advanced cutaneous squamous cell carcinoma (CSCC): the Roswell Park experience and a review of the literature. *Am J Clin Oncol*. 2016;39:545–548.
88. Bander TS, Nehal KS, Lee EH. Cutaneous squamous cell carcinoma: updates in staging and management. *Dermatol Clin*. 2019;37:241–251.
89. Jerjes W, Hamdoon Z, Rashed D, Sattar AA, Hopper C. In vivo optical coherence tomography in assessment of suspicious facial lesions: a prospective study. *Photodiagnosis Photodyn Ther*. 2021;36:102493.
90. Goyal U, Suszko J, Stea B. The feasibility of using ultrasound during follow-up for superficial non-melanoma skin cancers after electronic brachytherapy. *J Contemp Brachytherapy*. 2017;9:535–539.
91. Goyal U, Pan J, Cui H, Stea B. Does ultrasound measurement improve the accuracy of electronic brachytherapy in the treatment of superficial non-melanomatous skin cancer? *J Contemp Brachytherapy*. 2017;9:14–19.
92. Allison RR, Mota HC, Bagnato VS, Sibata CH. Bio-nanotechnology and photodynamic therapy–state of the art review. *Photodiagnosis Photodyn Ther*. 2008;5: 19–28.
93. Allison RR, Sibata CH. Photodiagnosis for cutaneous malignancy: a brief clinical and technical review. *Photodiagnosis Photodyn Ther*. 2008;5:247–250.

10

Photodynamic Therapy of Basal Cell Carcinoma

Theresa Hommel, Rolf-Markus Szeimies

KEY POINTS

- Basal cell carcinoma (BCC) is the most common human malignant tumor.
- The treatment options for BCC include surgical excision, Mohs surgery, and photodynamic therapy (PDT).
- PDT is an alternative for superficial or nodular BCCs up to a tumor thickness of ≤2 mm, large surface area, an aesthetically disfiguring anatomic location, and in the setting of concomitant diseases.
- PDT of superficial BCCs of the trunk shows the best clinical results.

OBJECTIVES

- Recognize basal cell carcinoma (BCC) cases that would benefit most from photodynamic theory (PDT).
- Discuss the value of PDT for BCC in view of evidence-based clinical guidelines and regulatory updates.
- Identify the risks and benefits of PDT in BCC variants other than nodular and superficial subtypes.
- Select the right candidates for PDT in combination with other treatment options.

INTRODUCTION

In recent years, photodynamic therapy (PDT) has become increasingly important in everyday dermatological practice. The main indication for PDT is still the treatment of actinic keratoses (AK). In addition, PDT is also being used to treat superficial and nodular basal cell carcinomas (BCC) and Bowen's disease. Especially in elderly, multimorbid patients or very large, inoperable tumors, PDT can be a good and effective alternative to classical surgery.

Conflict of interest: TH: TH has participated as an investigator in clinical studies in the indication area of the companies Almirall, Biofrontera, Galderma, and Leo, as well as received lecture and consulting fees from Biofrontera and Galderma. **RMS:** RMS has participated as an investigator in clinical studies in the indication area of the companies Almirall, Biofrontera, Galderma, and Leo, received lecture and consulting fees from the aforementioned companies as well as Photonamic and is a member of the advisory boards of Almirall, Biofrontera, Galderma, ISDIN, Leo, Photonamic, and Pierre-Fabre. RMS was also involved in the development of an ALA-containing TTS and an LED lamp for PDT.

BASAL CELL CARCINOMA

Basal cell carcinoma (BCC) is the most common human malignant tumor in Central Europe.[1] It is a slow-growing, epithelial neoplasia characterized by infiltrating and locally destructive growth. Metastasis is rarely observed. The incidence is currently given as 200 per 100,000 inhabitants per year, with a steady increase.[2,3] In Europe, for example, an annual increase of 5% in incidence has been observed over the last 10 years.[4] The average age of onset is 70 years.[1,2] However, it has been shown that the incidence of BCC also increases in younger people under 40 years of age. Especially in young women, an increase in BCCs is seen, which is attributed to increased UV exposure and the

TABLE 10.1 **Clinical Variants of Basal Cell Carcinoma**

Clinical Variants of BCC
Superficial BCC
Nodular BCC
Sclerosing/morphoeic BCC
Ulcerated BCC
Pigmented BCC

use of artificial UV sources (solarium).[5] For example, UV-exposed areas such as the head and neck area, subsequently the trunk and extremities represent the predilection sites of BCC.[3,6–8] The clinical presentation is diverse. A distinction is made between nodular BCC (nBCC) and superficial BCC (sBCC), sclerodermic BCC, ulcerated BCC, and pigmented BCC (see Table 10.1). The classic nodular BCC impresses as a yellowish-erythematous papule with a bead-like marginal wall that is crisscrossed by telangiectasias. It is not uncommon for central ulceration to be observed.[9] Superficial BCC presents as a sharply defined, erythematous plaque and is often found on the trunk ("trunk skin basal cell carcinoma") and extremities, while sclerodermic BCC impresses as whitish atrophy reminiscent of a sunken scar. Sclerodermic or morphoeic BCC is mainly observed in UV-exposed areas (face, nose, and periorbital).[8] It is often clinically difficult to delineate and is characterized by branched, infiltrative growth. Besides, it is prone to recurrence and responds poorly to nonsurgical interventions.[10]

The gold standard of therapy is still surgery with the aim of complete removal of the tumor.[11] In recent years, however, other nonsurgical treatment options have also been established that can be a good alternative for BCCs with a low risk of recurrence. In addition to cryotherapy, treatments with the locally applied cytostatic drug 5-fluorouracil and local immunomodulator imiquimod should be mentioned here.[11,12] Another option for topical treatment is PDT, especially if there are contraindications to surgery. However, it may be helpful for the therapy decision to carry out a risk stratification to be able to better assess the recurrence tendency of the BCC (see Table 10.2). BCCs that have a high probability of recurrence are referred to as high-risk BCCs, while those with a low probability are referred to as low-risk BCCs. While high-risk BCCs should primarily be treated surgically or, in the case of contraindications, radiotherapy, low-risk BCCs can be treated using the above-mentioned nonsurgical procedures. Risk factors for a high tendency to recur

TABLE 10.2 **Risk Stratification of Basal Cell Carcinoma**

	Low-risk BCC	High-risk BCC
Localization	H-Zone (<6 mm) M-Zone (<10 mm) L-Zone (<20 mm)	H-Zone (>6 mm) M-Zone (>10 mm) L-Zone (>20 mm)
Tumor diameter	<6 mm	>6 cm
Subtype	Superficial BCC Nodular BCC	Morphoeic BCC Infiltrative BCC Metatypic BCC
Other		Local recurrence Tumor on radioderma Perineural invasion

From Lang BM, Balermpas P, Bauer A, et al. S2k guidelines for cutaneous basal cell carcinoma–part 2: treatment, prevention and follow-up. *J Dtsch Dermatol Ges.* 2019;17(2):214–230.

include localization, maximum tumor diameter, histological subtype, BCCs on a radioderma, and recurrences.[11,13] Several studies have shown that tumors in the so-called H-zone (nose, periorbital, temples, lips, jaw angles, ears, genitals, hands, and feet) are more prone to recurrence than tumors in the rest of the face (M-zone) or on the trunk/extremities (L-zone).[14,15] A horizontal tumor diameter of >6 mm in the area of the H-zone and >10 mm in the area of the M-zone also seems to entail a higher risk of recurrence.[16,17] It should be noted, however, that the latest US guidelines no longer make this division into H, M, and L zones. Here, only the trunk and extremities are classified as low-risk areas, provided that the BCC is <20 mm.[18] It is undisputed that a larger horizontal tumor diameter is associated with frequent recurrences. Breuninger and colleagues were able to show that the probability of subclinical tumor residuals after surgery increases with increasing tumor diameter and thus the risk of recurrence is higher.[19] In addition, recent studies have shown that larger tumors are associated with a higher risk of perineural invasion.[20] The histopathological subtype also plays a decisive role. Numerous histopathological variants of BCC are known. Studies have shown that especially sclerodermic, infiltrative, and metatypic BCCs are associated with a higher risk of recurrence, while superficial and nodular BCCs have a lower risk of recurrence.[21] As mentioned earlier, the risk assessment serves the therapy decision and enables the practitioner to select suitable patients for nonsurgical interventions, such as PDT (see Fig. 10.1).

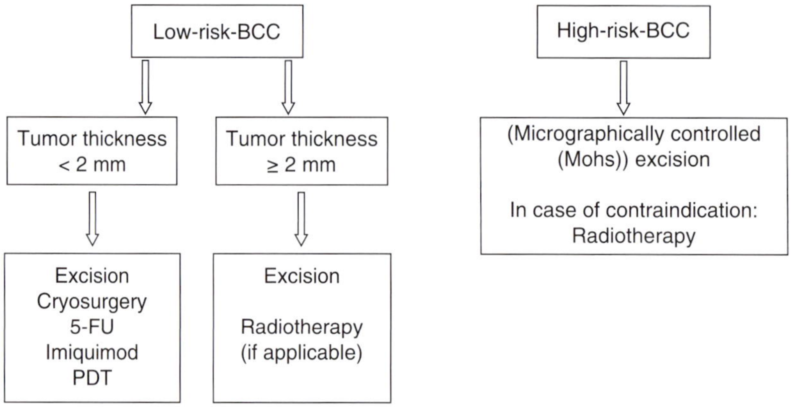

Fig. 10.1 Therapy algorithm for the treatment of basal cell carcinoma (Modified from Lang BM, Balermpas P, Bauer A, et al. S2k guidelines for cutaneous basal cell carcinoma–part 2: treatment, prevention and follow-up. *J Dtsch Dermatol Ges.* 2019;17(2):214–230.)

TABLE 10.3 Indications for PDT In Basal Cell Carcinomas

Indications for PDT in BCC	
Histological subtype	superficial BCC nodular BCC
Tumor thickness	≤2 mm
Localization	M-zone of the face Trunk Extremities

PHOTODYNAMIC THERAPY OF BASAL CELL CARCINOMA

Basics

PDT is approved in Europe for the treatment of superficial and nodular BCCs with a tumor thickness of ≤2 mm. Tumors in the H-zone as well as sclerodermic, ulcerated, and pigmented BCCs should not be treated with PDT (see Table 10.3).[18,22,23]

As early as 1990, initial studies on 80 BCCs showed that PDT with topically applied ALA (5-aminolevulinic acid) is effective. Thus in 90% of cases, complete healing occurred after a single treatment.[24] The principle of PDT in BCC is based on the selective accumulation of so-called photosensitizers in the tumor cells. In BCC, these are primarily stem cells of the hair follicles and the interfollicular epidermis.[25,26] Two photosensitizers or their precursors are currently available for PDT in BCCs: on the one hand, a 5-aminolevulinic acid-containing nanoemulsion as a gel (Ameluz, Biofrontera) and its methyl ester as a cream (Metvix, GALDERMA). While Metvix has been approved for PDT since 2006, a multicenter, randomized phase III study showed that PDT with the 5-ALA-containing nanoemulsion Ameluz was not inferior to PDT with the ALA methyl ester (Metvix, MAL) in nonaggressive BCCs (response rates of 93.4% vs. 91.8%), which led to a corresponding approval extension of Ameluz in Europe in 2017.[27] Recent 5-year follow-up data confirmed these findings (personal communication, Dr. Morton). Due to their low molecular weight, both photosensitizers penetrate well into the epidermis, where they are converted to the actual photosensitizer protoporphyrin IX (PpIX). This is followed by exposure to red light with a wavelength of 635 nm. There is a formation of reactive oxygen species in the affected cells, which leads to necrosis and apoptosis. In addition, studies have shown that in BCC, PDT can lead to an immunomodulating response with activation of neutrophils, macrophages, and Langerhans cells.[28,29] In addition, it has been shown that PDT in patients with BCC leads to an increased immune response to the tumor antigen *Hip1* (hedgehog-interacting protein 1), and thus tumor growth can be suppressed. This effect was more pronounced in superficial BCCs than in nodular BCCs.[29,30] Heat-related damage to the tumor tissue as a result of PDT could be ruled out in one study.[31] In total, the thermal effect of PDT was investigated in 40 BCCs and it could be seen that most of the energy released was used for the photodynamic effect and not for local heating of the tissue.[29,31] While the exact mechanism of action of PDT in BCCs is repeatedly the subject of numerous studies, the efficacy and clinical added benefit are considered undisputed.

PDT IN SUPERFICIAL AND NODULAR BCCs

As early as 1990, Kennedy and colleagues were able to demonstrate response rates of 90% after performing PDT in BCCs. These results were confirmed in later studies. Szeimies and colleagues investigated the efficacy of MAL-PDT compared to excision in 196 patients with superficial BCCs. They were able to show that after 3 months, the response rates were 92.2% (MAL-PDT) versus 98.2% (excision).[32] Similar results could be presented for the treatment of nodular BCCs (91% vs. 98%).[33] Other studies, however, show that PDT seems to be less effective in nodular BCCs than in superficial BCCs. For example, Fantini and colleagues performed PDT on a total of 194 BCCs. There was a complete healing of all lesions at 62%, with a significant difference between superficial BCCs (healing rate of 82%) and nodular BCCs (healing rate of 33%).[34] In the study by Cosagera and colleagues, the difference in response rates between superficial and nodular BCCs after PDT was smaller, but it was also shown that nodular BCCs respond worse to PDT than superficial BCCs.[35,36] The frequency of recurrence after PDT also appears to be higher in nodular BCCs. Zou and colleagues were able to show that, especially in the case of nodular BCCs, the probability of recurrence over the years is significantly higher than after surgical excision.[37] Szeimies and colleagues reported a recurrence rate of 9% after one year for superficial BCCs, while Lindberg-Larsen and colleagues were able to present a recurrence rate of 16% after 12 months.[32,38] This study also showed that nodular BCCs have a higher risk of recurrence than superficial BCCs.[38] The main reason for the poorer response and the higher recurrence rate in nodular BCCs is the tumor thickness. The red light, which is usually used in the context of standardized PDT protocols, shows a maximum penetration depth of 2–3 mm into the epidermis. Therefore according to the approval, PDT should only be performed on tumors with a tumor thickness ≤2 mm.[22] Furthermore, it is recommended to carry out a so-called "debulking" before PDT, especially in the case of nodular BCCs. In this case, the upper part of the tumor is removed tangentially with a curette, thus reducing the tumor thickness to be treated.[36,39] Studies have shown that pretreatment with curettage leads to significantly better results.[22,40,41] Another advantage of "debulking" is that it removes the stratum corneum. This is considered to be the main barrier with regard to the penetration of MAL or the 5-ALA nanoemulsion.[42] Studies have shown that pretreatment with ablation of the stratum corneum leads to significantly better uptake of these photosensitizers, thereby improving clinical outcomes.[43,44]

PDT IN OTHER BCC VARIANTS

There is currently no evidence for the performance of PDT in other histopathological subtypes of BCC. Nevertheless, studies with smaller case numbers or case reports are published again and again, in which PDT is used for other forms of BCC. As early as 2005, Kaviani and colleagues conducted initial studies on the effectiveness of PDT in pigmented BCCs, among other things. Here, response rates of 14% were found.[45] However, it must be mentioned that the study protocol provided for an intravenous injection of the photosensitizer photoheme, so that a comparison with the currently performed form of topical PDT with standardized photosensitizers is only possible to a limited extent.[45] Nevertheless, a possible explanation for the poorer response of PDT in pigmented lesions seems to be the fact that there is less penetration of photoactivating light due to the melanin deposits in the epidermis. Various studies have shown that pretreatment with ablation of the macroscopically visible pigment before PDT can significantly improve response rates.[46–48] In a study by Itoh and colleagues, 14 out of 16 cases resulted in complete healing of the pigmented BCC after pigment removal and PDT was performed three times.[46] Salvio and colleagues were able to show complete healing 4 weeks after PDT in a total of 30 pigmented lesions. Even after 24 months, there were no recurrences. In this study design, PDT was performed on pigmented BCCs after prior "debulking" in two sessions on the same day with MAL.[48] Overall, however, the study situation is weak and the study protocols are too variable to be able to make a generally valid statement. Therefore further clinically randomized studies must follow to prove a possible benefit of PDT in pigmented BCCs after prior "debulking."

A recommendation for the performance of PDT in sclerodermic BCCs or other high-risk BCCs cannot be given due to the infiltrative growth and the high risk of recurrence.[22] In these cases, surgical excision is still considered the therapy of choice and superior to PDT.[49,50] However, PDT can also be useful in the case of sclerodermic BCC before an excision is performed to reduce the size of the tumor and thus achieve better surgical conditions (debulking).[51] However, these are certainly special individual cases of a few patients.

SIDE EFFECTS

One of the challenges of PDT is a pronounced discomfort during light exposure. This is often the reason why treatment is discontinued or patients are dissatisfied afterward.[52,53] From our experience, however, PDT appears to be less painful in BCC than in field cancerization with AK. One reason for this is certainly the much smaller area that is being treated. Nevertheless, in addition to a detailed explanation of the patient, adequate pain management during exposure is necessary. There is controversy as to whether the choice of photosensitizer plays a role in this. In a study by Kessels and colleagues, PDT with 5-ALA was perceived as more painful compared to conventional PDT with MAL.[54] Kuijpers and colleagues, on the other hand, saw no difference in pain after PDT with MAL versus PDT with 5-ALA.[55] Ibbotson and colleagues also investigated the perception of pain during PDT in 40 patients with superficial BCC using a visual analog scale. Here it was shown that PDT with MAL was perceived as slightly less painful than with PDT with 5-ALA (median VAS score 3.5 vs. 4.5). However, this difference was not significant.[56] Rather, modified exposure protocols seem to be useful in order to reduce the sensation of pain without jeopardizing the success of the therapy.[53] The use of cold sprays is also recommended.[52] However, this seems to lead to a poorer clinical outcome, especially in the treatment of BCCs. Thus it could be shown that the application of cold sprays during exposure led to a poorer photochemical reaction and a lower healing rate.[57] A possible explanation could be the vasoconstriction by the cold thus leading to a lower intradermal oxygen supply necessary for the photodynamic effect.

Other typical side effects of PDT such as erythema, crusting, or blistering are observed but are generally mild.[42] Further, there are reports of the occurrence of allergic contact dermatitis to the photosensitizer. However, this seems to be rarely the case overall and represents a low risk for patients who have already received numerous PDT treatments in mostly large areas.[53] Analogous to PDT in AK, PDT in BCCs is also associated with excellent cosmetic results. There are no scars or pigmentary changes after the treatment.[42,58] Thus the cosmetic result is significantly better than after a surgical procedure.[59] This aspect is important in that a study could show that the cosmetic result is very important to patients in the treatment of BCC in addition to the healing of the findings. This is especially true for lesions in the facial area.[60] Interestingly, patients with a BCC recurrence stated that the cosmetic result of the treatment was more important to them than minimizing the risk of recurrence.[60] Thus despite higher recurrence rates, PDT is a very good therapeutic alternative to excision, which should be discussed with the patient.

PRACTICAL APPROACH

As mentioned above, PDT should only be performed on superficial and nodular BCCs with a maximum tumor thickness of ≤2 mm. Therefore a histological confirmation by means of a sample biopsy should be carried out before planning the therapy. After the patients have been properly informed, the current recommendation is to perform PDT twice at intervals of 7 days.[11,61] After 3 months, a clinical control should be carried out. In the event of incomplete healing, a new course of therapy can then be carried out.[61] In everyday practice, it can sometimes prove impractical for patients to have to consult the doctor twice within 7 days. This is particularly challenging for elderly, immobile patients. Therefore Salvio and colleagues investigated the effectiveness of a so-called "one-day PDT" compared to the standard protocol. A total of 120 BCC lesions were treated, with half receiving standard PDT with two sessions within a week and the other half receiving two PDT sessions in 1 day. After 1 month, a histological check was carried out and the findings were completely healed in 85% according to standard protocol and in 93.3% according to "one-day PDT." The results of the "one-day PDT" were also successful in terms of recurrence rates and superior to the standard protocol (freedom from recurrence after 60 months: 80.6% vs. 69.0%).[62] The results are promising. However, this is a study with a relatively small patient population. So further studies should follow to verify these results. However, this could simplify the practical implementation of PDT on BCCs in the future. The possibility of Daylight PDT (DL-PDT) for the treatment of BCCs is also discussed. This simple and less painful procedure is already being used successfully in the treatment of AK.[63–65] Wiegell and colleagues already conducted investigations on DL-PDT in BCCs in 2014. So far 32 lesions were treated with MAL using DL-PDT and the procedure was repeated after 7 days. After 3 months, 94% of the lesions had healed, after 12 months it was still 74%.[66] Despite these promising results, the study situation is sparse in this regard so DL-PDT cannot currently be recommended for the treatment of BCCs.[18,22,23,50] Rather, the currently implemented and recognized protocol provides for the following procedure:

1. Educate the patient and exclude contraindications (porphyria, allergies to the photosensitizer, etc.)

2. Exact definition and demarcation of the treatment area after histological confirmation
3. "Tumor debulking": Mild removal of prominent tumor parts and "roughening" of the area with the help of a curette
4. Application of the photosensitizer (MAL/5-ALA as a nanoemulsion) in the area of the tumor and approximately 0.5–1 cm beyond the visible tumor boundaries
5. Application of an occlusive film for better penetration of the photosensitizer
6. Cover with an opaque film
7. After the incubation period of 3 h, remove the foils and expose them to red light (635 nm, 37 J/cm^2)
8. Inform the patient about possible side effects and the need for UV protection of the treated area, re-presentation in case of signs of inflammation or bacterial infection
9. Repetition of the procedure after 7 days and clinical controls after 3 months

PDT AS A COMBINATION THERAPY

PDT can also be used in combination with other forms of therapy to increase effectiveness. Often, combination therapy leads to improved penetration of the photosensitizer, which is associated with a more pronounced response and better healing rates. Studies have shown that fractional laser pretreatment with either Er:YAG-, CO_2–, or Thulium lasers leads to increased fluorescence and better clearance rates.[67] Choi and colleagues were able to demonstrate this observation by performing pretreatment using fractional Er:YAG laser in patients with nBCCs before PDT. Cosmetically, the picture was similarly as good as after conventional PDT.[68] On the other hand, however, there is a study by Haak and colleagues that could not show any difference after fractional laser pretreatment before PDT compared to conventional PDT.[69] Combination treatments of PDT with imiquimod have also been investigated several times. In a study by Logan and colleagues, 17 patients with a total of 21 BCC lesions were first subjected to two cycles of MAL-PDT and then a 5% imiquimod cream was applied to the lesions for 6 weeks, 5 days a week. During a 24-month follow-up period, two patients showed recurrences (10%). The cosmetic result was rated as excellent in 57% and as good in 38%.[70] A placebo-controlled study has also shown that the use of 5% imiquimod following PDT can promote healing. In patients who applied 5% imiquimod twice a week for 5 weeks 72 h after PDT, the lesions healed completely in 75% of cases. Patients who applied a placebo for 5 weeks after PDT showed complete healing of the lesions in 60%.[71] However, side effects such as redness, crusting, burning, and itching were significantly more pronounced and long-lasting in the group treated with 5% imiquimod. Although these healed without scarring and showed very good cosmetic results after 14 months, it is still necessary to critically consider which patients benefit from such a combination therapy and are willing to accept the longer and more pronounced side effects.[71] In the treatment of BCCs, it can also be useful to combine PDT with surgical procedures. For example, it may be useful to perform neo-adjuvant PDT for large lesions. Al-Niaimi and colleagues were able to show that PDT performed in accordance with guidelines 2–10 weeks before micrographically controlled surgery led to a reduction in the size of the tumor to be operated on and that the number of post-excisions in the context of micrographically controlled surgery averaged 1.85. Patients who underwent micrographically controlled surgery without prior PDT had to be operated on an average of 2.5 times before tumor-free surgery could be achieved.[72] Only BCC lesions in the facial area were included in this study and it makes it clear that PDT before surgery in the facial area can be helpful, especially for large lesions, to avoid large defects that are difficult to close. In addition, the risk of frequent and unpleasant post-excisions for the patient can be reduced.[72] However, PDT can also be performed postoperatively if post-excision is to be avoided. Bu and colleagues investigated the extent to which PDT can be an alternative to surgical post-excision as a follow-up treatment for initially R_1-resected BCCs. A total of 20 patients received either PDT or post-excision after R_1 resection of BCC. After 8 months, there was no difference in the frequency of recurrence in both groups.[73] Reddy and colleagues published a case in which, despite six times post-excision in the course of micrographically controlled surgery, parts of a superficial BCC were found in over 50% of the peripheral area. To avoid further post-excision and defect enlargement, they performed MAL-PDT with two sessions within a week and waited for the secondary wound healing of the defect. After 4 weeks, the wound was healed. In addition, there was no evidence of residues of the superficial BCC described earlier.[74] This case not only shows the effectiveness of PDT in the treatment of BCCs but also shows that PDT leads to faster re-epithelialization and wound healing, which is particularly interesting for large defects. This seems to be due to an increased expression of the matrix metalloproteinases MMP-1, MMP-9, and the growth factor TGF-β3.[75] However, further studies must follow to prove this effect.

CONCLUSION

In summary, it can be said that surgery is still the therapeutic gold standard for BCCs. However, PDT is a good alternative for superficial or nodular BCCs up to a tumor thickness of ≤2 mm, especially if lesions are large, for example in terms of surface extension, an aesthetically disturbing scar on the part of the patient is to be avoided or surgery is not possible due to numerous concomitant diseases. Superficial BCCs of the trunk show the best clinical results.[34] A good and conscientious selection of patients who are suitable for PDT is therefore essential to avoid frustrating treatments and frequent recurrences.

REFERENCES

1. Ciążyńska M, Kamińska-Winciorek G, Lange D, et al. The incidence and clinical analysis of non-melanoma skin cancer. *Sci Rep*. 2021;11:15705.
2. Lang BM, Balermpas P, Bauer A, et al. S2k guidelines for cutaneous basal cell carcinoma – part 1: epidemiology, genetics and diagnosis. *J Dtsch Dermatol Ges*. 2019;17(1):94–103.
3. Asgari MM, Moffet HH, Ray GT, Quesenberry CP. Trends in basal cell carcinoma incidence and identification of high-risk subgroups, 1998–2012. *JAMA Dermatol*. 2015;151:976–998.
4. Dika E, Scarfi F, Ferracin M, et al. Basal cell carcinoma: a comprehensive review. *Int J Mol Sci*. 2020;21(15):5572.
5. Christenson LJ, Borrowman TA, Vachon CM, et al. Incidence of basal cell and squamous cell carcinomas in a population younger than 40 years. *JAMA*. 2005;294:681.
6. Lobeck A, Weiss C, Orouji A, et al. Observation of the dermatosurgical patient collective at a skin tumor center in Germany. *Dermatologist*. 2017;68:377–384.
7. Rubin AI, Chen EH, Ratner D. Basal-cell carcinoma. *N Engl J Med*. 2005;353:2262–2269.
8. Bauer A, Haufe E, Heinrich L, et al. Basal cell carcinoma risk and solar UV exposure in occupationally relevant anatomic sites: do histological subtype, tumor localization and Fitzpatrick phototype play a role? A population-based case-control study. *J Occup Med Toxicol*. 2020;15:28.
9. Kossard S, Epstein EH, Cerio J, et al. Basal cell carcinoma. In: LeBoit PE, Burg G, Weedon D, Sarasin A, eds. *Skin Tumours: Pathology and Genetics. World Health Organization Classification of Tumours*. IARC Press; 2006:13–20.
10. Husein-ElAhmed H. Sclerodermiform basal cell carcinoma: how much can we rely on dermatoscopy to differentiate from non-aggressive basal cell carcinomas? Analysis of 1256 cases. *An Bras Dermatol*. 2018;93(2):229–232.
11. Lang BM, Balermpas P, Bauer A, et al. S2k guidelines for cutaneous basal cell carcinoma–part 2: treatment, prevention and follow-up. *J Dtsch Dermatol Ges*. 2019;17(2):214–230.
12. Krieter M, Schultz ES. Current management of basal cell carcinoma. *Aktuelle Derm*. 2022;48(04):131–140.
13. Ramelyte E, Nägeli MC, Hunger R, et al. Swiss recommendations for cutaneous basal cell carcinoma, *Dermatology*, 2023;239(1):122–131.
14. Kornevs E, Apse IA, Safronovs TJ, et al. Basal cell carcinoma. Analysis of 395 cases localized in the neck, ear and nose region. *Stomatologija*. 2020;22(1):9–16.
15. Bernardini N, Skroza N, Zuber S, et al. Face and scalp basal cell carcinoma treatment: a review of the literature. *Acta Dermatovenerol Croat*. 2019;27(1):22–27.
16. Bichakjian CK, Olencki T, Aasi SZ, et al. Basal cell skin cancer, version 1.2016, NCCN clinical practice guidelines in oncology. *J Natl Compr Canc Netw*. 2016;14(5):574–597.
17. Silverman MK, Kopf AW, Grin CM, et al. Recurrence rates of treated basal cell carcinomas. Part 2: curettage-electrodesiccation. *J Dermatol Surg Oncol*. 1991;17(9):720–726.
18. Seidl-Philipp M, Nina Frischhut N, Höllweger N. Known and new facts on basal cell carcinoma. *J Dtsch Dermatol Ges*. 2021;19(7):1021–1041.
19. Breuninger H, Dietz KJ. Prediction of subclinical tumor infiltration in basal cell carcinoma. *Dermatol Surg Oncol*. 1991;17(7):574–578.
20. Pyne JH, Myint E, Hou R. Basal cell carcinoma with perineural invasion: a prospective study examining subtype, tumor surface diameter, invasion depth, and anatomic site in 3005 consecutive cases. *J Cutan Pathol*. 2020;47(11):1033–1038.
21. Di Stefani A, Chimenti S. Basal cell carcinoma: clinical and pathological features. *G Ital Dermatol Venereol*. 2015;150(4):385–391.
22. Morton CA, Szeimies RM, Basset-Seguin N, et al. European Dermatology Forum guidelines on topical photodynamic therapy 2019 part 1: treatment delivery and established indications - actinic keratoses, Bowen's disease and basal cell carcinomas. *J Eur Acad Dermatol Venereol*. 2019;33(12):2225–2238.
23. Peris K, Fargnoli MC, Garbe C, et al. Diagnosis and treatment of basal cell carcinoma: European consensus-based interdisciplinary guidelines. *Eur J Cancer*. 2019;118:10–34.
24. Kennedy JC, Pottier RH, Pross DC. Photodynamic therapy with endogenous protoporphyrin IX: basic principles and present clinical experience. *J Photochem Photobiol B*. 1990;6:143–148.
25. Youssef KK, Van Keymeulen A, Lapouge G, et al. Identification of the cell lineage at the origin of basal cell carcinoma. *Nat Cell Biol*. 2010;12(3):299–305.
26. Peterson SC, Eberl M, Vagnozzi AN, et al. Basal cell carcinoma preferentially arises from stem cells within hair follicle and mechanosensory niches. *Cell Stem Cell*. 2015;16(4):400–412.
27. Morton CA, Dominicus R, Radny P, et al. A randomized, multinational, noninferiority, phase III trial to evaluate

the safety and efficacy of BF-200 aminolaevulinic acid gel vs. methyl aminolaevulinate cream in the treatment of nonaggressive basal cell carcinoma with photodynamic therapy. *Br J Dermatol.* 2018;179(2):309–319.

28. Adamek M, Kawczyk-Krupka A, Mostowy A, et al. Topical ALA-PDT modifies neutrophils' chemiluminescence, lymphocytes' interleukin-1beta secretion and serum level of transforming growth factor beta1 in patients with nonmelanoma skin malignancies a clinical study. *Photodiagn Photodyn Ther.* 2005;2:65–72.
29. Collier NJ, Rhodes LE. Photodynamic therapy for basal cell carcinoma: the clinical context for future research priorities. *Molecules.* 2020;25(22):5398.
30. Kabingu E, Oseroff AR, Wilding GE, et al. Enhanced systemic immune reactivity to a basal cell carcinoma associated antigen following photodynamic therapy. *Clin Cancer Res.* 2009;15:4460–4466.
31. Stringasci MD, Salvio AG, Moriyama LT, et al. Energy analysis of PDT using thermography during the treatment of basal cell carcinoma. *Photodiagn Photodyn Ther.* 2020;29:101586.
32. Szeimies RM, Ibbotson S, Murrell DF, et al. A clinical study comparing methyl aminolevulinate photodynamic therapy and surgery in small superficial basal cell carcinoma (8–20 mm), with a 12-month follow-up. *J Eur Acad Dermatol Venereol.* 2008;22:1302–1311.
33. Rhodes LE, de Rie M, Enström Y, et al. Photodynamic therapy using topical methyl aminolevulinate vs surgery for nodular basal cell carcinoma: results of a multicenter randomized prospective trial. *Arch Dermatol.* 2004;140:17–23.
34. Fantini F, Greco A, Del Giovane C, et al. Photodynamic therapy for basal cell carcinoma: clinical and pathological determinants of response. *J Eur Acad Dermatol Venereol.* 2011;25(8):896–901.
35. Cosgarea R, Susan M, Crisan M, et al. Photodynamic therapy using topical 5-aminolaevulinic acid vs surgery for basal cell carcinoma. *J Eur Acad Dermatol Venereol.* 2013;27:980–984.
36. Savoia P, Deboli T, Previgliano A, et al. Usefulness of photodynamic therapy as a possible therapeutic alternative in the treatment of basal cell carcinoma. *Int J Mol Sci.* 2015;16(10):23300–23317.
37. Zou Y, Zhao Y, Yu J, et al. Photodynamic therapy versus surgical excision to basal cell carcinoma: meta-analysis. *J Cosmet Dermatol.* 2016;15(4):374–382.
38. Lindberg-Larsen R, Sølvsten H, Kragballe K. Evaluation of recurrence after photodynamic therapy with topical methylaminolaevulinate for 157 basal cell carcinomas in 90 patients. *Acta Derm Venereol.* 2022;92(2):144–147.
39. Christensen E, Mjønes P, Grimstad Ø. Comparison of clinical and histopathological evaluations of basal cell carcinoma thickness. *Br J Dermatol.* 2015;173(2): 578–580.
40. Roozeboom MH, van Kleef L, Arits AHMM, et al. Tumor thickness and adnexal extension of superficial basal cell carcinoma (sBCC) as determinants of treatment failure for methylaminolevulinate (MAL)-photodynamic therapy (PDT), imiquimod, and 5-fluorouracil (FU) capsule summary. *J Am Acad Dermatol.* 2015;73:93–98.
41. Thissen MR, Schroeter CA, Neumann HA. Photodynamic therapy with delta-aminolaevulinic acid for nodular basal cell carcinomas using a prior debulking technique. *Br J Dermatol.* 2000;142:338–339.
42. Gómez C, Pilar Cobos P, Alberdi E. Methyl aminolevulinate photodynamic therapy after partial debulking in the treatment of superficial and nodular basal cell carcinoma: 3-years follow-up. *Photodiagnosis Photodyn Ther.* 2021;33:102176.
43. Marjukka Suhonen T, Bouwstra JA, Urtti A. Chemical enhancement of percutaneous absorption in relation to stratum corneum structural alterations. *J Control Release.* 1999;59:149–161.
44. Braathen LR, Paredes BE, Saksela O, et al. Short incubation with methyl aminolevulinate for photodynamic therapy of actinic keratoses. *J Eur Acad Dermatol Venereol.* 2009;23:550–555.
45. Kaviani A, Ataie-Fashtami L, Fateh M, et al. Photodynamic therapy of head and neck basal cell carcinoma according to different clinicopathologic features. *Lasers Surg Med.* 2005;36:377–382.
46. Itoh Y, Henta T, Ninomiya Y, et al. Repeated 5-aminolevulinic acid-based photodynamic therapy following electro-curettage for pigmented basal cell carcinoma. *J Dermatol.* 2000;27(1):10–15.
47. Gracia-Cazaña T, Gonzalez S, Juarranz A, et al. Methyl aminolevulinate photodynamic therapy combined with curettage debulking for pigmented basal cell carcinoma. *Photodermatol Photoimmunol Photomed.* 2017;33(4):228–232.
48. Salvio AG, Requena MB, Stringasci MD, et al. Photodynamic therapy as a treatment option for multiple pigmented basal cell carcinoma: long-term follow-up results. *Photodiagnosis Photodyn Ther.* 2021;33:102154.
49. Ceilley RI, Del Rosso JQ. Current modalities and new advances in the treatment of basal cell carcinoma. *Int J Dermatol.* 2006;45:489–498.
50. Collier NJ, Haylett AK, Wong TH. Conventional and combination topical photodynamic therapy for basal cell carcinoma: systematic review and meta-analysis. *Br J Dermatol.* 2018;179(6):1277–1296.
51. Torres T, Fernandes I, Costa V, Selores M. Photodynamic therapy as adjunctive therapy for morpheaform basal cell carcinoma. *Acta Dermatovenerol Alp Pannonica Adriat.* 2011;20(1):23–25.

52. Wang B, Shi L, Zhang Y, et al. Gain with no pain? Pain management in dermatological photodynamic therapy. *Br J Dermatol.* 2017;177(3):656–665.
53. Ibbotson SH, Wong TH, Morton CA, et al. Adverse effects of topical photodynamic therapy: a consensus review and approach to management. *Br J Dermatol.* 2019;180(4):715–729.
54. Kessels JP, Kreukels H, Nelemans PJ, et al. Treatment of superficial basal cell carcinoma by topical photodynamic therapy with fractionated 5-aminolaevulinic acid 20% vs. two-stage topical methyl aminolaevulinate: results of a randomized controlled trial. *Br J Dermatol.* 2018;178(5):1056–1063.
55. Kuijpers DI, Thissen MR, Thissen CA, Neumann MH. Similar effectiveness of methyl aminolevulinate and 5-aminolevulinate in topical photodynamic therapy for nodular basal cell carcinoma. *J Drugs Dermatol.* 2006;5(7):642–645.
56. Ibbotson SH, Valentine R, Hearn R. Is the pain of topical photodynamic therapy with methyl aminolevulinate any different from that with 5-aminolaevulinic acid? *Photodermatol Photoimmunol Photomed.* 2012;28(5):272–273.
57. Tyyrell J, Paterson C, Curnow A. Regression analysis of protoporphyrin IX measurements obtained during dermatological photodynamic therapy. *Cancers (Basel).* 2011;11(1):72.
58. Szeimies RM. Methyl aminolevulinate-photodynamic therapy for basal cell carcinoma. *Dermatol Clin.* 2007; 25(1):89–94.
59. Wang BC, Fu C, Qin L, et al. Photodynamic therapy with methyl-5-aminolevulinate for basal cell carcinoma: a systematic review and meta-analysis. *Photodiagnosis Photodyn Ther.* 2020;29(3):101667.
60. Martin I, Schaarschmidt ML, Glocker A, et al. Patient preferences for treatment of basal cell carcinoma: importance of cure and cosmetic outcome. *Acta Derm Venereol.* 2016;96(3):355–360.
61. Morton CA, Szeimies RM, Sidoroff A, et al. European dermatology forum guidelines on topical photodynamic therapy. *Eur J Dermatol.* 2015;25:296–311.
62. Salvio AG, Veneziano DB, Moriyama LT, et al. A new photodynamic therapy protocol for nodular basal cell carcinoma treatment: effectiveness and long-term follow-up. *Photodiagnosis Photodyn Ther.* 2022;37:102668.
63. Wiegell SR, Haedersdal M, Philipsen PA, et al. Continuous activation of PpIX by daylight is as effective as and less painful than conventional photodynamic therapy for actinic keratoses; a randomized Röwert-Huiber´rzed, controlled, single-blinded study. *Br J Dermatol.* 2008;158:740–746.
64. Hommel T, Szeimies RM. Actinic keratoses. *Hautarzt.* 2016;67:867–875.
65. Morton CA, Braathen LR. Daylight photodynamic therapy for actinic keratoses. *Am J Clin Dermatol.* 2018;19(5):647–656.
66. Wiegell SR, Skødt V, Wulf HC. Daylight-mediated photodynamic therapy of basal cell carcinomas - an explorative study. *J Eur Acad Dermatol Venereol.* 2014; 28(2):169–175.
67. Lippert J, Smucler R, Vlk M. Fractional carbon dioxide laser improves nodular basal cell carcinoma treatment with photodynamic therapy with methyl 5-aminolevulinate. *Dermatol Surg.* 2013;39(8):1202–1208.
68. Choi SH, Kim KH, Song KH. Er:YAG ablative fractional laser-primed photodynamic therapy with methyl aminolevulinate as an alternative treatment option for patients with thin nodular basal cell carcinoma: 12-month follow-up results of a randomized, prospective, comparative trial. *J Eur Acad Dermatol Venereol.* 2016;30(5):783–788.
69. Haak CS, Togsverd-Bo K, Thaysen-Petersen D, et al. Fractional laser-mediated photodynamic therapy of high-risk basal cell carcinomas–a randomized clinical trial. *Br J Dermatol.* 2015;172(1):215–222.
70. Logan IT, Kulakov EL, Perrett CM. Sequential treatment of superficial basal cell carcinomas with topical methyl aminolevulinate photodynamic therapy and imiquimod 5% cream: a retrospective study of clinical and cosmetic outcomes. *Dermatol Surg.* 2020;46(10):1272–1278.
71. Osiecka B, Jurczyszyn K, Ziolkowski P. The application of Levulan-based photodynamic therapy with imiquimod in the treatment of recurrent basal cell carcinoma. *Med Sci Monit.* 2012;18(2):PI5–PI9.
72. Al-Niaimi F, Sheth N, Kurwa HA, et al. Photodynamic therapy followed by Mohs micrographic surgery compared to Mohs micrographic surgery alone for the treatment of basal cell carcinoma: results of a pilot single-blinded randomised controlled trial. *J Cutan Aesthet Surg.* 2015;8(2):88–91.
73. Bu W, Zhang M, Zhang Q, et al. Preliminary results of comparative study for subsequent photodynamic therapy versus secondary excision after primary excision for treating basal cell carcinoma. *Photodiagnosis Photodyn Ther.* 2017;17(3):134–137.
74. Reddy KK, Hanke CW, Tierney EP. Rapid wound re-epithelialization and basal cell carcinoma clearance after Mohs micrographic surgery with postoperative photodynamic therapy. *J Drugs Dermatol.* 2010;9(2):143–148.
75. Mills SJ, Farrar MD, Ashcroft GS. Topical photodynamic therapy following excisional wounding of human skin increases production of transforming growth factor-beta3 and matrix metalloproteinases 1 and 9, with associated improvement in dermal matrix organization. *Br J Dermatol.* 2014;171(1):55–62.

11

Photodynamic Therapy for Mycosis Fungoides

David Weiner, Joi B. Carter

KEY POINTS

- PDT is a second-line treatment option for localized mycosis fungoides.
- The most common PDT regimen is MAL 20%, occlusion for 3 h, 630 nm light, and 37.5 J/cm^2 dosage.
- PDT is particularly useful for isolated recalcitrant plaques, skin folds, and the face.

OBJECTIVES

- Summarize the rationale and suggested indications for photodynamic therapy as a treatment for early stage mycosis fungoides.
- Review current protocols and clinical outcomes using different photosensitizers, with a focus on aminolevulinic acid, methylaminolevulinate, and hypericin.
- Identify limitations of existing studies and highlight the need for more rigorous clinical trials to standardize protocols.

INTRODUCTION

Mycosis fungoides (MF) is the most common type of cutaneous T-cell lymphoma (CTCL), a non-Hodgkin lymphoma of skin-homing T-cells. Early stage MF typically present with erythematous scaly patches or plaques in sun-protected areas. In more advanced stages, erythroderma and tumors can develop, as well as lymph node and blood involvement.

As early MF (stages IA–IB) is usually skin-limited and has an excellent prognosis, skin-directed therapies are preferred such as topical steroids, phototherapy with narrowband UVB or psoralen with UVA, local radiation, topical chemotherapy, and topical immunomodulators. All these treatments have associated adverse events, especially with long-term use. For example, topical steroids can cause skin thinning over time and topical mechlorethamine can cause contact dermatitis.[1]

Photodynamic therapy (PDT) is an alternative skin-directed treatment option for early MF. PDT involves the use of a topical photosensitizer gel such as aminolevulinic acid (ALA) or methylaminolevulinate (MAL) followed by activation by a light source, typically coherent light in the red (approximately 635 nm) or blue (approximately 400 nm) spectrum.[2] These photosensitizers are metabolized into protoporphyrin IX (PpIX) within cells, generating reactive oxygen species that eventually cause cell apoptosis (via the intrinsic mitochondrial pathway) and necrosis as well as inhibition of cell proliferation.[3] In general, neoplastic cells take up more porphyrins than normal cells, leading to preferential cell death in neoplastic cells. MF is thought to be susceptible to PDT due to increased uptake of porphyrins in lymphoma cells as well as enhanced photosensitizer penetration of an abnormal stratum corneum and slower metabolism of protoporphyrin into heme by malignant T-cells.[4] A combination of direct tumor cell destruction, production of an inflammatory response, and inhibition of T-cell proliferation have been observed in in vitro studies of MF samples after PDT.[5,6] Apoptosis triggered by PDT is mediated by the intrinsic apoptosis pathway, a useful treatment mechanism for MF, which may have defects in the extrinsic apoptosis pathway.[7]

The photosensitizer ALA was discovered in 1990, and the first case report on ALA-PDT for MF was published by Svanberg and colleagues in 1994.[8] Since the discovery of ALA, MAL has also been introduced as a PDT prodrug that is available for usage in Europe and Asia. MAL, the methyl ester derivative of ALA, has enhanced penetration of the epidermis due to increased lipophilicity.[9] Hypericin, an alternative photosensitizer that can be activated by visible fluorescent light, has also been developed for MF and studied in clinical trials.[10,11]

With its non-mutagenic mechanism of action and lower risk of burns, PDT may be safer than narrowband UVB therapy for long-term use in MF patients. Furthermore, the visible light wavelengths used in PDT may provide enhanced penetration into the skin compared to nbUVB. PDT can also help treat “sanctuary sites” not effectively targeted by phototherapy, such as inguinal or axillary skin folds. PDT is typically conducted weekly to monthly and can therefore be a useful alternative for patients who do not want to apply topical therapies every day or who cannot travel for narrowband UVB or psoralen plus ultraviolet-A radiation (PUVA) multiple times per week.

Thus far, there are a few small case series regarding PDT in MF, and more research is needed to fully evaluate the efficacy of PDT in MF and determine the optimal protocol. In this chapter, we review the current data regarding PDT in MF and discuss the potential clinical indications.

TABLE 11.1 Studies of Mycosis Fungoides Treated with Photodynamic Therapy With 5-aminolevulinic Acid

Study	No. of Patients (Total No. of Lesions/No. Lesions Per Patient)	Patient Characteristics	MF Characteristics	PDT Protocol
Coors et al.[12] (Germany)	4 (7/1–3)	41–65/3M1F/ 14–18 months	cMF(2), ALCL(1), CD8+ CTCL (1)/PUVA (4), IFN-alpha (3), acitretin (2), TSEBT (1)	20% ALA/6h/Visible light source/72–144 J/cm²/60–160 mW/ cm²/15–20 min/2–7/q2w
Edstrom et al.[13] (Sweden)	10 (12/1–2)	58–81yo/6M4F/ 71–82 months	cMF/IA–IIB/plaque, tumor/PUVA (6), TCS (1), XR (1)	20% ALA/5–6h/600–730 nm/80–180 J/cm²/ q1–2w/2–11
Han et al.[14] (China)	3 (3/1)	45–46yo/1M2F/ 8–17 months	cMF/all plaque/PUVA (3), IFN (3)	20% ALA/4h/635 nm/60 mW/cm²/20 min/ q2w/2–3
Severson et al.[15] (USA)	11 (30/1–3)	22–82/6M5F	cMF (6), fMF (5)/TCS (11), nbUVB (5), MCI (5), IMQ (4), XR (3), BX (2), acitretin (1)	20% ALA/2–4 h/417 nm/10 J/cm²/16.7 min/1–6/ monthly

Patient characteristics: age range/#male#female/follow-up average (range).
MF characteristics: type of MF/stage(s)/morphology of targeted lesion(s)/prior treatments.
PDT protocol: photosensitizing agent/occlusion time/light source/light intensity/light exposure time/interval between treatments/ total number of treatments (range).
Response: a. clinical response rate (# CR, # PR), b. if post-treatment biopsies done: histologic response rate (# histologic remission), c. # of any recurrences (time to recurrence).

CURRENT APPLICATIONS

PDT Protocols

Tables 11.1 and 11.2 summarize the published case series in which three or more patients were treated with PDT for MF. Standard protocols have not yet been developed. While initial studies used ALA as the photosensitizer, ALA has limited tissue penetration and therefore reduced efficacy in thick plaques or tumors. ALA also requires a longer occlusion period of 4–16 h, which can be cumbersome for patients.[2] MAL, the methyl ester derivative of ALA, has enhanced lipophilic properties that result in deeper penetration throughout the skin as well as shorter required occlusion times (about 3 h).[2] MAL has therefore been used as the photosensitizer in more recent case series on PDT in MF; however, MAL is not easily acquired in the United States. Hypericin is an alternative photosensitizer for MF that was recently evaluated in phase II and phase III clinical trials.[10,11] Hypericin can be activated by visible light (500–650 nm) and therefore could potentially be used by patients at home.[10] Hypericin also may be more specific for malignant T-cells compared to MAL and ALA.[11]

Several light sources are available for PDT, including visible blue or red light, as well as non-coherent light or coherent laser light. Most studies have used red light (approximately 630 nm) for MF, as longer wavelengths maximize tissue penetration. The optimal light fluence and intensity have not yet been determined. One study found that higher fluence (>75 J/cm²) and higher intensity (>150 mW/cm²) results in less epidermal damage and more clinical efficacy.[16] However, in other studies higher fluence has resulted in more skin pain.[17] The ideal number of treatments and the treatment interval

Locations of Lesions	Response	Adverse Events	Reason for PDT	Notes
Intergluteal cleft (1) Scalp/face (2) Forearm (1)	a. 100% (4/4 CR) b. Unknown c. 2 (3 months)	Pain, blisters	Single lesions after PR to conventional MF therapies	One relapsed patient had disseminated lesions treated with PUVA, with CR in 6 months One relapsed patient treated with PDT; CR again with no relapse after 14 months.
Trunk (6) Legs (3) Gluteal (2) Arm (1)	a. 75% (9/12 CR) b. 75% (9/12 hCR) c. 3	Pain	Localized MF	3 patients developed tumor-stage MF and died; timing and treatments not reported
Legs (2) Trunk (1)	a. 100% (2/3 CR) b. Unknown c. n/a	Pain, blisters, ulceration	Localized MF who failed prior therapy	
Legs (4) Trunk (2) Arm (4) Face (1)	a. 36% (1/11 CR) b. Unknown c. Unknown	Bullous dermatitis, pain, ulceration, pruritus	Patients refractory to conventional therapy (at least two skin-directed or one systemic) or folliculotropic MF	Insurance coverage unknown

Notes: treatment of any recurrences, concurrent treatments, other unique study features.
ALCL, Anaplastic Large Cell Lymphoma; *BX*, bexarotene; *cMF*, classic MF; *CR*, complete response; *fMF*, folliculotropic MF; *hCR*, histologic complete response; *IMQ*, imiquimod; *MCI*, mechlorethamine gel; *nbUVB*, narrowband UVB; *PUVA*, psoralen + ultraviolet-A; *TCS*, topical corticosteroids; *tIM*, topical immunomodulator; *tR*, topical retinoid; *TSEBT*, total skin electron beam therapy; *uMF*, unilesional MF; *XR*, local radiation.

TABLE 11.2 Studies of Mycosis Fungoides Treated With Photodynamic Therapy With Methyl Aminolevulinate

Study	No. of Patients (Total No. of Lesions/No. Lesions Per Patient)	Patient Characteristics	MF Characteristics	PDT Protocol
Zane et al.[18] (Italy)	5 (5/1)	31–65yo/3M2F/ 12–34 months	uMF/all IA/patch/ TCS (5), PUVA (5)	20% MAL/3 h/635±18 nm/37.5 J/cm^2/86 mW/ cm^2/weekly/1–9
Debu et al.[17] (France)	3 (8)	54–68/2M1F	fMF/IA, IIB, unknown/patch, plaque	16.8% MAL/3 h/630 nm/37 J/cm^2/10 min/ q1–2 w/1–10
Fernandez-Guarino et al.[19] (Spain)	12 (24/1–4)	30–63/3M9F/ 4–33 months	All plaque/TCS (12), PUVA (5), tR (1), tIM (2)	MAL/3 h/630 nm/37 J/ cm^2/8 min/5–6/monthly
Kim et al.[20] (South Korea)	10 (16)	26–68yo/5M5F/ (8–31 months)	cMF/IA(9), IB(1)/ patch, plaque/ TCS(6), acitretin (2), PUVA (2)	16.8% MAL/3 h/630 nm/37.5 J/cm^2/75 mW/cm^2/8.3 min/ weekly/2–6
Calzavara-Pinton et al.[21] (Italy)	19 (19)	60.6 ± 12.5 yo/ 8M11F/ 10+/−10.5 months	cMF(10), uMF(9)/all plaque	20% MAL/3–4h/635± 18 nm/37 J/cm^2/ average 16 days/1–7
Quereux et al.[22] (France)	12 (21/1–2)	43–82yo/5M5F/ 12 months (6–35)	cMF/IA(6), IB(6)/ patch, plaque/ BCNU (11), HN2 (7), IFNa (7), PUVA (4), BX (4), XR (3), IMQ (2), UVB (2)	20% MAL/3 h/630 nm/37 J/cm^2/ monthly/2–6
Pileri et al.[23] (Italy)	4 (4/1)	53–74/3M1F/6– 120 months	cMF (1), fMF (1), PR (1)/all patch/TCS (4), PUVA (2), UVB (1), acitretin (1), systemic steroids (1)	16% MAL/3 h/630 nm/37 J/cm^2/9 min/4– 9/monthly
Jang et al.[24] (South Korea)	4 (4+; number unknown)	32–68yo/3M1F/36 months	fMF/all IA/patch, papule, plaque/ PUVA (2), IFNa (2)	16.8% MAL/3 h/630 nm/37.5 J/cm^2/75 mW/ cm^2/8.3 min/monthly/3

Locations of Lesions	Response	Adverse Events	Reason for PDT	Notes
Trunk (2) Legs (3)	a. 100% (4/5 CR) b. Unknown c. n/a	Erythema, edema, pain	Unilesional MF that had not responded to several treatments	
Face (8)	a. 100% (7/8 CR) b. 100% (6/7 hCR) c. n/a	Local pain	Face (area where treatment options limited); refractory or not	Facial fMF One patient received concurrent MTX 25 mg weekly Unknown: prior treatments
Unknown	a. 92% (6/12 CR) b. Unknown c. n/a	Eczema	Lack of response to at least one conventional treatment; localized plaque-stage MF	
Face/scalp (4) Trunk (4) Palm (1) Leg (7)	a. 70% (5/10 CR) b. 63% (5/8 hCR) c. 1 (9 months)	Erythema, pain	Treat localized MF	Relapsed patient received six more PDT sessions; had PR after 2nd session
"major body folds" (10)	a. 68% (5/19 CR) b. Unknown c. 2	Pain, erythema	Folds that could not be reached by phototherapy (10) Localized/unilesional MF (9)	Unknown timing of relapse, etc.
Trunk (11) Arms (3) Legs (7)	a. 75% (6/12 CR) b. 67% (1/12 hCR) c. 2 (12 months)	Erythema, burning pain, crusting	Treat localized MF (paucilesional <5 lesions)	Responses were reported in targeted skin lesions per patient. However, five patients had new patches/plaque develop (overall PD even though targeted lesions responded). Unknown treatment of relapsed patients
Plantar (2) Leg (1) Pubic area (1)	a. 100% (2/4 CR) b. Unknown c. n/a	Burning sensation	Difficult to treat anatomical areas	
Face (3) Trunk (1)	a. 100% (4/4 CR) b. n/a biopsies c. n/a	N/a reported	Treat localized MF	Missing data

Continued

TABLE 11.2 **Studies of Mycosis Fungoides Treated With Photodynamic Therapy With Methyl Aminolevulinate—cont'd**

Study	No. of Patients (Total No. of Lesions/No. Lesions Per Patient)	Patient Characteristics	MF Characteristics	PDT Protocol
Dairi et al.[25] (France)	4 (4/1)	54–77 yo/2M2F/ (6–18 months)	cMF/all IA/ all plaques/all clobetasol	16% MAL/3 h/"red light"/37 J/cm²/ monthly/4–12

Patient characteristics: age range/#male#female/follow-up average (range).
MF characteristics: type of MF/stage(s)/morphology of targeted lesion(s)/prior treatments.
PDT protocol: photosensitizing agent/occlusion time/light source/light intensity/light exposure time/interval between treatments/total number of treatments (range).
Response: a. clinical response rate (# CR, # PR), b. if post-treatment biopsies done: histologic response rate (# histologic remission), c. # of any recurrences (time to recurrence).

are unknown. Most patients require at least two treatments to achieve a response, and the total number of sessions depends on whether a response occurs and the duration of response. Prior studies have administered PDT monthly or twice monthly, which provides sufficient time for any skin irritation to resolve.

As the studies on PDT in MF are limited, the parameters used are adapted from more commonly approved indications such as actinic keratosis. In general, the most common published protocol is MAL 20% with occlusion for 3 h, activation by red light (630 nm) at a dose of 37.5 J/cm^2. However, MAL is not easily acquired in the US. The most common ALA-based protocol is 20% ALA with occlusion for 6 h, activation by red light (630 nm), and a light fluence ranging from 60 to 180 J/cm^2. Multiple cycles of PDT are typically required to achieve clinical benefit; about two to six treatments in total, with a dosing interval of 2–4 weeks.

General contraindications to PDT include a known photosensitivity disorder or use of photosensitizing drug, known hypersensitivity to the topical photosensitizer, and pregnancy or breastfeeding.[2] PDT is also not suitable for treatment of MF tumors due to insufficient depth of penetration.[26]

CLINICAL DATA

Overall, there is promising evidence for use of PDT in patch and plaque-stage MF that is confined to a limited area. However, more extensive study of PDT is necessary and standard protocols have not yet been established for MF. It is currently challenging to evaluate the efficacy of PDT for MF as there are mainly case series available and a variety of techniques have been used.

A literature review showed 13 case series with three or more patients who were treated with ALA or MAL-based PDT for MF.[15,17] There were 101 patients in total, with approximately 157 treated skin lesions. The majority of studies (69%) used MAL (16.8% or 20%) as the photosensitizer, with shorter occlusion time (3 h for MAL vs. 4–6 h for ALA) due to the enhanced lipophilicity and skin penetration of MAL. The number of PDT sessions ranged from 1 to 12 and the timeframe between sessions ranged from weekly to monthly. Most studies also used red light (92%) rather than blue light, as longer wavelengths are thought to enhance penetration of thicker plaques. To our knowledge, all but one patient received PDT as monotherapy. Overall response rates ranged from 36% to 100%. Histologic response to PDT was typically concordant with clinical response; histologic response rates ranged from 67% to 100% in studies that did post-PDT biopsies. Adverse events were overall mild and did not result in cessation of therapy. The most frequent adverse events were skin irritation, pain, blistering, and post-inflammatory hyperpigmentation. Good cosmetic results were usually obtained, with limited scarring, hair loss, or dyspigmentation. In studies that reported whether relapses occurred, 10 of 90 total patients (11%) relapsed in treated areas about 3–12 months after an initial response to PDT.[15] Two relapsed patients were retreated with PDT; one had a PR, and one had a CR.[12,27] Another relapsed patient had a CR

Locations of Lesions	Response	Adverse Events	Reason for PDT	Notes
Inguinal fold (1) Buttock (1) Cheek (1) Thigh (1)	a. 100% (4/4 CR) b. 100% (3/3 hCR) c. n/a	Local irritation, pain, PIH	Treat localized MF (w/ laser enhancement)	Laser-assisted drug delivery with fractional CO_2 laser was used to improve photosensitizer penetration.

Notes: treatment of any recurrences, concurrent treatments, other unique study features.
BCNU, Carmustine; *BX*, bexarotene; *cMF*, classic MF; *CR*, complete response; *fMF*, folliculotropic MF; *HN2*, nitrogen mustard; *hCR*, histologic complete response; *IMQ*, imiquimod; *MCl*, mechlorethamine gel; *nbUVB*, narrowband UVB; *PUVA*, psoralen + ultraviolet-A; *tIM*, topical immunomodulator; *tR*, topical retinoid; *TCS*, topical corticosteroids; *TSEBT*, total skin electron beam therapy; *uMF*, unilesional MF; *XR*, local radiation.

with PUVA. The treatment courses of the other seven relapsed patients are unknown.[12]

Most patients had classic MF ($n = 70$). However, some studies included patients with folliculotropic MF ($n = 13$), unilesional MF ($n = 14$), pagetoid reticulosis ($n = 1$), and CD8 + CTCL ($n = 1$). Reasons for usage of PDT included (1) treatment of isolated lesions (some of which were refractory to previous therapies; 11 studies), (2) treatment of lesions in areas not accessible by phototherapy (eight studies), and (3) treatment of facial lesions when a good cosmetic outcome is desired (1 study). As examples: (1) Coors and colleagues successfully treated four patients (100% ORR; all CR) with ALA-PDT who had residual lesions after partial response to conventional MF therapies such as PUVA and interferon-alpha,[12] (2) Pileri and colleagues reported 100% ORR with MAL-PDT for patients with MF in anatomical areas that are challenging to treat with phototherapy such as the plantar feet and inguinal folds,[23] and (3) Debu and colleagues had a 100% ORR with MAL-PDT for folliculotropic MF located on the face, with good cosmetic results.[17]

In general, patients appreciated that they could use PDT as an intermittent monotherapy rather than daily application of creams or frequent phototherapy appointments. Quereux and colleagues conducted a patient perception survey, finding that patients considered PDT more convenient than topical chemotherapy with nitrogen mustard or carmustine.[28] Furthermore, 82% of patients preferred to receive PDT to topical chemotherapy in the future.[28]

OTHER PDT PROTOCOLS

Alternative photosensitizers have also been studied in MF. Hypericin, a photodynamic agent naturally found in plants such as St. John's wort, may mediate more targeted destruction of malignant T-cells compared to ALA/MAL. Hypericin has been studied in a phase II trial by Rook and colleagues as well as a recent multicenter phase III clinical trial (the FLASH study) by Kim and colleagues.[10,11] The FLASH study included 169 total patients with stage IA–IIA classic MF. The treatment protocol consisted of twice-weekly 0.25% hypericin, a visible light source ranging from 500 to 650 nm, and a light dosage of 5 J/cm^2 that was increased by 1 J/cm^2 with each treatment session to a maximum of 12 J/cm^2. Response rates in individual lesions were 16% ($n = 19/116$) after one 6-week cycle, 40% ($n = 44/110$) after two cycles, and 44% ($n = 38/78$) after three cycles, which were more effective than placebo. The most common adverse events were mild skin pain, pruritus, and irritation.

The silicon phthalocyanine Pc4 is another photosensitizer with a longer peak absorption wavelength (approximately 675 nm) compared to ALA and MAL, providing deeper tissue penetration. A phase I clinical trial of Pc4-PDT had a response rate of 40% ($n = 14$) in 35 total patients with classic MF stage IA–IIB.[29]

Epigenetically enhanced PDT consisting of ALA-PDT with concurrent methotrexate has also been studied in MF cell lines.[3] Methotrexate has been shown to augment the sensitivity of lymphoma cells to PDT by inducing expression of apoptotic factors such as the death receptor FAS, thus triggering the extrinsic caspase-8-mediated apoptosis pathway. Epigenetically enhanced PDT has not yet been evaluated in clinical studies of MF.

DISCUSSION

Early MF is usually managed with one or more skin-directed therapies. First-line therapies include topical corticosteroids, topical chemotherapy (nitrogen mustard), topical retinoids (bexarotene), topical imiquimod, local radiation, or phototherapy (UVB or PUVA). However, these therapies do not always produce consistent or durable responses, and each can result in adverse effects. For example, topical steroids have a complete response rate of 25%–63%, with treatment-limiting side effects such as skin atrophy.[26] Topical bexarotene, an expensive medication, had an overall response rate of 44% in a phase III trial.[30] Mechlorethamine causes contact dermatitis in about 40% of patients.[1] Phototherapy with UVB or PUVA is effective for diffuse early patch and plaque-stage MF but cannot access skin folds and may cause an increased long-term risk of skin cancer. PUVA is also limited by nausea and phototoxic reactions. There is therefore a need for additional skin-directed therapies for early MF.

Overall, there is sufficient evidence that PDT is an effective and well-tolerated second-line option for selected cases of localized early MF. Based on the current data and understanding of MF, the following are the most appropriate indications for PDT in early stage MF (stage IA–IB):

- Isolated patch or plaque that has not responded to prior therapies.
- Isolated patch or plaque in a location that cannot be effectively targeted by phototherapy (e.g., skin fold).
- Patch or plaque located on the face when a good cosmetic outcome is desired.
- Patients who do not want to apply creams daily or have difficulty with travel to frequent phototherapy appointments.
- Patch or plaque located on the feet when risk of poor healing is a concern.

Published case series have demonstrated the utility of PDT in all of the above clinical scenarios. For example, PDT had a 68% objective response rate (ORR) when used to treat residual lesions in body folds of patients who had previously received phototherapy.[27] Most patients received PDT as second-line or later monotherapy for residual localized patches or plaques, with treatment intervals ranging from weekly to monthly. MAL-PDT may also be efficacious for folliculotropic MF since the enhanced lipophilicity of MAL enables penetration into the pilosebaceous unit. However, more study in this patient population is necessary.

PDT is not useful as monotherapy for diffuse patch or plaque-stage MF, which is better suited to phototherapy or systemic treatment. PDT is also ineffective for tumor-stage MF because red light penetrates approximately 1–2 mm into the skin, which is too superficial for most tumors.[31] Certain areas such as the hands and feet may be difficult to treat by PDT because photosensitizer occlusion can be disrupted by frequent movement. PDT is also generally avoided in the eyelid area due to the need for occlusion for several hours after photosensitizer application and the increased risk of skin irritation and phototoxic damage. MAL is also expensive and not easily accessible in the United States.

PDT has many potential advantages for treatment of MF, including the ability to target specific areas, the low risk of serious adverse events, and the efficiency of monthly or twice-monthly treatments. However, controlled clinical trials are lacking and protocols have not yet been standardized. Furthermore, a major limitation of most published studies is that they report responses to treatment in individual targeted lesions but do not report overall outcomes in patients. Therefore it is possible that patients responded to the patch or plaque treated by PDT but had disease progression overall. PDT can also theoretically be combined with other skin-directed or systemic treatments to target specific sites in patients with more advanced MF. However, the efficacy of PDT in combination with other treatments has not yet been studied.

Future research is necessary to determine the optimal treatment protocol for PDT based on lesion type (e.g., patch vs. plaque) and location (e.g., face vs. trunk). Future studies should also combine PDT with other treatments, as in clinical practice PDT will likely be used as an adjunct measure to target specific refractory plaques. PDT could also be trialed as a first-line treatment for patients with localized MF. Lastly, most skin-directed treatments for CTCL achieve a peak clinical response after several months, so it may be useful to try more extended PDT regimens in patients with a partial response.

CONCLUSION

In conclusion, PDT is a promising but under-researched second-line treatment option for localized MF plaques. The most common PDT regimen for MF is MAL 20%, occlusion for 3 h, 630 nm light, and 37.5 J/cm^2 dosage. However, protocols have varied across studies. PDT is particularly useful for isolated plaques that have been recalcitrant to prior therapies, for targeted treatment of specific sites such as the skin folds, or for treatment of sensitive areas such as the face. PDT is not suited to treatment of large or disseminated plaques or tumors. Additional large-scale prospective clinical studies are needed to clarify the most effective treatment regimens for PDT.

REFERENCES

1. Vonderheid EC, Tan ET, Kantor AF, Shrager L, Micaily B, Van Scott EJ. Long-term efficacy, curative potential, and carcinogenicity of topical mechlorethamine chemotherapy in cutaneous T cell lymphoma. *J Am Acad Dermatol.* 1989;20(3):416–428.
2. Hasan T, Ortel B, Solban N, Pogue B. Photodynamic therapy of cancer. *Cancer Med.* 2003;7:537–548.
3. Salva KA, Wood GS. Epigenetically enhanced photodynamic therapy (ePDT) is superior to conventional photodynamic therapy for inducing apoptosis in cutaneous T-cell lymphoma. *Photochem Photobiol.* 2015;91(6):1444–1451.
4. Fien SM, Oseroff AR. Photodynamic therapy for non-melanoma skin cancer. *J Natl Compr Canc Netw.* 2007;5(5):531–540.
5. Boehncke WH, König K, Rück A, Kaufmann R, Sterry W. In vitro and in vivo effects of photodynamic therapy in cutaneous T cell lymphoma. *Acta Derm Venereol.* 1994;74(3):201–205.
6. Rittenhouse-Diakun K, Van Leengoed H, Morgan J, et al. The role of transferrin receptor (CD71) in photodynamic therapy of activated and malignant lymphocytes using the heme precursor δ-aminolevulinic acid (ALA). *Photochem Photobiol.* 1995;61(5):523–528.
7. Wu J, Nihal M, Siddiqui J, Vonderheid EC, Wood GS. Low FAS/CD95 expression by CTCL correlates with reduced sensitivity to apoptosis that can be restored by FAS upregulation. *J Invest Dermatol.* 2009;129(5):1165–1173.
8. Svanberg K, Andersson T, Killander D, et al. Photodynamic therapy of non-melanoma malignant tumours of the skin using topical δ-amino levulinic acid sensitization and laser irradiation. *Br J Dermatol.* 1994;130(6):743–751.
9. Calzavara-Pinton PG, Venturini M, Sala R. Photodynamic therapy: update 2006 part 1: photochemistry and photobiology. *J Eur Acad Dermatol Venereol.* 2007;21(3):293–302.
10. Rook AH, Wood GS, Duvic M, Vonderheid EC, Tobia A, Cabana B. A phase II placebo-controlled study of photodynamic therapy with topical hypericin and visible light irradiation in the treatment of cutaneous T-cell lymphoma and psoriasis. *J Am Acad Dermatol.* 2010;63(6):984–990.
11. Kim EJ, Mangold AR, DeSimone JA, et al. Efficacy and safety of topical hypericin photodynamic therapy for early-stage cutaneous T-cell lymphoma (Mycosis Fungoides): the FLASH phase 3 randomized clinical trial. *JAMA Dermatol.* 2022;158(9):1031–1039.
12. Coors EA, von den Driesch P. Topical photodynamic therapy for patients with therapy-resistant lesions of cutaneous T-cell lymphoma. *J Am Acad Dermatol.* 2004;50(3):363–367.
13. Edström DW, Hedblad M-A. Long-term follow-up of photodynamic therapy for mycosis fungoides. *Acta dermato-venereologica.* 2008;88(3):288–290.
14. Han D, Xue J, Wang T, Liu Y. Observation of clinical efficacy of photodynamic therapy in 3 patients with refractory plaque-stage mycosis fungoides. *Photodiagnosis and Photodynamic therapy.* 2016;16:9–11.
15. Severson KJ, Cumsky HJL, Brumfiel CM, et al. Blue light photodynamic therapy with 5-aminolevulinic acid in refractory mycosis fungoides: a prospective, open-label study. *J Am Acad Dermatol.* 2021;85(4):969–971.
16. Oseroff AR, Whitaker J, Conti C, et al. Effects of fluence and intensity in PDT of cutaneous T-cell lymphoma with topical ALA: high intensities spare the epidermis. *J Investig Dermatol.* 1996;106(4):950.
17. Debu A, Girard C, Kluger N, Guillot B. Dereure O. "Topical methyl aminolaevulinate–photodynamic therapy in erosive facial mycosis fungoides. *Br J Dermatol.* 2010;163(4):884–885.
18. Zane C, et al. Photodynamic therapy with methylaminolevulinate as a valuable treatment option for unilesional cutaneous T-cell lymphoma. *Photodermatology, photoimmunology & photomedicine.* 2006;22(5):254–258.
19. Fernandez-Guarino M, et al. Plaque-phase mycosis fungoides treated with photodynamic therapy: results from 12 patients. *Actas Dermo-Sifiliográficas (English Edition).* 2010;101(9):785–791.
20. Kim ST, et al. Photodynamic therapy with methyl-aminolaevulinic acid for mycosis fungoides. *Acta dermato-venereologica.* 2012;92(3):264–268.
21. Calzavara-Pinton PG, Rossi MT, Sala R. A retrospective analysis of real-life practice of off-label photodynamic therapy using methyl aminolevulinate (MAL-PDT) in 20

Italian dermatology departments. Part 2: oncologic and infectious indications. *Photochemical & Photobiological Sciences.* 2012;12(1):158–165.
22. Quéreux G, et al. Photodynamic therapy with methyl-aminolevulinic acid for paucilesional mycosis fungoides: a prospective open study and review of the literature. *Journal of the American Academy of Dermatology.* 2013;69(6):890–897.
23. Pileri A, Sgubbi P, Agostinelli C, Infusino SD, Vaccari S, Patrizi A. Photodynamic therapy: an option in mycosis fungoides. *Photodiagnosis Photodyn Ther.* 2017;20:107–110.
24. Jang MS, et al. Folliculotropic mycosis fungoides in 20 Korean cases: clinical and histopathologic features and response to ultraviolet A-1 and/or photodynamic therapy. *Annals of Dermatology.* 2018;30(2):192–201.
25. Dairi M, et al. Localized mycosis fungoides treated with laser-assisted photodynamic therapy: a case series. *Clinical and Experimental Dermatology.* 2019; 44(8):930–932.
26. Tarabadkar ES, Shinohara MM. Skin directed therapy in cutaneous T-cell lymphoma. *Front Oncol.* 2019;9:260.
27. Kim ST, Kang DY, Kang JS, Baek JW, Jeon YS, Suh KS. Photodynamic therapy with methyl-aminolaevulinic acid for mycosis fungoides. *Acta Derm Venereol.* 2012;92(3):264–268.
28. Quéreux G, Brocard A, Saint-Jean M, et al. Photodynamic therapy with methyl-aminolevulinic acid for paucilesional mycosis fungoides: a prospective open study and review of the literature. *J Am Acad Dermatol.* 2013;69(6):890–897.
29. Baron ED, Malbasa CL, Santo-Domingo D, et al. Silicon phthalocyanine (Pc 4) photodynamic therapy is a safe modality for cutaneous neoplasms: results of a phase 1 clinical trial. *Lasers Surg Med.* 2010;42(10):728–735.
30. Heald P, Mehlmauer M, Martin AG, et al. Topical bexarotene therapy for patients with refractory or persistent early-stage cutaneous T-cell lymphoma: results of the phase III clinical trial. *J Am Acad Dermatol.* 2003;49(5):801–815.
31. Röder B. Photodynamic therapy. In *Encyclopedia of Analytical Chemistry: Applications, Theory and Instrumentation*; Wiley. 2006.

12

Photodynamic Therapy for Cutaneous Vascular Lesions

Kristen M. Kelly, Rachel Elsanadi

KEY POINTS

- Pulsed-dye laser (PDL) is currently the first-line treatment for port-wine birthmarks (PWB).
- Photodynamic therapy (PDT) is widely studied and may be as useful as PDL or an effective option for PDL-resistant lesions.
- PDT for PWB is associated with a photosensitive period duration of a week or more.
- In angiosarcoma, PDT is investigative but may be considered in life-threatening cases.

OBJECTIVES

- Learn how PDT has been used for cutaneous vascular conditions especially port-wine birthmarks and angiosarcoma.
- Acquire knowledge about studies evaluating PDT and comparing PDT and PDL for port-wine birthmarks.
- Learn about side effects observed with PDT for cutaneous vascular lesions.

INTRODUCTION

Photodynamic therapy (PDT) involves administration of a photosensitizer followed by irradiation with visible light, which results in excitation of the photosensitizer and subsequent formation of reactive oxygen species (ROS) (Fig. 12.1).[1,2] PDT has been utilized to treat a variety of benign, premalignant, and malignant conditions.[3] These conditions commonly include actinic keratoses and skin cancers.[3] PDT has also been evaluated for the treatment of vascular conditions, such as port-wine birthmarks (PWB), infantile hemangiomas (IHs), and angiosarcoma.

The ROS form free radicals which, when targeting vascular lesions, can achieve endothelial cell destruction and vessel wall damage.[1,4] This method of tissue injury is different from heat-induced tissue injury, such as pulsed-dye laser (PDL)-mediated selective photothermolysis, which is currently the gold-standard treatment for cutaneous vascular conditions such as PWB in the United States (US).[5] While laser-based treatment, especially PDL, can often achieve excellent results, some patients have resistant conditions, multiple treatments are required, and maintenance is needed. In addition, PDL is less effective and has a higher risk of adverse effects in more melanated skin types because light is also absorbed by melanin at the dermal-epidermal junction.[1,4] Therefore PDT may be a useful alternative to PDL in such patients.[4]

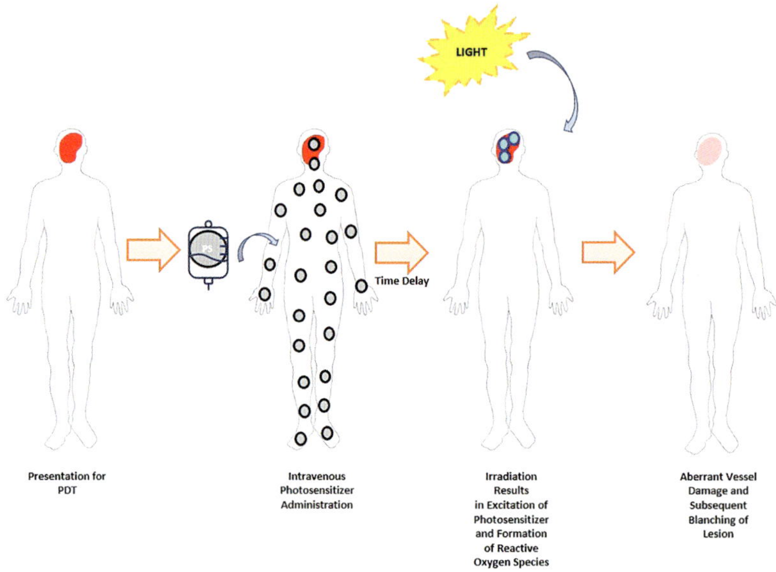

Fig. 12.1 Photodynamic therapy (PDT) protocol.

PDT photosensitizers may be applied topically or delivered systemically (orally or intravenously).[1,2] However, PDT for treatment of cutaneous vascular lesions often involves systemic administration of photosensitizers to achieve peak concentrations in the vessels and induce vascular thrombosis and vessel closure.[1–5] This chapter will review PDT for cutaneous vascular lesion treatment.

PORT-WINE BIRTHMARKS

PWB are congenital capillary malformations occurring in 0.3%–0.5% of infants.[1,2] They are often found on the face and neck but can occur anywhere on the body.[2,4] Without treatment, PWB may evolve over time, darkening or thickening with age, and developing nodules.[2,4] This can cause a decrease in quality of life for patients, due to psychosocial issues and social stigma.[1,2,4] Moreover, hypertrophy and hyperplasia of PWB can be associated with medical complications, such as spontaneous bleeding and impairment of essential functions, including eating.[2]

PDL is the current standard-of-care intervention for PWB in the US; however, less than 20% completely resolve with PDL and up to 30% have been reported in some studies to be unresponsive to treatment.[2,4] Furthermore, some recurrence following PDL treatment of PWB is common.[1] PDL is also known to be less effective in darker skin types due to dermal-epidermal junction melanin absorption inhibiting penetration of therapeutic light to the targeted vessels.[1,6]

PDT is a treatment both under investigation and in use for PWB. Most clinical studies of PDT have been carried out in Southeast Asia (predominately, China). The premise for efficacy of PDT is that photosensitizer in vessels, especially the dilated and ectatic vessels of PWB, when irradiated with the appropriate wavelengths of light, generates ROS.[4] These cause injury to dermal vessels, diminishing the characteristic lesion erythema.[4]

Numerous studies of PDT for PWB have been conducted. The vast majority of clinical studies involve systemic administration of photosensitizer. Hematoporphyrin monomethyl ether (HMME) has been used most commonly and was approved by the National Medical Products Administration (formerly known as the Chinese Food and Drug Administration) for treatment of PWB in 2016.[4] Prior to approval of HMME, a number of other photosensitizers were investigated and this will be reviewed very briefly.

Topical ALA-PDT is used commonly in dermatology to treat skin cancers and precancerous lesions; however, as noted earlier, topical ALA does not concentrate in the vessels, limiting its utility for treatment of vascular lesions. In an animal model study performed on the rooster comb by Lai and colleagues, topical red-light PDT resulted in erosion and scabs, while systemic red-light PDT with ALA resulted in epidermal necrosis and scar formation.[7] It was concluded that both topical and systemic ALA are not suitable options for PWB treatment.[7]

Photocarcinorin (PsD-007), a first-generation photosensitizer, was investigated for PWB treatment and found to be moderately efficacious; however, it has a very long half-life (>30 h), resulting in significant treatment reactions and requiring patients to avoid direct sunlight for around 4–8 weeks after treatment.[4,8] Han and colleagues conducted long-term follow-up of PsD-007 (4–7 mg/kg) PDT (532 nm laser, 80–90 mW/cm^2) for 13 patients of skin types III and IV ranging between 1 and 23 years old (mean 10.1 years) with facial PWB.[9] In the average follow-up period of 7.1 years, it was found that 30.77% experienced "excellent" (>75% clearance) color blanching, and 23.08% experienced "good" improvement (51%–75% clearance) with no evidence of recurrence.[8]

Half-life of HMME is much shorter (1.5 h) and HMME is reported to be better tolerated by patients.[4] Efficacy of HMME in animal models has been documented both in vitro and in vivo. Mei and colleagues used human umbilical vein endothelial cells (HUVECs) incubated both with and without HMME and irradiated with a 532 nm light source and found that phototoxicity was dose-dependent. They also documented that apoptotic factors were induced and pro-angiogenic factors were reduced, and hypothesized that PDT could result in less recurrence of PWB.[10]

A retrospective study by Ma and colleagues of PDT for PWB comparing PsD-007 (5 mg/kg, intravenously over 5 min; 532 nm laser applied continuously starting as soon as the injection started for 25–30 min at an energy density of 80–90 mW/cm^2) to HMME (5 mg/kg, intravenously over 20 min; 532 nm laser applied continuously starting 10 min after infusion of HMME initiated at an energy density of 80–90 mW/cm^2) found no significant difference in efficacy (assessed visually and by chromometer) or adverse effects.[4] However, patients were required to avoid "strong light exposure" to prevent photosensitivity for 30–60 days in the PsD-007 group compared to 14–30 days in the HMME group.[4] Mild-to-moderate hyperpigmentation (but no hypopigmentation) occurred irrespective of group which resolved within 2 months and there were no cases of scarring reported.[4]

Current Clinical Protocols for Utilization of HMME-PDT to Treat PWB

There is no established or agreed-upon PDT treatment protocol for PWB (Table 12.1) and PDT is currently not performed routinely and actually, rarely if at all, in the US. In studies from China, a number of protocols have been reported. We summarize some guidelines as follows: On treatment day, prior to intravenous administration of photosensitizer, some treatment protocols

TABLE 12.1 Ranges of Reported PDT Settings Over the Past Decade in Studies Using 532 nm Irradiation of PWB[1–4,6,8,11–26]

Type of Photosensitizer	Dosage	Duration of Administration of Photosensitizer	Administration Method	Energy	Fluence	Duration of Irradiation
HMME	2.5–7.5 mg/kg[a,b]	5–20 min	Intravenous	75–110 mW/cm^2[c]	80–190 J/cm^2[d]	15–30 min
PsD-007	4–7 mg/kg	2–20 min	Intravenous	80–100 mW/cm^2	96–180 J/cm[d]	20–60 min[e]

[a]5 mg/kg is typically used.
[b]2.5 mg/kg utilized as the "low dose" in one phase IIb clinical trial to compare to "high dose" of 5 mg/kg. Dosage of HMME was increased by 0.5 mg/kg each to a maximum of 7.5 mg/kg in one study if patients did not respond initially to 5 mg/kg.
[c]Typically 80–100 mW/cm^2, although some studies use a range of 75–95 mW/cm^2.
[d]1 Watt = 1 Joule/second.
[e]Typically 25–30 min. 60 min in only one study.

require negative skin allergy test to photosensitizer.[7,11–15] Laboratory tests, such as hepatic and renal function tests, and electrocardiogram (ECG) may be performed. Areas of the lesion to be irradiated are typically marked and the surrounding normal skin is covered with black cloth. Photosensitizer is then administered intravenously; as discussed previously, various photosensitizers have been documented, however, HMME (typically at a dose of 5 mg/kg) is most commonly utilized (Table 12.1). The delineated lesion area is then continuously irradiated, in some cases after a brief delay between conclusion of photosensitizer administration and initiation of light. Irradiation occurs for a set period of time, most commonly with a 532 nm green light laser as the source (Table 12.1). Duration of irradiation is variable. Active cooling during treatment, sometimes with skin temperature monitoring, and cool compresses or ice immediately following the conclusion of irradiation have been utilized and may help prevent skin damage.[8] There is no well-defined observable endpoint of treatment, and this limits safety. In some studies, skin swelling or darkening, color fading, or appearance of petechiae have reportedly been used as an endpoint.[6,13]

Treatments require pain control. Studies have reported use of topical anesthetics, such as lidocaine, or general anesthesia for children and other populations with difficulty tolerating pain.[11]

Side effects can occur, and patients should be monitored in postoperative weeks as the treatment site is healing. Skin swelling, color fading, or darkening of treatment area, and petechiae may occur during treatment, while post-treatment reactions may most commonly include edema and scabbing.[13] Phototoxicity occurs in all patients and blistering may occur in the interim after treatment. Long-term adverse effects, though reported less commonly, may include permanent pigmentation changes or scarring.[13]

Clinical Data of PWB Treatment With PDT

A number of published studies from China looked at the safety and efficacy of PDT for PWB. We summarize several studies below which exemplify the body of work.

Zhao and colleagues performed the first large phase 3 randomized, double-blind, placebo-controlled clinical trial investigating the efficacy and safety of HMME-PDT in 440 adolescent and adult patients of skin types III and IV with PWB. Patients were randomized to receive either HMME (5 mg/kg, intravenously) or normal saline (placebo, intravenously) in a 3:1 ratio.[1] Ten minutes after the initiation of the infusion of photosensitizer, clinicians administered 532 nm laser irradiation (96–120 J/cm^2) to a 7 cm diameter area or less for 20 min.[1] A second treatment with HMME was performed in all subjects 2 months after the initial intervention.[1] Follow-up occurred within a week after each treatment and 2 months after the second treatment.[1] At 8 weeks, the PDT-HMME group had significantly higher rates of efficacy compared to the placebo group: 89.7% of HMME subjects showed "at least some improvement" (defined as ≥20% color blanching) versus 24.5% of patients in the placebo group, 43.5% of HMME subjects showed "at least great improvement" (defined as ≥60% color blanching) versus 0.9% of placebo patients, and 11.2% of patients' PWB "completely resolved" (defined as ≥90% color blanching) versus 0.0% of placebo patients.[1] Patients who received two successive HMME-PDT treatments compared with patients who received one placebo and one HMME treatment also had significantly higher efficacy at 16 weeks: "at least some improvement," 97.4% versus 90.1%, "at least great improvement," 64.0% versus 42.6%, and "complete resolution," 28.1% versus 6.9%.[1] At week 8, the hypertrophic type of PWB was significantly less likely to achieve "at least some improvement."[1] Patients in the HMME group were significantly more likely to rate their appearance as "good" to "excellent" at both 8 and 16 weeks.[1] Edema was the most common treatment reaction in the HMME group, and there were significantly higher levels of edema in patients treated twice and significantly lower levels of crusting.[1] There were also significantly higher levels of hyperpigmentation (22.99%) in the HMME group, which did not occur in any of the placebo group patients; however, this resolved in all patients.[1] There was no significant difference in hypopigmentation (1.9% vs. 0%, HMME and placebo, respectively) or scarring (0.5% vs. 0%, respectively) between the groups.[1]

Wu and colleagues conducted a phase IIb randomized, double-blind clinical trial to study optimal dosing of HMME in PDT in 100 subjects.[6] In the first stage, patients were randomized at a 2:2:1 ratio to receive either high-dose HMME (5 mg/kg), low-dose HMME (2.5 mg/kg), or placebo (normal saline) intravenously over a 20-min period.[6] Ten minutes after photosensitizer infusion, investigators delivered 20 min of irradiation with a 532 nm Nd-YAG laser (80–100 mW/cm^2).[6] In the second stage, 8 weeks after initial treatment, patients, including those who had received placebo, were randomized to receive a second PDT treatment with either high- or low-dose HMME. Assessment of photographs to determine efficacy (color blanching) was performed 8 weeks after each treatment.[6] Efficacy results for the high-dose, low-dose, and placebo groups at 8 weeks after the first treatment were are as follows, respectively: "no improvement" (defined as <20% color blanching), 25.0% versus 60.0% versus 85.0%; "some improvement" (defined as 20%–59% color blanching), 35.0% versus 37.5% versus 15.0%; "great improvement" (defined as 60%–89% color blanching); 35.0% versus 2.0% versus 0%; and "complete resolution" (defined as ≥90% color blanching), 5% versus 0% versus 0%.[6] Patients in the high-dose group experienced a significantly higher incidence of reaching "at least some" or "at least great improvement" (≥20% or ≥60% improvement, respectively) compared to the low-dose group.[6] In the low-dose group, there were no statistically significant differences in efficacy from control. In the high-dose group, pink-type PWB experienced a higher (but non-statistically significant) level of improvement compared to purple or hypertrophic types.[6] Patients and investigators subjective satisfaction was significantly higher in the high-dose group as compared to low-dose and control groups after the first stage of treatment.[6] Low-dose satisfaction was also higher than in the control group.[6] There were also significantly higher levels of adverse events in the high-dose group compared to the low-dose group, with hyperpigmentation being the most common (46.0% vs. 14.3%).[6] Most cases are resolved within 3–6 months.[6] Only one patient in the high-dose group experienced hypopigmentation, and none in the low-dose group.[6] Scarring incidence was not reported.[6]

Another phase IIb study was performed by Tang and colleagues to evaluate associations between treatment efficacy and adverse reactions.[2] Fifty adolescent and adult patients were randomized to receive either 5 mg/kg HMME ($n = 38$) or placebo (normal saline, $n = 12$) intravenously over 20 min, followed by irradiation with a 532 nm laser light source (80–100 mw/cm^2) starting 10 min after the onset of the injection of photosensitizer and continuing until the administration of photosensitizer was finished.[2] Then, all patients, whether or not they had previously been administered placebo, received HMME for a second treatment 8 weeks later.[2] Patients were seen for follow-up both twice within the first week and once 8 weeks following each treatment.[2] There were significantly higher rates of treatment reactions in the HMME group, although some patients in the placebo group who had received normal saline followed by laser irradiation did experience pain (8.33%) and burning (16.67%) during treatment.[2] Younger patients tended to have significantly worse swelling, and, after the first treatment, the incidence of pruritis and scabbing were significantly higher, the further the treatment area was from the face.[2] Significantly less burning sensation was experienced by patients during the second HMME-PDT treatment, and scabs formed significantly less and healed significantly faster than after the first HMME-PDT treatment.[2] Pain peaked at 20 min after irradiation.[2] Onset of treatment site reaction was the same between the first and second treatments.[2] In terms of efficacy, scab, and pain severity at 5 min were positively correlated with treatment efficacy.[2] Pruritis, which only occurred in the HMME-PDT group, was positively correlated with scabbing and investigators hypothesized this may lead to scarring.[2] Incidence of hyperpigmentation, hypopigmentation, and scarring were not reported.[2]

PDT has also been studied in pediatric patients.[11] Chun-hua and colleagues retrospectively investigated outcomes in 439 children aged 1–14 years who received HMME-PDT (5 mg/kg, intravenously over an undefined period of time).[11] Up to 10 × 10 cm of affected skin was subsequently continuously irradiated with a 532 nm laser light source (96–115 J/cm^2) for 20–25 min, not exceeding a temperature of 40°C, and energy density was increased by 5 J/cm^2 each session if no response was produced.[11] Topical lidocaine was applied to the area to be irradiated; however, if patients were anxious, general anesthesia was offered and 80% was accepted.[11] Patients were followed up by telephone or in-person within the first 2 weeks, and again at 8 weeks in-person following treatment.[11] Efficacy was assessed by color blanching: 34.2% of PWB "completely resolved" (defined as ≥90% fading), 40.1% showed "great improvement" (defined as 60%–89% improved), and 20.9% showed "some improvement" (defined as 20%–59% improved), and PDT was "ineffective" in 4.8% (defined as <20% improvement).[11] There were significantly higher levels of efficacy on the face and neck compared to trunk and limbs.[11] There was no difference in response between medial and lateral cheek.[11] Red and pink lesions and multiple treatments were associated with significantly higher levels of efficacy.[11] Receiving more than one treatment also resulted in higher efficacy.[11] Edema occurred in 98% of patients with head and neck as compared to 78% of trunk and extremity PWB, and resolved by 3–5 days post treatment.[11] Pigmentation changes (hyper or hypopigmentation) affected two-thirds of patients but were reported to resolve within 2–6 months.[11] Atrophic scars occurred in eight patients with an onset of 2–4 weeks post treatment and were reported to improve over time.[11]

Li and colleagues retrospectively investigated HMME-PDT (5 mg/kg, intravenously) for treatment of 19 PWB in Sturge-Weber Syndrome patients and 33 patients with large segmental facial PWB (defined in this study as a PWB that encompassed at ≥75% of the hemifacial V1 or V2 distribution).[17] Photosensitizer was administered over a period of 20 min; then, patients were irradiated with a 532 nm light source for 20–25 min (80–95 mW/cm^2) approximately 10 min into the intravenous administration of photosensitizer.[17] Two treatments were given and follow-up occurred in-person 8 weeks after each.[17] Efficacy assessed from photographs by three independent investigators in patients with SWS versus patients with large segmental facial PWB was as follows: "poor" (defined as ≤24% color blanching), 47.4% versus 30.3%; "fair" (defined as 25%–49% color blanching), 36.8% versus 27.3%; "good" (defined as 50%–74% color blanching), 5.3% versus 24.2%; and "excellent" (defined as ≥75% color blanching), 10.5% versus 18.2%.[13] There were no significant differences in efficacy in patients with SWS compared to large segmental PWB.[17] Edema and pain were extremely common treatment reactions among both groups, occurring in most patients (edema, 100% of SWS patients and 98.5% of large segmental patients; pain, 100% of patients in both groups).[17] Hyperpigmentation occurred in 57.9% of SWS patients and 53.0% of patients with large segmental facial PWB and took on the order of months to improve; scarring occurred in one patient in the SWS group.[17]Hypopigmentation incidence was not reported.[17]

HMME-PDT for PWB With Alternative Light Sources Other Than 532 nm

Although the vast majority of recent studies of HMME-PDT for the treatment of PWB have investigated a 532 nm laser as a source of irradiation, other light sources have been tested, including a copper vapor laser and 535 nm laser.[13,27] A retrospective study of treatment reactions and adverse effects in 700 patients who had been treated with HMME-PDT (3.5 mg/kg in children, 4–5 mg/kg in adults; intravenously), with either a copper vapor (wavelength peaks at 510.6 and 578.2 nm; 80–100 mW/cm^2, $n = 606$) or with a 532 nm laser (80–100 mW/cm^2, $n = 94$) as the therapeutic light source, was performed by Yuan and colleagues.[13] The duration over which the photosensitizer was administered was unspecified. Irradiation occurred for 20–25 min immediately after photosensitizer injection.[13] In the 532 nm compared to the copper laser group, a non-statistically significant lower incidence of scarring (1% vs. 3%) and blistering (2% vs. 5%) was observed in the 532 nm group at 2-month follow-up post treatment.[13] Edema occurred in all patients, reaching a maximum on day 2 and resolving by day 3–5.[13] Hyperpigmentation and hypopigmentation occurred in 5% and 1% of patients, respectively, and resolved without treatment within a reported 3–6 month period.[13] Scarring also occurred in 1%–3% of patients; scars were primarily hypertrophic and hypothesized to be due to overtreatment (photosensitizer and/or light) and improper scab handling.[13]

Another case series utilizing HMME (5 mg/kg, intravenously over an unknown duration) and a 535 nm green light laser (20 min of irradiation, 95 mW/cm^2) in two pediatric patients (1.5 and 3 years) to treat pink facial PWB was reported by Zhang and colleagues.[27] The duration between photosensitizer administration and irradiation was not stated.[27] Authors detailed complete clearance of lesions after 2–3 treatments with no evidence of recurrence two years post treatment and with no long-term adverse effects.[27]

PDT Versus PDL for Treatment of PWB

PDL is currently the gold-standard treatment of PWB in the US and there have been studies in China that have directly compared PDL and PDT to evaluate respective efficacies.[28,29] Gao and colleagues ($n = 15$) performed a side-by-side comparison of PDL and PDT by splitting each PWB into two parts.[28] A 585 nm PDL (pulse duration of 300–450 μs, spot size 5 mm, no dynamic epidermal cooling and ice bag for 30 min after treatment) was used to treat one-half of the PWB and HMME-PDT (5 mg/kg, intravenous over an unknown duration; irradiation for 20 min after completion of the injection; 510.6 and 578.2 nm, 100 mW/cm^2) was used to treat the other half.[28] It is important to note that PDL without epidermal cooling is suboptimal and results must be interpreted with this in mind.[28] Colorimetric evidence at 2-month follow-up, performed by chromometer, indicated that there were statistically significant differences in the blanching rate 2 months post initial treatment in all PWB: For red, blanching rates for PDL were between −11% and 24% and between 22% and 55% for PDT after a single session.[28] In $n = 6$ purple PWB, four patients had an 8%–33% blanching rate with PDL and 30%–45% with PDT; two patients of skin type IV did not respond to either treatment.[28] Visual evaluation of photographs by independent evaluators only found statistically higher significant difference in response to PDT versus PDL (measured as blanching) in red PWB 2 months after treatment.[28] Scoring scale for clearance response was as follows: 1 = no clearance; 2, poor (<25% clearance); 3, fair (25%–50% clearance); 4, good (51%–75% clearance); 5, excellent (>75% clearance).[28] In red PWB, 33.3% of PWB responded to PDL (score 2) while 100% responded to PDT (score 2–3.7), while in purple PWB, 50% of PWB responded to PDL (score 1.4–2) and 66.7% responded to PDT (score 2–3).[28]

Zhang and colleagues ($n = 260$) retrospectively evaluated blanching rate in 532 nm (80–100 mW/cm^2) HMME-PDT (3.5 mg/kg, intravenously; irradiation delivered for 20–25 min immediately after injection of photosensitizer) and 585 nm PDL without dynamic cooling (fluence between 4.8 and 6.5 J/cm^2; pulse duration unspecified; spot size between 5 and 7 mm) for flat facial PWB in pediatric patients.[29] Post-treatment cooling was conducted with an "ice-cold bag" placed on skin for an undefined duration of time.[29] Efficacy results for PDL compared to PDT were as follows: "no response," 2.3% versus 2.3%; "poor" (defined as blanching <25%), 8.6% versus 7.6%; "fair" (defined as 25%–50% blanching), 32.8% versus 19.7%; "good" (defined as blanching 51%–75%), 45.3% versus 45.5%; and "excellent" (defined as >75% blanching), 10.9% versus 25.0%. They found that the rate of "excellent" blanching (defined as >75% color blanching) was significantly higher in the PDT compared to the PDL group (25.0% vs. 10.9%, respectively), although there was no overall statistically significant difference in response (89.1% vs. 90.2%, respectively).[29] Overall response was significantly higher in purple lesions in the PDT group.[29] There was also an overall significantly lower incidence of scarring, hyperpigmentation, and hypopigmentation in the PDT group (21.1% in PDL group and 8.3% in PDT group).[29] To elaborate, there were 14 cases (10.9%) of hyperpigmentation in the PDL group and five (3.8%) in the PDT group; seven cases (5.5%) of hypopigmentation in the PDL group and two (1.5%) in the PDT group; and there were six cases (4.7%) of scarring in the PDL group and four (3%) in the PDT group.[29] When analyzed by color of PWB, both purple and red lesions had significantly higher incidence of adverse effects in the PDL group compared to PDT, however, within the PDL group, there was no significant difference in incidence by color of PWB.[29] Authors of this study hypothesized that these results indicate that PDL may indeed result in greater risk of adverse effects, although again, it is very important to note that suboptimal epidermal cooling was used with PDL.[29]

Combination of PDT and PDL for Treatment of PWB

Our center has conducted research on combination of PDT and PDL (PDT + PDL) for PWB treatment.[30] Four test sites were treated in each subject. One site was a control that was not treated, the second site was treated with PDL (585 nm, 7 mm spot size, 8 J/cm^2, 30 ms cryogen spurt with a 20 ms delay), the third site was treated with PDT, and the fourth with PDT + PDL.[30] For PDT in site 3, liposomal benzoporphyrin derivative monoacid ring A (BPD-MA) photosensitizer was intravenously administered (6 mg/m^2 delivered in a total volume of 30 mL) over a 10-min period, followed by irradiation with an argon pumped dye laser (576 nm, 100 mW/cm^2) 15 min after the start of the 10-min infusion.[30] Radiant exposures varied by subjects: two subjects each received 15, 30, 45, 60, and 75 J/cm^2; one subject received 90 J/cm^2 (Table 12.2). For the fourth site, PDT was performed first, then PDL.[30] Visually, there was increased efficacy (blanching) of the PDT + PDL group compared to PDL alone, specifically at exposures of 75 J/cm^2 and above, but no long-term improved efficacy was clearly achieved with the combined treatment.[30] BPD-MA has a photosensitivity period of 5 days in humans, and no photosensitive reactions were reported.[30] Treatment reactions included fine scabbing and mild temporary hyperpigmentation at locations treated with PDL.[30] PDT + PDL may offer a synergistic and safe blanching effect on PWB but further research is required.[30]

PDT for Treatment of PDL-Resistant PWB

Multiple studies have been conducted on efficacy of PDT for treating PDL-resistant PWB.[3,16] Zhang and colleagues conducted two sessions of PDT (HMME, 5 mg/kg intravenously over 20 min; irradiation with

TABLE 12.2 Data on Settings from a Proof-Of-Concept, Tolerance, and Safety Dose-Ranging Study Comparing Treatment With Pulsed-Dye Laser (PDL), Photodynamic Therapy (PDT), and Combination PDL + of PDT for Skin Affected by Port-Wine Birthmark[30]

PULSED-DYE LASER PARAMETERS							
Wavelength	**Spot Size**	**Radiant Exposure**	**Cooling**				
585 nm	7 mm	8 J/cm^2	30 ms cryogen spurt with a 20 ms delay				
PHOTODYNAMIC THERAPY PARAMETERS							
Type of Photosensitizer	**Dosage**	**Duration of Administration of Photosensitizer**	**Administration Method**	**Wavelength**	**Energy**	**Fluence**	**Duration of Irradiation**
Verteporfin[a]	6 mg/m^2	10 min	Intravenous	576 nm	100 mW/cm^2	Increasing exposures by increasing duration of laser exposure[b]	Dependent on goal fluence

[a]Liposomal benzoporphyrin derivative monoacid ring A.

[b]Two subjects each received increasing radiant exposure of 15, 30, 45, 60, and 75 J/cm^2 while one subject received a radiant exposure of 90 J/ cm^2.

532 nm LED green light performed 10 min after start of HMME infusion for 20–25 min; mean power density of 80–95 mW/cm^2) for 31 adult patients with facial PWB with history of at least five PDL treatments who had not experienced further blanching since their last treatment.[16] Patients were majority (90.3%) skin type IV, and the remainder were type III.[16] After two treatments compared to one treatment, responses were as follows: "no improvement" (defined as <20% fading), 0% versus 4%; "some improvement" (defined as 20–59% fading), 38.7% versus 58.1%; "great improvement" (defined as 60%–89% fading), 61.3% versus 29.0%; and "almost cured" (defined as ≥90% fading), 0% versus 0%. Two treatments had significantly greater efficacy than one session.[16] Treatment reactions included pruritus (88.7%), burning (100%), edema (100%), purpura (80.6%), and crusting (77.4%).[16] Hyperpigmentation (41.9%) faded after 3–6 months, and hypopigmentation and scarring did not occur.[16] Investigators hypothesized that repeated treatments of lesions refractory to PDL may result in improvement, although no lesions were completely cured.[16]

PDT for PDL-resistant PWB has also been investigated in children.[3] Zhang and colleagues performed one treatment of PDT (HMME, 5 mg/kg intravenously over 20 min; irradiation with 532 nm LED green light 5–10 min after photosensitizer administration for 20 min; power density of 80–100 mW/cm^2) for 107 children and two treatments for 65 patients (average age 4.82 years).[3] All patients had been previously treated with at least five PDL sessions and had not improved with the most recent two treatments.[3] After two treatment sessions compared to one treatment session, visually assessed efficacy was as follows: "no improvement" (defined as color fading <20%), 2% versus 12%; "moderate improvement" (defined as color fading 20%–59%), 30% versus 60%; "good improvement" (defined as color fading 60%–89%), 19% versus 25%; and "excellent improvement" (defined as color fading ≥90%), 14% versus 10%.[3] The difference was statistically significant.[3] Younger-aged children experienced better levels of efficacy, along with patients with lateral facial and pink PWB.[3] After a mean follow-up duration of 21.3 months, no patients had recurrence.[3] Edema occurred in all patients, along with thin crusting (36.4%), one hypertrophic scar (0.9%), and hyperpigmentation (9.3%) which resolved within 3–6 months.[3] There were no cases of hypopigmentation reported.[3]

Adverse Effects of PDT in PWB Treatment

PDT for PWB may result in significant treatment reactions and adverse effects.[13] Post-treatment edema is the most commonly reported treatment reaction.[13] In most studies, it has been reported to onset by day 2–3 and resolve by days 3–7.[13,31] Other commonly reported treatment reactions include scabbing, crusting, congestion, pain, burning, pruritis, color change, and petechiae. Per Yuan and colleagues short-term complications included blistering, eczema, and phototoxicity, and long-term scarring and hyper/hypopigmentation were seen.[13]

A major difficulty in utilizing PDT for treating PWB is the prolonged photosensitive period. Depending on the photosensitizer, patients may need to avoid sunlight and strong indoor light for up to 2 months in PsD-007 and two weeks in HMME. Exposure to sunlight too soon following treatment may result in swelling, redness, and itching.[17]

PDT can have dangerous results if cooling is not employed immediately after treatment.[32] Therefore patients who are unable to tolerate cold compresses immediately after treatment may make poor candidates for PDT.[32] A case report (reported by Chen and colleagues) of a 5-year-old male patient with Sturge-Weber Syndrome and developmental delay described skin necrosis in the treated facial area following HMME-PDT, possibly due to the cold compress not being applied after treatment as was routine.[32] He eventually developed superimposed infection with methicillin-resistant *Staphylococcus aureus*, which required debridement and skin grafting and significant scarring resulted.[32]

PDT FOR INFANTILE HEMANGIOMAS

Infantile hemangiomas (IH) occur in up to 5% of infants. Their typical course involves appearance within the first few weeks of life, followed by rapid proliferation.[9,33] Maximal size is generally achieved by 3–6 months, with a reported 80% of size obtained by 3 months.[9,34] The proliferative phase may last up to 9 months. The lesion typically stabilizes and involutes thereafter, a process that may last several years.[33] Lesions may ulcerate, result in cosmetic deformity after involution, or impair critical functions including breathing, eating, or seeing.[33,34] Beta blockers are the standard of care when treatment is advantageous.

This treatment is generally well-tolerated but there is the potential for side effects. PDT has been explored as an alternative treatment option, although it is not extensively investigated in the literature. However, the authors would like to emphasize that this should only be considered in cases where standard-of-care treatment has not been effective, and benefits outweigh risks.

Jerjes and colleagues reported on the use of ultrasound-guided interstitial PDT (iPDT) in a variety of vascular anomalies, including IHs.[38] iPDT involves needle and thin optical fiber insertion into the anomaly rather than surface irradiation to allow greater tissue irradiation.[35] It can be supplemented by imaging methods before and after the procedure, such as magnetic resonance imaging (MRI) or computed tomography (CT).[35] Meta-tetra-hydroxyphenyl chlorine (mTHPC) was used as the photosensitizer (0.15 mg/kg, intravenously, administered on average 96 h prior to irradiation).[35] During this time, patients needed to be kept in a dim room to avoid photosensitization.[35] Multiple spinal needles were inserted into the lesion (ultrasound-guided) 7–9 mm apart (18 Gauge 70 mm) and 1 cm from vessels if there were any nearby.[35] A four-channel 652 nm diode laser with polished tip diffuse fibers with a goal of 20 Joules per site was utilized.[38] Patients were required to avoid sunlight or bright light for 15 days following the procedure.[35] Clinical follow-up occurred at 6 weeks for evaluation of improvement in size and symptoms of the lesion.[35] Forty-three patients with vascular anomalies were evaluated (n = 13 had IHs).[35] About 80% of patients with pain associated with their conditions had significant improvement in pain at follow-up, and 87.5% of patients who had previously experienced bleeding had significant improvement in bleeding.[35] Significant improvement in swelling and disfigurement were also reported by patients (80% and 86.1%, respectively).[35] Improvement in patients with previous difficulty swallowing was significant (75%), and breathing improvement was also significantly improved in patients with previous difficulty (77.8%).[35] Clinically, evaluation revealed 51.2% of patients had a “good response” (no definition provided) and 30.2% of patients had a “moderate response” (no definition provided).[35] Compared to prior treatment, MRI 5–6 weeks after treatment was unchanged in 9.3% of patients, “minimally responsive” (defined as <25% size reduction) in 27.9% of patients, “moderately responsive” (defined as 50%–75% size reduction) in 25.6% of patients, and “significantly responsive” (defined as 50%–75% size reduction) in 34.9% of patients.[35] Data of efficacy in IH specifically was not provided; however, in the study, investigators reported that generally, lymphatic and arterio-venous malformations responded best to treatment.[35] Inflammation surrounding the lesion following treatment occurred in all patients and pain was experienced by a reported 27.9% of patients.[35] Two marginal mandibular nerves were injured, which was hypothesized to be due to needle insertion; motor function recovered in both patients.[35] Two other patients had sensory dysfunction which also recovered.[35] Five patients had postoperative infection treated with antibiotics, three patients had ulceration/necrosis, and six patients experienced “skin burn.”[35] Incidence of scarring, hyperpigmentation, and hypopigmentation was not noted.[35]

PDT FOR ANGIOSARCOMA

Introduction

Angiosarcoma, a rare malignancy, originates from endothelial cells in blood or lymphatic vessels.[33,34] Comprising 1%–4% of soft tissue sarcomas, it typically appears as a bruise-like, poorly demarcated ulcerated lesion with satellites on the head and neck, especially the scalp.[33,34] Radiation may be a risk factor, and prognosis is typically poor, with a reported 5-year survival of 35%.[33] Treatment may include a combination of surgical excision, although recurrence is common, and chemotherapy. PDT has been investigated as an alternative option for patients with angiosarcoma.[33]

Clinical Cases

Liu and colleagues reported a case of a 49-year-old woman who presented with six scattered, ulcerated red masses on the head, up to 3 × 2 cm in size, diagnosed as cutaneous angiosarcoma by histopathology and immunohistochemistry.[36] The patient received five rounds of chemotherapy and refused radiation due to potential side effects.[36] Due to lack of improvement in skin lesions, PDT was attempted and the patient received five treatments separated by 1-week intervals.[36] For photosensitizer, 20% 5-aminolaevulinic acid (5-ALA) cream was applied; 4 h later, lesion irradiation with 633 nm red light (irradiation dose, 80 mW/cm^2) was implemented for 20 min.[36] After the five treatments, the size of two of the lesions was reduced by four-fifths, boundaries were clear, color was lighter, there was less firmness, and ulceration resolved.[36] Surgery was performed on the lesions after the PDT with a 2 cm margin with no local recurrence after 6 months.[36] The authors hypothesize that presurgical PDT in combination with chemotherapy may be helpful in treating cutaneous angiosarcoma.[36]

Topical ALA-PDT may also be part of a post-surgical PDT treatment regimen for angiosarcoma.[37] Gao and colleagues reported on an 81-year-old male with several lesions at the right medial angle of the eye consistent with epithelioid angiosarcoma.[37] The patient had reportedly been treated with excision 10 days prior to presentation but returned due to recurrence.[37] The tumor was excised again with a 2 mm margin, then, 10% 5-ALA emulsion was applied topically prior to treatment, and after 4 h of incubation, the patient's lesions were irradiated with an XD-635AB 635 nm laser with an energy density of 120 J/cm^2 for 15 min.[37] The patient received four treatments.[37] They also received a skin graft after the first two treatments.[37] There was no visually observable recurrence at 1 year following treatment.[37] Side effects included mild edema and redness around the treated area which resolved within 2 days of treatment.[37]

Thong and colleagues reported on a case of cutaneous angiosarcoma treated with PDT and improvement of distant metastases.[38] A 64-year-old Chinese man with biopsy-proven multifocal angiosarcoma of the head and neck had previously been treated with chemotherapy and had recurrence.[38] PDT was performed with chlorin e6 and polyvinylpyrrolidone as photosensitizers.[38] Since the patient had several lesion areas across the head and neck, locations were treated at different times.[38] Photosensitizer dose was 2.0–5.7 mg/kg administered over 10–20 min, with irradiation with a 665nm (± 3 nm) light source for 65–200 J/cm^2 (80–150 mW/cm^2).[38] No adverse effects except local pain during treatment were noted.[38] Ten months after initial treatment, right arm lesions were noted; some were treated with PDT and some spontaneously resolved.[38] Also, 14 months after treatment, some of the head and neck lesions recurred and a right-sided occipital lesion was treated with PDT at that time (21 months).[38] Forty-eight hours after this treatment, initial biopsy of a left occiput tumor revealed a perilesional T-cell infiltrate, which was predominately composed of CD4+ (95%) cells.[38] However, a repeat biopsy 1 month later was predominately composed of CD8+ infiltrate and no further evidence of cancer.[38] Investigators hypothesize that a common antigen in the widespread tumors may have led to a tumor-specific cell-mediated response against all lesions after PDT.[38]

CONCLUSION

PDT is a potentially efficacious treatment for cutaneous vascular lesions that continues to be under investigation. While it has been widely studied in China for PWB, there has been less utilization in other parts of the world due to the potential for adverse effects. Although PDL is currently the first-line treatment for PWB in much of the world, PDT may be as useful as PDL or an effective option for PDL-resistant lesions. The long photosensitive period requiring light avoidance on the order of a week or more may make PDT a less appealing option for some patients and their families. In angiosarcoma, treatment is still under investigation, and less evidence is available to assess whether this is a safe treatment for the stated conditions. However, given that there are limited treatment options, PDT may be considered in life-threatening cases. With further studies, PDT may become another effective treatment option for cutaneous vascular lesions.

REFERENCES

1. Zhao Y, Tu P, Zhou G, et al. Hemoporfin photodynamic therapy for port-wine stain: a randomized controlled trial. *PLoS One*. 2016;11(5):e0156219. doi:10.1371/journal.pone.0156219.
2. Tang Y, Xie H, Li J, Jian D. The association between treatment reactions and treatment efficiency of Hemoporfin-photodynamic therapy on port wine stains: a prospective double blind randomized controlled trial. *Photodiagnosis Photodyn Ther*. 2017;18:171–178. doi:10.1016/j.pdpdt.2017.02.005.
3. Zhang LC, Yang J, Huang YB, Bi MY. Efficacy of hemoporfin photodynamic therapy for pulsed dye laser-resistant facial port-wine stains in 107 children: a retrospective study. *Indian J Dermatol Venereol Leprol*. 2022;88(2):275. doi:10.25259/IJDVL_976_20.
4. Ma G, Han Y, Ying H, et al. Comparison of two generation photosensitizers of PsD-007 and hematoporphyrin monomethyl ether photodynamic therapy for treatment of port-wine stain: a retrospective study. *Photobiomodul*

Photomed Laser Surg. 2019;37(6):376–380. doi:10.1089/photob.2018.4593.

5. Brightman LA, Geronemus RG, Reddy KK. Laser treatment of port-wine stains. *Clin Cosmet Investig Dermatol.* 2015;8:27–33. doi:10.2147/CCID.S53118.
6. Wu Q, Tu P, Zhou G, et al. A dose-finding study for hemoporfin in photodynamic therapy for port-wine stain: a multicenter randomized double-blind phase IIb trial. *Photodermatol Photoimmunol Photomed.* 2018;34(5):314–321. doi:10.1111/phpp.12384.
7. Zhang XY, Al-Odaini N, Fan RG, et al. The efficacy of hematoporphyrin monomethyl ether photodynamic therapy in adult patients with port-wine stains: a retrospective study. *Dermatol Ther (Heidelb).* 2022;12(4):861–869. doi:10.1007/s13555-022-00699-w.
8. Han Y, Yu W, Wang L, et al. Histological characteristics of port-wine stains with complete regression after photodynamic therapy treatment: a 7-year follow-up. *Photobiomodul Photomed Laser Surg.* 2022;40(3):159–162. doi:10.1089/photob.2021.0111.
9. Leonardi-Bee J, Batta K, O'Brien C, Bath-Hextall FJ. Interventions for infantile haemangiomas (strawberry birthmarks) of the skin. *Cochrane Database Syst Rev.* 2011;(5):CD006545. doi:10.1002/14651858.CD006545.pub2. Update in: *Cochrane Database Syst Rev.* 2018;4:CD006545.
10. Mei Y, Xiao X, Fan L, et al. In vitro photodynamic therapy of endothelial cells using hematoporphyrin monomethyl ether (hemoporfin): relevance to treatment of port wine stains. *Photodiagnosis Photodyn Ther.* 2019;27:268–275. doi:10.1016/j.pdpdt.2019.06.003.
11. Chun-Hua T, Li-Qiang G, Hua W, et al. Efficacy and safety of hemoporfin photodynamic therapy for port-wine stains in paediatric patients: a retrospective study of 439 cases at a single centre. *Photodiagnosis Photodyn Ther.* 2021;36:102568. doi:10.1016/j.pdpdt.2021.102568.
12. Zhang Y, Yang Y, Zhang Z, et al. Clinical study on hemoporfin PDT for infant facial port-wine stains. *Photodiagnosis Photodyn Ther.* 2019;25:106–110. doi:10.1016/j.pdpdt.2018.09.012.
13. Yuan KH, Gao JH, Huang Z. Adverse effects associated with photodynamic therapy (PDT) of port-wine stain (PWS) birthmarks. *Photodiagnosis Photodyn Ther.* 2012;9(4):332–336. doi:10.1016/j.pdpdt.2012.03.007.
14. Li DC, Nong X, Hu ZY, et al. Efficacy and related factors analysis in HMME-PDT in the treatment of port wine stains. *Photodiagnosis Photodyn Ther.* 2020;29:101649. doi:10.1016/j.pdpdt.2020.101649.
15. Zhang Y, Zou X, Chen H, Yang Y, Lin H, Guo X. Clinical study on clinical operation and post-treatment reactions of HMME-PDT in treatment of PWS. *Photodiagnosis Photodyn Ther.* 2017;20:253–256. doi:10.1016/j.pdpdt.2017.09.013.
16. Zhang M, Wu Q, Lin T, et al. Hematoporphyrin monomethyl ether photodynamic therapy for the treatment of facial port-wine stains resistant to pulsed dye laser. *Photodiagnosis Photodyn Ther.* 2020;31:101820. doi:10.1016/j.pdpdt.2020.101820.
17. Li X, Diao P, Liu L, et al. Hematoporphyrin monomethyl ether photodynamic therapy for the treatment of Sturge-Weber syndrome and large segmental facial port-wine stain. *Dermatol Ther.* 2022;35(5):e15404. doi:10.1111/dth.15404.
18. Li Y, Wang X, Liu Y, Tao J. Dermoscopy predicts outcome in hemoporfin-mediated photodynamic therapy of port-wine stains: a prospective observational study. *J Am Acad Dermatol.* 2020;83(6):1765–1767. doi:10.1016/j.jaad.2020.03.063.
19. Lin Y, Gong W, Kang J, et al. Hemoporfin-mediated photodynamic therapy for port-wine stains: multivariate analysis of clinical efficacy and optical coherence tomography appearance. *Front Med (Lausanne).* 2022;9:800836. doi:10.3389/fmed.2022.800836.
20. Khalaf AT, Sun Y, Wang F, Sheng M, Li Y, Liu X. Photodynamic therapy using HMME for port-wine stains: clinical effectiveness and sonographic appearance. *Biomed Res Int.* 2020;2020:6030581. doi:10.1155/2020/6030581.
21. Liu J, Zhou J, Hu D, et al. Retrospective analysis of Hemoporfin-mediated photodynamic therapy in the treatment of naïve port-wine stains. *Photodiagnosis Photodyn Ther.* 2022;39:103003. doi:10.1016/j.pdpdt.2022.103003.
22. Zhao Y, Tao J, Tu P. Quantitative evaluation of efficacy of photodynamic therapy for port-wine stains using erythema index image analysis. *Photodiagnosis Photodyn Ther.* 2013;10(2):96–102. doi:10.1016/j.pdpdt.2012.10.001.
23. Li-Qiang G, Hua W, Si-Li N, Chun-Hua T. A clinical study of HMME-PDT therapy in Chinese pediatric patients with port-wine stain. *Photodiagnosis Photodyn Ther.* 2018;23:102–105. doi:10.1016/j.pdpdt.2018.06.006.
24. Wang Y, Zuo Z, Liao X, Gu Y, Qiu H, Zeng J. Investigation of photodynamic therapy optimization for port wine stain using modulation of photosensitizer administration methods. *Exp Biol Med (Maywood).* 2013;238(12):1344–1349. doi:10.1177/1535370213505958.
25. Ren J, Li P, Zhao H, et al. Assessment of tissue perfusion changes in port wine stains after vascular targeted photodynamic therapy: a short-term follow-up study. *Lasers Med Sci.* 2014;29(2):781–788. doi:10.1007/s10103-013-1420-4.
26. Huang N, Zeng J, Liang J, Qiu H, Wang Y, Gu Y. A randomized, double-blind, placebo-controlled study of oral

oxycodone plus acetaminophen for the treatment of pain in photodynamic therapy on port wine stains. *Photodiagnosis Photodyn Ther.* 2014;11(2):134–140. doi:10.1016/j.pdpdt.2014.03.004.

27. Zhang Y, Jiang S, Chen H, Zou X. Hemoporfin-mediated photodynamic therapy for the treatment of port-wine stain birthmarks in pediatric patients. *An Bras Dermatol.* 2017;92(4):559–561. doi:10.1590/abd1806-4841.20176431.
28. Gao K, Huang Z, Yuan KH, Zhang B, Hu ZQ. Side-by-side comparison of photodynamic therapy and pulsed-dye laser treatment of port-wine stain birthmarks. *Br J Dermatol.* 2013;168(5):1040–1046. doi:10.1111/bjd.12130.
29. Zhang B, Zhang TH, Huang Z, Li Q, Yuan KH, Hu ZQ. Comparison of pulsed dye laser (PDL) and photodynamic therapy (PDT) for treatment of facial port-wine stain (PWS) birthmarks in pediatric patients. *Photodiagnosis Photodyn Ther.* 2014;11(4):491–497. doi:10.1016/j.pdpdt.2014.06.004.
30. Tournas JA, Lai J, Truitt A, et al. Combined benzoporphyrin derivative monoacid ring photodynamic therapy and pulsed dye laser for port wine stain birthmarks. *Photodiagnosis Photodyn Ther.* 2009;6(3–4):195–199. doi:10.1016/j.pdpdt.2009.10.002.
31. Zhang LC, Yang J, Huang YB, Huang Z, Bi MY. Post treatment care in photodynamic therapy (PDT) of large facial port-wine stain (PWS) birthmarks. *Photodiagnosis Photodyn Ther.* 2021;36:102604. doi:10.1016/j.pdpdt.2021.102604.
32. Chen Y, Zhang L, Zhang C, Pan L, Wu S. Skin necrosis due to post-treatment care failure after photodynamic therapy of facial port-wine stain in Sturge-Weber syndrome - a case report. *Photodiagnosis Photodyn Ther.* 2021;36:102546. doi:10.1016/j.pdpdt.2021.102546.
33. Valdebran M, Martin B, Kelly KM. State-of-the-art lasers and light treatments for vascular lesions: from red faces to vascular malformations. *Semin Cutan Med Surg.* 2017;36(4):207–212. doi:10.12788/j.sder.2017.044.
34. Patel AM, Chou EL, Findeiss L, Kelly KM. The horizon for treating cutaneous vascular lesions. *Semin Cutan Med Surg.* 2012;31(2):98–104. doi:10.1016/j.sder.2012.02.001.
35. Jerjes W, Upile T, Hamdoon Z, et al. Interstitial PDT for vascular anomalies. *Lasers Surg Med.* 2011;43(5):357–365. doi:10.1002/lsm.21058.
36. Liu D, Li B, Shi W, Chen X, Zhao S. A case report of cutaneous angiosarcoma treated by photodynamic therapy with chemotherapy and surgery. *Photodiagnosis Photodyn Ther.* 2019;25:317–318. doi:10.1016/j.pdpdt.2018.12.012.
37. Gao Y, Wang WS, Wang HL, Liu J, Lu YG. Treatment of Epithelioid angiosarcoma with topical ALA-PDT in the course of surgery. *Photodiagnosis Photodyn Ther.* 2017;19:153–155. doi:10.1016/j.pdpdt.2017.05.009.
38. Thong PS, Ong KW, Goh NS, et al. Photodynamic-therapy-activated immune response against distant untreated tumours in recurrent angiosarcoma. *Lancet Oncol.* 2007;8(10):950–952. doi:10.1016/S1470-2045(07)70318-2.

PART IV

PDT for Rejuvenation

13

Photodynamic Photorejuvenation

Macrene Alexiades

KEY POINTS

- PDT for photorejuvenation involves the topical application of photosensitizing agents, such as aminolevulinic acid (ALA) or methyl aminolevulinate (MAL), which selectively accumulate in target cells.
- Light sources commonly used in photodynamic photorejuvenation (PDP) include lasers, broadband light devices, or light-emitting diodes (LEDs) with wavelengths that match the absorption peak of the photosensitizer (PS).
- The activated PS generates reactive oxygen species (ROS) when exposed to light, which selectively destroys photodamaged skin cells.
- PDT can stimulate the production of collagen, contributing to smoother, firmer skin, and may help reduce the appearance of wrinkles.
- PDT is effective in addressing sun damage, including sunspots, age spots, and uneven skin tone, in wrinkle reduction, and in the treatment of acne, reducing inflammation and improving skin appearance.

OBJECTIVES

- Understand the rationale and strategy of treating photoaging.
- Learn the PDT protocols demonstrated to rejuvenate photoaged skin.
- Identify the photosensitizers and light sources shown to photorejuvenate skin.
- Recognize the ideal patient for photodynamic photorejuvenation.

INTRODUCTION

Photodynamic therapy (PDT) is a first-line treatment for field cancerization of actinic keratosis (AK) that has been associated with concurrent improvement in photoaging, including telangiectasiae, lentigines, and skin texture.[1–5] The appropriateness of PDT as an aesthetic treatment depends upon skin type, the presence of actinic damage, alternative treatment considerations, and customized treatment planning.

Photorejuvenation is specifically defined as the use of laser or light-based devices to reverse the signs of aging and improve skin quality. Photodynamic photorejuvenation (PDP) pairs lasers or light-based devices with a photosensitizer (PS) to more effectively target damaged skin structures and stimulate a renewal process. PDP improves the appearance of the skin by targeting lentigines, dyspigmentation, telangiectasia, and AK, and by inducing epidermal and dermal remodeling that correlates clinically with improvement in rhytids and skin texture.[6,7] This chapter delves into the strategy and implementation of PDP, exploring its mechanisms, applications, and the evolving landscape of research and clinical outcomes.

BACKGROUND

Mechanisms of PDT

PDT combines the use of a photosensitizing agent, light, and oxygen to target a specific tissue or material and achieve a therapeutic effect.[8] The process begins with the administration of a PS, often a topical agent such as aminolevulinic acid (ALA) or methyl aminolevulinate (MAL). Once applied, the PS selectively accumulates in target tissues, specifically accumulating in actively metabolizing cells such as dyskeratotic or neoplastic cells found in the skin. Upon exposure to specific wavelengths of light highly absorbed by the PS, the PS undergoes a photochemical reaction, generating reactive oxygen species (ROS).[8] These ROS induce localized cellular damage, targeting structures like blood vessels, pigmentation, and dysplastic cells. In the context of photorejuvenation, PDT aims to eliminate these targets in the skin to improve dyspigmentation, erythema, and texture, while stimulating collagen production to reduce fine lines and wrinkles.

Applications in Photorejuvenation

PDT has demonstrated efficacy in addressing various dermatological concerns associated with aging and sun damage. PDT has been employed for the treatment of AK, a precursor to squamous cell carcinoma (SCC), inflammatory skin conditions such as acne and rosacea, and has been shown to improve lentigines, dyspigmentation, telangiectasia, scars, and skin texture.[2,6,7]

PDT Photorejuvenation Protocols

The PS, light sources, standard approved PDT protocols, and published PDP protocols are presented in the following sections.

Topical PDP Photosensitizers

Topical photosensitizers (PSs), including ALA or MAL, selectively accumulate in target structures, including sun-damaged cells, telangiectasia, lentigines, and scars.

Approved PS

- In the United States (US) and Canada: A 20% ALA solution (Levulan Kerastick, DUSA Pharmaceuticals, MA, USA) and Ameluz gel (nanoemulsion at 78 mg of ALA/g, Biofrontera, Leverkusen, Germany) are available.[9–12]
- In the European Union (EU): Four topical PSs are approved for PDT: Metvix cream and Luxera cream (160 mg MAL/g, Galderma, Paris, France), Ameluz gel (nanoemulsion at 78 mg of ALA/g, Biofrontera, Leverkusen, Germany), and a 4-cm^2 patch containing 8 mg of ALA (Alacare; Galderma).[13–15]

Alternative compounded PS are in use, but unapproved by regulatory agencies.

PDP Light Sources

Specific wavelengths of light, most commonly in the red or blue spectrum, are used to activate the PS and induce the photochemical reaction. PDT can utilize both natural and artificial light sources if their emitted spectrum aligns with the absorption spectrum of the PS and the light intensity is sufficient for a reasonable exposure duration.[16] An irradiance lower than 100–150 mW/cm^2 is typically advised to avoid photothermal effects.[16] The PpIX absorption spectrum spans the visible range, therefore a variety of light sources are suitable for MAL/ALA-PDT. Acceptable light sources emit a range of the visible spectrum, such as intense-pulsed light (IPL), or selective wavebands matching the strong absorption peak (Soret band) at 406 nm, or the four minor peaks (the Q-bands) at 506, 542, 577, and 630nm.[3,16,17] Longer wavelengths penetrate deeper; therefore light sources with an emission peak at 630 nm are preferred to reach epidermal and dermal targets in photorejuvenation.[6,16] Light sources emitting in the entire visible spectrum include daylight or natural sunlight, fluorescent lamps, IPL, and broadband light-emitting diodes (LEDs). Lamps emitting selected wavebands are defined as coherent (e.g., lasers, particularly the dye laser) and noncoherent (e.g., IPL, selected fluorescent lamps, filtered metal halide lamps, and narrowband LEDs).[18–20] The light sources employed in PDP include approved and unapproved light sources in combination with approved PSs as detailed in the following sections.

Approved Light Sources

The following are the EU- and US-approved light sources for topical PDT:

Blue Light

- Blu-U is a blue light source emitting 417 (±5) nm and maximum power output of 10 J/cm^2 at 1000 s, which corresponds to 16 m 40 s; dosage requires that the patient's lesions are within 2–4 inches of the device.[20]

Red Light

- Aktilite is a narrow output spectrum red light with a peak at 630 nm and a spectral half-width of approximately 20 nm at a light dose of 37 J/cm^2 in 7–10 min session. The illumination surface is 18 × 8 cm = 144 cm^2.[21]

- BF-RhodoLED lamp is a red light source with a narrow spectrum and a peak at 635 nm, delivering a dose of approximately 37 J/cm^2 in a 10-min session.[10]

Approved Protocols

Approved ALA-PDT Protocols

Topical ALA 20% solution with blue light is FDA-approved in the US for the treatment of AK on the face and scalp. ALA is applied to individual AK lesions, followed 14–18 h later by 10 J/cm^2 of blue light exposure with the Blu-U device.[9,20]

Topical ALA 10% nanoemulsion gel with red light is FDA-approved in the US and licensed for use in the EU for the treatment of AK on the face and scalp. ALA is applied to AKs for 3 h followed by 37 J/cm^2 of red light exposure with the BF-RhodoLED lamp. In the EU it is also approved with 2 h of daylight.[10]

The ALA 2 mg/cm^2 patch is licensed for use in the EU for the treatment of AK on the face and scalp, applied for 4 h followed by 37 J/cm^2 of red light exposure with the BF-RhodoLED lamp.[15]

Approved MAL-PDT Protocols

In the US, topical MAL 16.8% cream is FDA-approved for AK on the face and scalp following curettage with an incubation period of 3 h under occlusion with 37 J/cm^2 red light using the Aktilite, two sessions 7 days apart.[11]

In the EU, topical MAL 16.8% cream is licensed for AK of face/scalp following curettage of the lesion, cream application for 3-h incubation under occlusion with 37 J/cm^2 red light using the Aktilite, and two sessions 7 days apart. It may also be illuminated with 2 h of daylight.[12]

PUBLISHED PDP STUDIES

The term "photodynamic photorejuvenation" was first published in 2002 in the context of the application of ALA-PDT in combination with IPL for rejuvenation, while the introduction of short incubation PS and alternative light sources including pulsed-dye laser (PDL), LEDs, and the observation of clinically visible improvements in dyspigmentation, erythema-telangiectasia scars, and skin texture were being developed and reported.[3,18,22]

Table 13.1 presents the numerous studies reporting PDP and the application of PDT variation protocols for the treatment of photoaging. While most studies are small, uncontrolled, and with limited follow-up, there are a few notable randomized controlled trials (RCTs) with split design and controls (Table 13.1). The randomized and controlled studies with objective measurement criteria for skin rejuvenation with better levels of evidence are reviewed in greater detail here.

ALA-PDP

BACKGROUND

Skin rejuvenation and photochemoprevention of skin cancers are treatments that fall on a PDT therapeutic spectrum, as cosmetic improvement in dyspigmentation, fine rhytids, and skin texture have been reported following AK treatment.[3] Patients with multiple AKs and signs of photoaging are ideal candidates for PDP (Fig. 13.1). Alongside treatment of AKs, PDT results in demonstrable improvements in dyspigmentation, including lentigines, erythema, telangiectasia, pores, and skin texture (Fig. 13.1). However, it is important to note that the PDP protocol is not standardized. Published studies differ in PS formulation, mode of application, incubation time, and light source, including emission spectrum, irradiance, dosage, and number and frequency of treatments (Table 13.1).

In the earliest reports of photorejuvenation following PDT, IPL and long-pulsed dye laser were employed in combination with 20% ALA at short incubation.[3,6,22] Ruiz-Rodriguez performed an uncontrolled prospective study in 17 subjects with AK and photoaging of ALA 4-h incubation followed by IPL (590–615 nm) 40 J/cm_2 double pulse.[22] Thirty-three of 38 AKs disappeared with two PDP treatments with IPL at 3 months follow-up and cosmetic results were reportedly excellent in all patients with no incidents of dyspigmentation or scarring.[22]

In the author's published study in 36 subjects and 3622 AKs, 20% ALA was applied for a 3-h incubation followed by LP PDL (595 nm) 4–7.5 J/cm_2 10 ms pulse duration.[3] AK clearance for AK was 90% for head lesions at 8 months, 70% for extremities at 4 months, and 65% for trunk at 4 months. Excellent post-treatment cosmesis with improved erythema-telangiectasia, rhytids, and photoaging was observed with no incidents of dyspigmentation, blistering, or scarring.[3] These studies were the first to transfer IPL and LP PDL, both proven efficacious monotherapies in treating photoaging, to serving as alternate light sources in PDT, providing both the rationale and scientific basis for PDP.

TABLE 13.1 Published Studies on Photodynamic Photorejuvenation

Author, Reference	PS	Light Source	# Sessions Interval/Follow-up	# Subjects	Outcomes/RR
Ruiz-Rodriguez et al.[22]	20% ALA x 4 h	IPL (590–615 nm); 40 J/cm²; double pulse 4 ms	2 monthly/ 3 months	17 photoaging; 38 AK	33/38 AK clearance; improved skin texture
Goldman[23]	20% ALA x 1 h	Blue Light (Blu-U)	1/6 months	32 photoaging	90% AK, 72% texture, 59% pigmentation
Alexiades and Geronemus[3]	20% ALA x 3 h	LP PDL (595 nm) 4–7.5 J/cm²; 10 ms; 2 passes	1/8 months	36 AK/ photoaging, 3622 AK	AK 90% AK head at 8 months, 70% extremities at 4 months, 65% trunk at 4 months, excellent post-treatment cosmesis improved rhytids, photoaging
Gold[24]	20% ALA 0.5–1 h	IPL	3 monthly	10 AK/ photoaging	85% pigmentation, 90% rosacea, 75% texture
Touma[25]	20% ALA 0.5–1 h	Blue Light (Blu-U);	1/NR	17 AK/ photoaging	Significant improvement in fine lines, texture, coarseness, pigmentation, erythema, edema
Avram[26]	20% ALA x 1 h	IPL (560 nm filter); 28–32 J/cm²	1/3 months	17 AK/ photoaging	68% AK, 55% telangiectasia, 48% pigmentation, 25% texture
Alster et al.[27,a]	20% ALA x 1 h	IPL (560 nm filter); 27–30 J/cm²	2 monthly/6 months	10 photoaging split face	PDP > IPL global score
Key[28]	20% ALA x 12 h	PDL (585 nm); 2–6 J/cm²; 40 ms; 3–4 passes	2 monthly/NR	14 photoaging split face	PDP > PDL texture, pigmentation, coarseness
Marmur[29]	20% ALA x 1 h	IPL	1/3 months	7 photoaging PDP vs. IPL control	PDP > IPL histology collagen
Dover et al.[30,a]	20% ALA x 0.5–1 h	IPL (515–1200 nm); 23–28 J/cm²; double pulse	3 × 3 weeks/ 1 month	20 split-face PDP vs. IPL control	PDP > IPL 80% vs. 45% global score, 95% vs. 60% pigmentation, 60% vs. 25% fine lines
Gold[31]	20% ALA x 0.5–1 h	IPL (550–570 nm); 34 J/cm²	3 monthly/ 3 months	13 split face	PDP > IPL 60%–80% vs. 30%–54%
Zane[32]	MAL x 3 h	Red (LED, Aktilite); 37 J/cm²	2 × 2–3 weeks/ 3 months	20 photoaging	88% AK; improved pigmentation, fine lines, coarseness

TABLE 13.1 Published Studies on Photodynamic Photorejuvenation—cont'd

Author, Reference	PS	Light Source	# Sessions Interval/Follow-up	# Subjects	Outcomes/RR
Babilas[33]	MAL x 3 h	IPL (610–950 nm); red LED	1/3 months	25 AK split-face IPL vs. LED	PDP IPL = PDP LED, no difference
Ruiz-Rodriguez[34]	MAL x 3 h	Red LED (Aktilite); 37 J/cm?	2 at 3 weeks/ 12 weeks	4; perioral zone; halfface; fractional-MAL- LED vs. fractional laser alone	Greater improvement with combined techniques; erythema, edema, crusts
Yang, 2010[35]	5% ALA x 1 h	IPL (560 nm filter); 34 J/cm^2; double pulse	4 monthly/	40 photoaging split face	PDP IPL > IPL alone in photoaging score reduction from 3.53 ± 0.60 to 2.82 ± 0.78 and 2.72 ± 0.82
Clementoni et al.[36]	20% ALA x 20 h	MN Red LED 630 p m; 75 J/cm?) vs. MN IPL (560 nm); 19–22 J/cm^2, double pulse	1/6 months	21 prospective, microneedling before ALA application	Significant improvement in global score, fine wrinkles, hyperpigmentation, complexion, coarseness, telangiectasia; no improvement in deep wrinkles; significant improvement greater than 6 months/3 months; erythema, edema, crusts (7 days)
Saclamente[37,a]	MAL x 3 h	Red Light (LED, Aktilite); 37 J/cm^2	2 × 2–3 weeks/ 1 month	48 photoaging split-face double-blind control	Significant improvement PDP side only global photoaging score (coarseness, pigmentations, fine wrinkles, yellowish complexion, erythema); patient satisfaction: 80.4%
Palm[38]	MAL x 3 h	Blue or Red Light	1/NR	18 photoaging split face	Blue = Red, no difference between groups
Szeimies[39]	MAL x 3 vs. 1.5 h	Red Light (LED, Aktilite); 37 J/cm^2	3 monthly/ 3 months	26 photoaging	AK: 89.5%; significant improvement global score, fine wrinkles, complexion, coarseness, erythema, vessels pigmentation; no improvement in deep wrinkles; IHC markers in favor of restoration

Continued

TABLE 13.1 **Published Studies on Photodynamic Photorejuvenation—cont'd**

Author, Reference	PS	Light Source	# Sessions Interval/Follow-up	# Subjects	Outcomes/RR
Togsverd- Bo[40]	MAL x 3 h	Red LED (Aktilite); 37 J/cm?	1/3 months	15 subjects	AFL-PDT > c-PDT for everything: photoaging; AK grade 1: 100% vs. 80%; AK grades 2–3: 88% vs. 59%; pain: 6.5 vs. 5.4; erythema, crusts, pigmentations
Torezan et al.[41,a]	MAL x 1.5 h	MN Red LED (Aktilite); 37 J/cm? vs. Red Alone	1/3 months	10 patients; microneedling; randomized: half face vs. c-PDT	AK disappearance: 88.3% (no difference); improvement in deeper wrinkles if MN-PDT: 1 case of bacterial infection (MN-PDTI)
Zhang et al.[42,a]	5% ALA x 2 h	PDP Red vs. Red vs. PDP IPL vs. IPL	1/NR	NR	PDP Red Light and PDP IPL > to Red and IPL Controls in photoaging scores, SC hydration, L(*) value, elasticity and thickness increases and in TEWL and MI value decreases. a(*) and EI value increased in red-light-PDT group only.
Lane et al.[43]	20% ALA x 1 h	Fx Er:YAG Daylight x 2.5 h + 15–30 min x 2–3 d	1 or 2 sessions/ NR	80 patients; fractional Er: YAG; face and off_face areas	Significant reduction in AKs and photoactinic damage (lentigines, signs of aging)
Alexiades[44,a]	20% ALA x 15 vs. 30 min	PDP $FxCO_2$ vs. $FxCO_2$ control + Blue (Blu-U)	1/8 weeks	20 AK/ photoaging RCT split-face RCT controlled	AK: 89% +$FxCO_2$ PDT vs. 71% PDT alone CR 30 min; 86% +$FxCO_2$ PDT vs. 69% PDT alone CR 15 min; cosmetic improvement rated excellent +$FxCO_2$ PDT vs. good PDT alone
Huang[45]	GlycoALA x 40 min	Red Light (LED, 633 nm)	3 x 3 weeks/ 4 weeks	6 photoaging	Mild improvement in skin texture, pigmentation, pores

[a]*RCT*, Randomized controlled trial.

AK, Actinic keratosis; CR, clearance rate; $FxCO_2$, fractional carbon dioxide laser; IPL, intense-pulsed light; LP, long pulsed; LED, light-emitting diode; MN, microneedling; NR, not reported; PDP, photodynamic photorejuvenation; PDL, pulsed-dye laser; PDT, photodynamic therapy; RR, response rate.

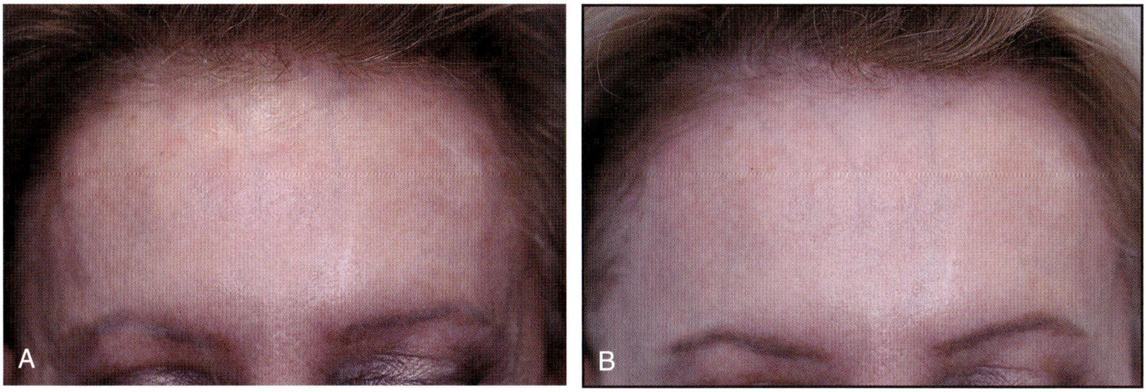

Fig. 13.1 Photodynamic photorejuvenation before and after images. Patient with photoaging at baseline (A) and at 1-month follow-up (B) after a single short incubation ALA-PDT with blue light. Dyspigmentation, including lentigines, erythema, telangiectasia, keratoses, pores, and skin texture are improved following treatment.

PUBLISHED PDP RCTS

In a split-face comparison, 20 subjects with photoaging were treated with 20% ALA plus IPL (560 nm) 27–30 J/cm^2 versus IPL (same settings) on the alternate side.[28] Each subject received two treatments at 1-month intervals with 6-month follow-up. PDP was reported to be more effective for facial rejuvenation as assessed by a global score.[28]

Dover and colleagues (2006) conducted a randomized split-face comparison of topical 20% ALA IPL versus IPL alone in 20 subjects with photodamage.[30] ALA incubation of 0.5–1 h followed by IPL (515–1200 nm) at 23–38 J/cm_2 double pulse was administered in three treatment sessions at 3-week intervals with 1-month follow-up. PDP was superior to IPL alone with comparative improvements of 80% versus 45% in global score, 95% versus 60% in pigmentation, and 60% versus 25% fine lines, respectively.[30]

A third double-blind split-face design RCT published in 2011 evaluated MAL at 3-h incubation and Red Light (LED, Aktilite) at 37 J/cm_2.[46] Two treatments at 2- to 3-week intervals and 1-month follow-up were performed. Significant improvement was reported on the PDP side for the global photoaging score, including coarseness, pigmentations, fine wrinkles, yellowish complexion, and erythema.[30] Patient satisfaction was high at 80.4%.[46]

Ten patients with multiple AKs and photodamage were randomized to receive conventional MAL-PDT with prior curettage on one side of the face and microneedling followed by MAL-PDT on the other side for a 90-min incubation and red LED.[47] At day 30, global scores for photodamage, mottled pigmentation, roughness, and sallowness improved on both sides ($p < .05$), but fine lines improved only on the MN-PDT side ($p = .004$). At day 90, facial erythema ($p = .04$) and coarse wrinkles ($p = .002$) also improved on the MN-PDT side, in addition to fine lines for conventional MAL-PDT ($p = .01$).[47] Erythema ($p = .009$), edema ($p = .01$), crusting ($p = .01$), and pain ($p = .004$) were more common and intense on the MN-PDT side. One patient developed a secondary bacterial infection on day 7 on the MN-PDT side. Average AK clearance was 88.3%, with no difference between the sides.[47]

A randomized comparison of PDP Red versus Red versus PDP IPL versus IPL was conducted using a 5% ALA preparation.[41] PDP Red Light and PDP IPL demonstrated greater improvements as compared to Red and IPL Controls in photoaging scores, SC hydration, L(*) value, elasticity, and thickness increases, and in TEWL and MI value decreases. a(*) and EI value increased in the red-light-PDT group only.[41]

In 2017, the author published an RCT of 20 AK and photoaging subjects in split-face controlled comparison of fractional carbon dioxide laser ($FxCO_2$) ALA-PDT versus ALA-PDT alone at 15- and 30-min incubations (Fig. 13.2).[42] Subjects were randomized to the 15-min versus 30-min incubation groups. Each subject was randomized to receive $FxCO_2$ ALA-PDT on one side of the head versus ALA-PDT on the other. After $FxCO_2$ on the randomized side, 20% ALA was applied for 15 versus 30-min incubation followed by Blue Light (Blu-U, SunPharma/DUSA). AK clearance was statistically significantly higher in the $FxCO_2$ ALA-PDT side versus ALA-PDT alone and higher in the 30-min versus

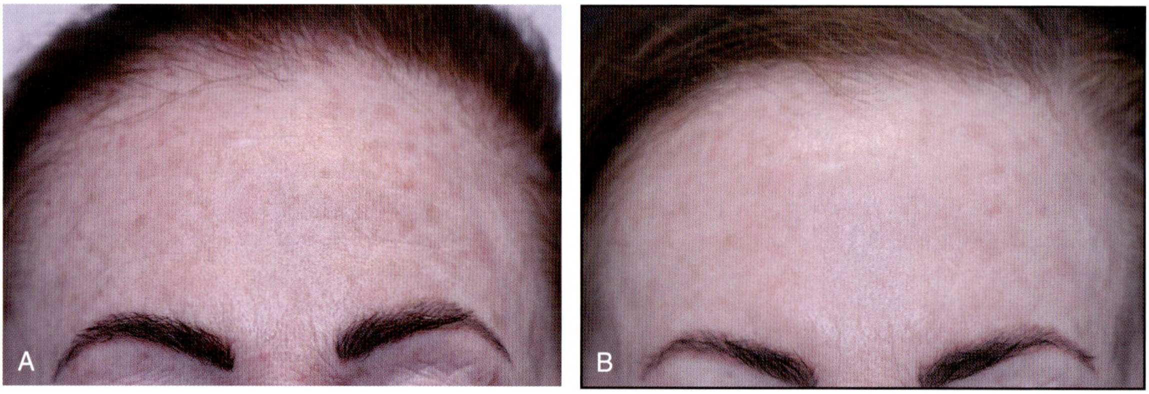

Fig. 13.2 Randomized comparison of fractional carbon dioxide laser and photodynamic photorejuvenation before and after images. Patient with photoaging and AKs at baseline (A) and at 2-month follow-up (B) after a single treatment with fractional carbon dioxide laser followed by short 15-min incubation ALA-PDT with blue light (left side) as compared to ALA-PDT alone (right side).[42] Dyspigmentation, including lentigines, erythema, telangiectasia, keratoses, pores, fine lines, and skin texture are improved following treatment alongside AK clearance. Improvements were rated higher on the combination treatment side.[42]

15-min incubation: 89% +$FxCO_2$ PDT versus 71% PDT alone at 30-min incubation, and 86% +$FxCO_2$ PDT versus 69% PDT alone at 15-min incubation. Cosmetic improvement was rated excellent for the $FxCO_2$ PDT side versus good for PDT alone (Fig. 13.2).[42] Alongside AK clearance, dyspigmentation, including lentigines, erythema, telangiectasia, keratoses, pores, fine lines, and skin texture improved following treatment. Improvements were rated higher on the combination treatment side (Fig. 13.2).[42]

DISCUSSION

Basic research studies and clinical trials have reported favorable outcomes in skin rejuvenation with improvements in skin texture, reduction in pigmentation irregularities, and increased collagen synthesis.[6,44,48] PDT has demonstrated effectiveness in improving skin texture by stimulating collagen production in photoaged mouse skin models and molecular assays.[44,48] Photorejuvenation with PDT has shown reproducible efficacy in reducing the appearance of fine lines and wrinkles in clinical trials, including several RCTs.[3,18,22,28,30,41,42,46,47] The targeted destruction of damaged skin cells and the subsequent stimulation of collagen appear to correlate clinically with reduction in the visible signs of aging.[2,6] PDT has been successful in addressing pigmentation irregularities and reducing redness associated with photodamage and rosacea with selective targeting of blood vessels and pigmented cells contributing to an overall improvement in skin tone.[3,19,30] PDT has been extensively studied and approved for the treatment of AK, by targeting and eliminating dysplastic cells, contributing to both cosmetic enhancement and the prevention of skin cancer.[2,3] Photochemoprevention is an application that is corroborated by findings obtained in mouse models where ALA-PDT protected against photocarcinogenesis by delaying ultraviolet induction of AK and SCC.[44,48] The mechanism of action is the destruction of dysplastic lesions at their early stages.

One of the advantages of PDT for photorejuvenation is the relatively minimal downtime compared to more invasive procedures.[6] Patients often experience mild redness or edema, but these side effects are generally temporarily resolving within several days.[6] While PDP has shown positive outcomes, responses can vary among individuals. Factors such as skin type, the specific condition being treated, and individual skin characteristics may influence the effectiveness of the treatment. Combining PDP with other cosmetic procedures, such as pretreatment with fractional laser resurfacing or microneedling radiofrequency, has enhanced overall outcomes.[36,40,42,43,49] Combination approaches may also provide synergistic effects, targeting multiple aspects of skin aging. Ongoing research is focused on optimizing PDP protocols, including variations in light parameters, PS formulations, and treatment intervals to improve efficacy.

CONCLUSIONS

In several RCTs, PDP has demonstrated statistically significant greater efficacy as compared to light- or laser-only controls in improvements in photoaging, particularly in the setting of AK. The most clinically studied protocols include ALA with IPL, blue light, and red light. Most recently, fractional carbon dioxide laser followed by PDT demonstrated greater efficacy in treating photoaging and rhytids in the setting of actinic damage. More studies will be helpful in optimizing treatment settings.

REFERENCES

1. Algorri JF, Ochoa M, Roldán-Varona P, Rodríguez-Cobo L, López-Higuera JM. Photodynamic therapy: a compendium of latest reviews. *Cancers (Basel)*. 2021;13(17):4447. doi: 10.3390/cancers13174447.
2. Tierney E, Barker A, Ahdout J, Hanke CW, Moy RL, Kouba DJ. Photodynamic therapy for the treatment of cutaneous neoplasia, inflammatory disorders, and photoaging. *Dermatol Surg*. 2009;35(5):725–746.
3. Alexiades-Armenakas MR, Geronemus RG. Laser-mediated photodynamic therapy of actinic keratoses. *Arch Dermatol*. 2003;139(10):1313–1320. doi:10.1001/archderm.139.10.1313.
4. Zhang L, Zhao Z, Wang P, et al. Long-term improvement on photoaging after ALA photodynamic therapy for actinic keratosis: a retrospective study. *Photodiagnosis Photodyn Ther*. 2021;33:102181.
5. Alexiades-Armenakas M. A quantitative and comprehensive grading scale for rhytides, laxity, and photoaging. *J Drugs Dermatol*. 2006;5(8):808–809.
6. Le Pillouer-Prost A, Cartier H. Photodynamic photorejuvenation: a review. *Dermatol Surg*. 2016;42(1):21–30.
7. Huang A, Nguyen JK, Austin E, et al. Facial rejuvenation using photodynamic therapy with a novel preparation of ALA and hyaluronic acid in young adults. *Arch Dermatol Res*. 2020;312:567–573.
8. Correia JH, Rodrigues JA, Pimenta S, Dong T, Yang Z. Photodynamic therapy review: principles, photosensitizers, applications, and future directions. *Pharmaceutics*. 2021;13(9):1332.
9. Levulan. https://www.accessdata.fda.gov/drugsatfda_docs/label/1999/20965lbl.pdf.
10. Ameluz US. https://www.accessdata.fda.gov/drugsatfda_docs/nda/2016/208081Orig1s000TOC.cfm.
11. Metvix US. https://www.accessdata.fda.gov/drugsatfda_docs/label/2005/021415s001lbl.pdf.
12. Metvix EU. https://www.medicines.org.uk/emc/product/6777.
13. Luxera. https://docetp.mpa.se/LMF/Luxera%20cream%20ENG%20PL_09001bee807a651e.pdf.
14. Ameluz EU. https://www.ema.europa.eu/en/medicines/human/EPAR/ameluz#authorisation details section.
15. Alacare. https://www.medicines.org.uk/emc/product/8958/smpc#gref.
16. Kim MM, Darafsheh A. Light sources and dosimetry techniques for photodynamic therapy. *Photochem Photobiol*. 2020;96(2):280–294. doi:10.1111/php.13219.
17. Alexiades-Armenakas M. Intense pulsed light-mediated photodynamic therapy. *J Drugs Dermatol*. 2005;4(5):657–658.
18. Alexiades-Armenakas M. Laser-mediated photodynamic therapy. *Clin Dermatol*. 2006;24(1):16–25. doi:10.1016/j.clindermatol.2005.10.027.
19. Xiang M, Zhou Q, Shi Z, et al. A review of light sources and enhanced targeting for photodynamic therapy. *Curr Med Chem*. 2021;28(31):6437–6457. doi:10.2174/0929867328666210121122106.
20. Blu U. https://www.accessdata.fda.gov/cdrh_docs/pdf/P990019C.pdf.
21. Aktilite. https://www.galderma.com/se/sites/default/files/inline-files/Produktblad_Aktilite_DK-NO-eng-2018_0.pdf.
22. Ruiz-Rodriguez R, Sanz-Sánchez T, Córdoba S. Photodynamic photorejuvenation. *Dermatol Surg*. 2002;28(8):742–744. discussion 744. doi:10.1046/j.1524-4725.2002.02018.x.
23. Goldman MP, Atkin D, Kincad S. PDT/ALA in the treatment of actinic damage: real world experience. *J Lasers Med Surg*. 2002;14(Suppl):24.
24. Gold MH. Intense pulsed light therapy for photorejuvenation enhanced with 20% aminolevulinic acid photodynamic therapy. *I Lasers Med Surg*. 2003;15(Suppl):47.
25. Touma D, Yaar M, Whitehead S, et al. Atrial of short incubation, broad area photodynamic therapy for t a c i a lactinic keratoses and diffuse photodamage. *Arch Dermatol*. 2004;140:33–40.
26. Avram DK, Goldman MP. Effectiveness and safety of ALA-IPL. ni treating actinic keratoses and photo damage. *J Drugs Dermatol*. 2004;3(1 Suppl):S36–S39.
27. Alster TS, Tanzi EL, Welsh EC. Photorejuvenation of facial skin with topical 20% 5-aminolevulinic acid and intense pulsed light treatment: a split-face comparison study. *J Drugs Dermatol*. 2005;4:35–38.
28. Key D . Aminolevulinic acid pulsed dye laser P U T for the treatment of photoaging. *Cosmet Dermatol* 2005;18:31–36.

29. Marmur ES, Phelps R, Goldberg DJ. Ultrastructural changes seen after ALA-IPL. photorejuvenation: a pilot study. *J Cosmet Laser Ther.* 2005;7:21–24.
30. Dover JS, Bhatia AC, Stewart B, Arndt KA. Topical 5-aminolevulinic acid combined with IPLi n the treatment of photoaging. *Arch Dermatol.* 2005;141:1247–1252.
31. Gold MH, Bradshaw VL, Boring MM, et al. Split-face comparison of PDT with 5-ALA and IPL versus IPL alone for photodamage. *DermatolSurg.* 2006;32:795–801 discussion 801-3.
32. Zane C, Capezzera R, Sala R, Venturini M, Calzavara-Pinton P. Clinical and echographic analysis of photodynamic therapy using methylaminolevulinate as sensitizer in the treatment of photodamaged facial skin. *Lasers Surg Med.* 2007 Mar;39(3):203–209. doi:10.1002/lsm.20470 PMID: 17311325.
33. Babilas P, Knobler R, Hummel S, et al. Variablepulsed light si less painful than LEDs for topical PDT of AKs: a prospective randomized controlled trial. *Br I Dermatol.* 2007;157:111–117.
34. Ruiz-Rodriguez R, Lopez L, Candelas D, Zelickson B. Enhanced efficacy of PDT after fractional resurfacing: fractional photodynamic rejuvenation. *J Drugs Dermatol.* 2007;6:818–820.
35. Yang G, Xiang LF, Gold MH. 5-Aminolevulinic acid-based photodynamic intense pulsed light therapy shows better effects in the treatment of skin photoaging in asian skin: a prospective, single-blinded, controlled trial. *J Clin Aesthet Dermatol.* 2010;3(3):40–43.
36. Clementoni MT, Röscher MB, Munavalli GS. Photodynamic photoreinvenation of the face with a combination of microneedling. Red light and broadband pulsed light. *Lasers Surg Med.* 2010;42:150–159.
37. Sanclemente G, Medina L, Villa JF, Barrera LM, Garcia HI. A prospective split-face double-blind randomized placebo-controlled trial to assess the efficacy of methyl aminolevulinate + red-light in patients with facial photodamage. *J Eur Acad Dermatol Venereol.* 2011 Jan;25(1):49–58. doi:10.1111/j.1468-3083.2010.03687.x.
38. Palm MD, Goldman MP. Safetyand efficacy comparison o fblue versus red light sources for photodynamic therapy using methylaminolevulinate ni photodamaged skin. *J Drugs Dermatol.* 2011;10:53–60.
39. Szeimies RM, Torezan L, Niwa A, et al. Clinical, histopathological and immunohistochemical assessment of human skin field cancerization before and after photodynamic therapy. *Br J Dermatol.* 2012;167(1):150–159. doi:10.1111/j.1365-2133.2012.10887.x.
40. Togsverd-Bo K, Haak CS, Thaysen-Petersen D, et al. Intensifiedphotodynamic therapy of actinic keratoses with fractional CO2 laser: a randomized clinical trial. *Br J Dermatol.* 2012;166:1262–1269.
41. Zhang HY, Ji J, Tan YM, et al. Evaluation of 5-aminolevulinic acid-mediated photorejuvenation of neck skin. *Photodiagnosis Photodyn Ther.* 2014;11(4):498–509.
42. Alexiades M. Randomized, controlled trial of fractional carbon dioxide laser resurfacing followed by ultrashort incubation aminolevulinic acid blue light photodynamic therapy for actinic keratosis. *Dermatol Surg.* 2017;43(8):1053–1064.
43. Lane KL, Hovenic W, Bal K, Zachary CB. Daylight photodynamic therapy: the Southern California experience. *Lasers Surg Med.* 2015;47:168–172.
44. Park JY, Jang YH, Kim YS, Sohn S, Kim YC. Ultrastructural changes in photorejuvenation induced by photodynamic therapy in a photoaged mouse model. *Eur J Dermatol.* 2013;23(4):471–477. doi:10.1684/ejd.2013.2050.
45. Huang A, Nguyen JK, Austin E, et al. Facial rejuvenation using photodynamic therapy with a novel preparation of ALA and hyaluronic acid in young adults. *Arch Dermatol Res.* 2020;312(8):567–573. doi:10.1007/s00403-020-02038-5.
46. Sanclemente G, Medina L, Villa JF, Barrera LM, Garcia HI. A prospective split-face double-blind randomized placebo-controlled trial to assess the efficacy of methyl aminolevulinate + red-light in patients with facial photodamage. *J Eur Acad Dermatol Venereol.* 2011;25(1):49–58. doi:10.1111/j.1468-3083.2010.03687.x.
47. Torezan L, Chaves Y, Niwa A, Sanches Jr JA, Festa-Neto C, Szeimies RM. A pilot split-face study comparing conventional methyl aminolevulinate-photodynamic therapy (PDT) with microneedling-assisted PDT on actinically damaged skin. *Dermatol Surg.* 2013;39(8):1197–1201. doi:10.1111/dsu.12233.
48. Wang P, Han J, Wei M, et al. Remodeling of dermal collagen in photoaged skin using low-dose 5-aminolevulinic acid photodynamic therapy occurs via the transforming growth factor-β pathway. *J Biophotonics.* 2018;11(6):e201700357. doi:10.1002/jbio.201700357.
49. Ruiz-Rodriguez R, Lopez L, Candelas D, Zelickson B. Enhanced efficacy of PDT after fractional resurfacing: fractional photodynamic rejuvenation. *J Drugs Dermatol.* 2007;6:818–820.

PART V

PDT for Infections

14

Photodynamic Therapy for Onychomycosis

Francelia J. Eckembrecher, Daphne G. Eckembrecher, Keyvan Nouri

KEY POINTS

- Onychomycosis is the most common nail disorder.
- Oral therapies are rarely used due to systemic toxicity such as hepatotoxicity and GI issues.
- The most common choice of treatment is topical therapy with a high recurrence rate. Photodynamic therapy is a valid treatment alternative for onychomycosis.

OBJECTIVES

- Understand the Epidemiology and Challenges of Onychomycosis.
- Provide an Overview of Photodynamic Therapy (PDT).
- Examine the Current Uses of PDT in Dermatology.
- Evaluate the Effectiveness of PDT for Onychomycosis.
- Assess the Future Potential of PDT for Onychomycosis.

INTRODUCTION

Onychomycosis comprises about 50% of nail disorders worldwide.[1] *Trichophyton rubrum* is the most common cause of onychomycosis.[2] The incidence of onychomycosis is growing, and although it predominantly affects adults, it can also affect individuals that are under the age of 18 years.[3] It is very prominent in old, diabetic, and immunocompromised individuals.[4] Due to the anatomy of the nail and its structure, it is difficult for antifungals to penetrate the lesion and effectively treat onychomycosis.[2] Moreover, systemic antifungal medications possess adverse effects with long-term use and have contraindications that add to their difficulty in treating the disease.[3] Due to this, advances in the treatment of onychomycosis are needed.[3] In recent years, photodynamic therapy (PDT), has been demonstrated to provide an effective alternative treatment for onychomycosis.[3] This chapter will provide insights into the use of PDT for the treatment of onychomycosis.

ONYCHOMYCOSIS

Background

Onychomycosis is the most common nail disorder that commonly affects the toenails, and it is caused by dermatophytes, nondermatophytes, and yeast.[5,6] The prevalence of onychomycosis is around 5.5% globally.[7] Common risk factors are advanced age, trauma, and tinea pedis. Comorbidities that are associated with increased risk are immunosuppression, malignancy, and diabetes.[8] Athletes are also at increased risk for onychomycosis as they may practice in warm environments, wear closed-toe shoes that can become sweaty and moist, can have trauma on their feet, and are in close quarters to others.[9]

Clinical Presentation

Clinically the nail may have discoloration, onycholysis, onychauxis, and subungual hyperkeratosis.[10] During a physical exam, a patient must have all their 20 nails evaluated. During the evaluation, hyperkeratosis can be seen on the nail bed along with onycholysis. When a patient has had a long-standing disease there can be ridging, crumbling, onychocryptosis, or nail loss.[8] It can also cause paresthesia, pain, and impaired social interactions.[6]

Diagnosis

Diagnosis is based on more than one technique, there is the KOH and fungal culture. The nail is clipped, and the subungual debris is scraped with a curette. KOH is used to dissolve the keratinocyte and then it is viewed under the microscope.[8] The other technique used is fungal culture, in which the nail is cleaned with isopropyl alcohol. The nail plate is clipped, and subungual debris is sent to the lab.[8] The medium that is used is Sabourad dextrose agar with an antibiotic, chloramphenicol, with or without cycloheximide.[7]

TREATMENT

For the treatment of onychomycosis, oral and topicals are the preferred treatment method. Although it is the preferred method of treatment, its efficacy is low and there is a 25%–30% relapse rate.[11] Topicals are also the most cost-effective and they have higher compliance. Topicals are also the most common choice of treatment because oral medications have greater side effects. Some of the side effects are hepatotoxicity and GI symptoms.[11] There are other drugs that have increased penetration, examples of these drugs are thioglycolic acid, sodium laurel sulfate, hydroxypropyl-β-cyclodextrin, N-acetylcysteine, and carbocysteine, among others. Even though PDT is very promising, its sustainability long-term has yet to be determined.[11]

PHOTODYNAMIC THERAPY

Principles of PDT

PDT is a noninvasive procedure that utilizes both a photosensitizer (PS) drug and a light source either red light, blue light, or laser light for treatment.[2] PDT functions by a light source to activate the photosensitizing agent that is either applied topically or systemically.[3] Once activated, the reactive oxygen species (ROS) are generated which induces the destruction of cells by apoptosis and necrosis.[3] There are a variety of PSs, the FDA-approved PSs include porfimer sodium (Photofrin), 5-aminolevulinic acid or ALA (Levulan, Ameluz, Alacare), and methyl aminolevulinate or MAL (Metvix).[3] In dermatologic PDT, ALA and MAL are most commonly utilized.[3] The mechanism of action of both PSs is due to their tissue metabolization, by heme pathway enzymes, to the potent photosynthesizer protoporphyrin IX (PpIX) in conjunction with the interaction of the molecular oxygen and light exposure.[3]

Current Uses of PDT

Current uses of PDT include dermatologic oncological conditions such as actinic keratosis, Bowen's disease, and superficial basal cell carcinoma.[4] Other dermatologic conditions that have effectively been treated with PDT include photo-aged skin, Hidradenitis Suppurativa (HS), and acne vulgaris.[4] PDT is also used for the treatment of infectious dermatosis such as viral warts, bacterial and fungal infections, and cutaneous leishmaniasis.[12]

Advantages and Disadvantages of PDT

There are several advantages to incorporating the use of PDT. PDT is a noninvasive procedure that can be performed in an outpatient setting. There are no long-term side effects when a PDT procedure has been performed compared to invasive surgical procedures.[13] Additionally, due to being able to apply the topical PSs to the lesion of interest, the solution will accumulate only in the area that will be treated.[13] Also, multiple sessions of PDT can be performed in the area of interest and there is minimal to no scarring on the treated area.[13]

The disadvantages that exist due to PDT consist of transient side effects.[14] Some of the more common side effects include burning, itching, or stinging on the area that was treated.[14] These symptoms begin when the procedure is initiated and terminate once the procedure has ended.[14] However, some patients have experienced this sensation for a few hours post procedure, but it diminishes with time.[14] Another symptom that is experienced post procedure is erythema and mild edema in the treated area.[14] Some of the more rare but severe adverse effects include blistering, ulceration, or excessive necrosis.[14] Noncompliance to PDT is also an issue due to frequency and length of visits; there are around 12 treatment sessions within 6 months and each session can last several hours.[15]

PDT for the Treatment of Onychomycosis

PDT is considered to be an effective alternative for the treatment of onychomycosis[16] due to the ability of fungi to absorb PSs.[1] PDT causes apoptosis by irritating specific wavelengths of light to the fungal cells that contain PSs; these PSs create ROS that cause apoptosis of the fungus.[7] Some of the most common PSs are ALA, MAL, and methylene blue (MB).[7] Additionally, PDT can be used on patients who have other comorbidities due to its lack of interactions with other medications.[3] A summary of the use of PDT for the treatment of onychomycosis is included in Table 14.1.

In an early case study, two patients with toe onychomycosis were treated with PDT and had successful results. One of the cases was a Japanese female that is 80 years old and had previously been treated with topical terbinafine. The patient was diagnosed with distal and lateral subungual onychomycosis. The second case was a Japanese female with distal and lateral subungual onychomycosis. Previously she was treated with oral itraconazole, but the patient discontinued her treatment due to gastric side effects. Both patients were treated with PDT using ALA. The procedure began with 20% urea applied to the nail and a plastic wrap for 10 h, then ALA was added to the nail and wrapped with a plastic film and aluminum foil for 5 h. The ALA-induced protoporphyrin IX fluorescence was confirmed and then the nail was treated horizontally and vertically with pulsed laser light with a wavelength of 630 nm at 100 J/cm^2 using an excimer-dye laser. The treatment was performed once a week. For case 1, the right first toenail was irradiated seven times (total dose, 700 J/cm^2) and the lesion improved. The dermatophyte was not detected on either KOH or culture. They used the second and third toenails as controls; they only received ALA or irradiation. They did not show clinical improvement after treatment. There was no recurrence clinically at a 6-month follow-up. In case 2, the right first toenail was irradiated six times (total dose, 600 J/cm^2) and the lesion improved. No dermatophyte was detected by KOH or culture. There was no recurrence clinically at a 3-month follow-up.[17]

In a clinical trial, there were 30 Caucasian patients enrolled who were between 41 and 81 years old. One toenail was treated per patient. The patients were treated with 20% urea ointment under occlusion for 10 consecutive nights. For the procedure, 20% 5-ALA was applied to the occlusive dressing topically on the entire nail bed (after the removal of subungual and nail plate hyperkeratosis). ALA-induced protoporphyrin IX fluorescence was confirmed by UV irradiation using a Woods light. The nail bed was treated with red light 3 h later (570–670 nm) from a noncoherent light source at a light dose of 40 J/cm^2 and a fluence rate of 40 mW/cm^2. Three treatments were performed at 2-week intervals. There were no systemic treatments or topicals allowed on the nail being treated during the study period. If a patient had more than one nail with onychomycosis, then it was treated with topicals to prevent reinfection on the PDT-treated nail. Clinical and mycological evaluations were done at 12 and 18 months after the last treatment. All the patients completed the study, and after 1 year, 13 (43.4%) of the patients were cured. Five (16.6%) patients showed complete absence of clinical signs, eight (26.6%) patients showed residual changes that affected less than 10% of the nail plate and negative mycological laboratory results. Four patients had dermatophyte infections covering more than 10% of the nail plate and a positive direct microscopic examination.[18]

In a blinded, randomized control trial there were two cases of women with onychomycosis. Case 1 was a 44-year-old female with a history of onychomycosis for 2 years of the fourth fingernail on the left hand. She had previously been treated with amorolfine and ciclopirox lacquers, oral terbinafine, and itraconazole but all were unsuccessful. Four of the nail samples were *Fusarium oxysporun*. The second case was a 60-year-old woman that has had onychomycosis on five of her nails for the past 5 years. Six different samples were taken and *Aspergillus terreus* was identified. The procedure used was as follows: 40% ointment urea was applied to the nail plate and periungual area under occlusion for 12 h, then 16% MAL cream was applied to the same area under occlusive dressing and protected from light for 4 h. A Wood lamp was used, and it showed light red fluorescence on paronychia areas. Later, the nails were illuminated with 635 nm LED. There were three sessions that were administered 2 weeks apart. Six months later, the patients were cured. Case 2 continued to show yellowing of the fourth and fifth nails. There were no recurrences detected.[19]

In a case report, a 59-year-old male has had onychomycosis for 30 years on the right great toe and 10 years on the left great toe. The patient had been treated with fluconazole and tested positive in the laboratory cultures. For the procedures, the patient applied an emollient of 20% urea for 10 min and 0.5 mm of nail thickness was removed. A PS, Photogem, was applied to the nail for 1 h. After an hour, a PS was checked using a digital camera Sony H50 coupled with a homemade device that emits

TABLE 14.1 **Studies on Photodynamic Therapy for the Treatment of Onychomycosis**

Author	Protocol	Result
Watanabe et al.[17]	Both patients were treated with PDT using ALA. The procedure began with 20% urea applied to the nail and a plastic wrap for 10 h, then ALA was added to the nail and wrapped with a plastic film and aluminum foil for 5 h. The ALA-induced protoporphyrin IX fluorescence was confirmed and then the nail was treated horizontally and vertically with pulsed laser light with a wavelength of 630 nm at 100 J/cm^2 using an excimer-dye laser. The treatment was performed once a week. Case 1: irradiated seven times Case 2: irradiated six times	No recurrence at follow-up.
Sotiriou et al.[18]	The patients were treated with 20% urea ointment under occlusion for 10 consecutive nights. For the procedure, 20% 5-ALA was applied to the occlusive dressing topically on the entire nail bed (after the removal of subungual and nail plate hyperkeratosis). ALA-induced protoporphyrin IX fluorescence was confirmed by UV irradiation using a Woods light. The nail bed was treated with red light 3 h later (570–670 nm) from a noncoherent light source at a light dose of 40 J/cm^2 and a fluence rate of 40 mW/cm^2. Three treatments were performed at 2-week intervals.	Thirteen (43.4%) of the patients were cured. Five (16.6%) patients showed complete absence of clinical signs, eight (26.6%) patients showed residual changes that affected less than 10% of the nail plate and negative mycological laboratory results. Four patients had dermatophyte infections covering more than 10% of the nail plate and a positive direct microscopic examination.
Gilaberte et al.[19]	The procedure used was as follows: 40% ointment urea was applied to the nail plate and periungual area under occlusion for 12 h, then, 16% MAL cream was applied to the same area under occlusive dressing and protected from light for 4 h. A Wood lamp was used, and it showed light red fluorescence on paronychia areas. Later, the nails were illuminated with 635 nm LED. There were three sessions that were administered 2 weeks apart.	No recurrence at follow-up.
Silva et al.[20]	The patient applied an emollient of 20% urea for 10 min and 0.5 mm of nail thickness was removed. A photosensitizer, Photogem, was applied to the nail for 1 h. After an hour, a photosensitizer was checked using a digital camera Sony H50 coupled with a homemade device that emits 405 nm. The area was then illuminated for 9 min with a total fluence of 54 J/cm^2 with an intensity of 100 mW/cm^2. The patients had a follow-up appointment for a clinical evaluation 7 days after the first illumination. There was a total of six sessions, one per week.	Complete healing after an irradiation over 6 weeks and they had a negative culture for fungi.
Figueiredo Souza et al.[21]	For a period of 24 weeks, group A received one placebo capsule per week and sessions of PDT. Group B received 300 mg oral fluconazole per week and sessions of placebo PDT. The PDT group received a session of MBLED every 15 days for 6 months. For the procedure, 2% aqueous solution was applied to the nail bed until it was saturated, followed by a 3-min rest period. Then the nail was illuminated with noncoherent red light (630 nm, 18 J/cm^2) from an LED device with a light intensity output of 3100 mW/cm^2 and optical intensity of 100 mW/cm^2.	Group A had a 90% cure rate, while group B responded poorly. At the 12-month post-treatment follow-up, group A had a clinical cure rate of 80%.

Continued

TABLE 14.1 Studies on Photodynamic Therapy for the Treatment of Onychomycosis—cont'd

Author	Protocol	Result
Souza et al.[22]	The procedure initiated with 2% aqueous MB solution was applied to the nail followed by irradiation with red light (630 nm, 36 J/cm^2) from an LED device with a light intensity output of 3100 mW/cm^2 and optical intensity of 100 mW/cm^2. Nails not penetrated by the dye had a nail abrasion. The treatment consisted of MBLED sessions for a total of 6 months. The sessions were conducted every 15 days.	All the patients were cured with mycological cure.
Souza LW et al.[23]	The patients received PDT for 6 months and they received sessions every 15 days. For the procedure, 2% aqueous methylene blue was applied to the nail then they received irradiation with red light (630 nm, 36 J/cm^2) from an LED device with a light intensity output of 3100 mW/cm and optical intensity of 100 mW/cm^2. If a patient had hyperkeratotic nails or dermatophytomas they were treated with an abrasive device.	All the patients were cured and showed clinical improvement.
da Silva et al.[24]	The study consisted of initially preparing the nail plate with a 40% urea emollient 2 h before the treatment. The urea was in contact with the nail for 1 h, once the excess product was removed, PSs either gel or emulsion was applied on the nail for 1 h before LED illumination. Patients were treated for 7 days, after the treatment was complete, the patients were evaluated for their clinical response through clinical evaluation, and it was documented by weekly images. Results depicted as follows: Patient 1 was treated with gel curcumin (1.5%), six PDT sessions were conducted. Patient 2 was treated with emulsion (1.5%), five PDT sessions were conducted.	Both patients had complete healing.
de Oliveira et al.[25]	For each patient, two sessions were conducted with 60-day intervals between them. The study consisted of the utilization of a fractional CO_2 laser 10.600 nm, 3rd overlap, 1.600 mJ energy and 0.6 mm density over the affected nail area. Then, methyl aminolevulinate hydrochloride 16% was applied over the area in which it was occluded by opaque material for 2 h. Afterwards, LED was applied to the area for 15 min. Both sessions were conducted following the same protocol.	Results depicted that 7/7 had mycological cure and 5/7 clinical cure at both follow-ups.
Tardivo et al.[26]	Afterwards, a 1:1 volume of the 2% methylene blue/2% toluidine blue mixture was added between the nail plate and the nail bed. Five minutes later a RL50 source was used to irradiate the nail initially at a 5 cm distance for 3 min at 18J/cm^2. After the procedure was complete, the site of treatment was assessed and photographed for 30 days, if necessary, the protocol was repeated. The patients attended from 1 to 22 sessions during a 1-month interval.	Complete clearance of 45% of the lesions and partial clearance of 40%.
Gilaberte et al.[27]	(1) MAL-PDT or (2) three weekly PDT placebo sessions. In both study groups, the patients' nail plates were treated with 40% urea ointment in order to enhance the penetration of the PSs. The 40% urea was applied every evening for 5 days before the PDT therapy. During the PDT treatment a 635 nm LED lamp was utilized, afterwards the area was protected from light for 24 h. The protocol was then repeated once a week for 3 weeks.	Results of the study indicated that there was a mycological cure of (PDT vs. Placebo) 32% vs. 11% and a clinical improvement indicated (PDT vs. Placebo) 41% vs. 17%.

TABLE 14.1 **Studies on Photodynamic Therapy for the Treatment of Onychomycosis—cont'd**

Author	Protocol	Result
Morgado et al.[28]	The study protocol consisted of pretreatment with 40% urea a week before the PDT treatment to increase PDT penetration. During treatment, the PSs was composed of an oil-in-water gel consistency nanoemulsion (NE) that contained a 65 μM of AlClPc and was applied to the affected area for 15 min. Afterwards, the AlClPc-NE-PDT illuminated with 660 nm with a light dose of 30.9 J/cm^2. The study consisted of a total of 69 total sessions (4.45 ± 1.76) at a 15-day interval.	Mycological cure occurred in 50% and a clinical cure occurred in 75%.
Houang et al.[29]	The study protocol included a urea ointment, nail abrasion, nail softening, or a plate removal if indicated for pretreatment. The treatment consisted of the application of the rose Bengal and afterwards the illumination with 532 nm for 5 mins. This protocol was repeated every 3 weeks until both mycological and clinical clearance was achieved.	Clinical clearance of 6/6.
Navarro-Bielsa et al.[16]	Protocol for this study consisted of pretreatment with 40% urea for 7 days, afterwards the patient was treated every 1–2 weeks for 3 h with 16% MAL and irradiation with red-light LED lamp (37 J/cm^2). There was an average of six sessions, and the range was between 3 and 15 sessions. There were 10 patients in this study who were treated simultaneously with systemic terbinafine, and three patients received topical terbinafine during the treatment protocol.	complete clinical response in 80% of cases and microbiological cure in 60%.

405 nm. The area was then illuminated for 9 min with a total fluence of 54 J/cm^2 with an intensity of 100 mW/cm^2. The patients had a follow-up appointment for a clinical evaluation 7 days after the first illumination. There was a total of six sessions, one per week. Patients experienced complete healing after an irradiation over 6 weeks and they had a negative culture for fungi.[20]

In a randomized control trial, there were 80 patients with onychomycosis on the distal and lateral subungual toenails that were diagnosed clinically and mycologically. The patients were between 18 and 85 years old and they were divided into two groups, A and B. For a period of 24 weeks, group A received one placebo capsule per week and sessions of PDT. Group B received 300 mg oral fluconazole per week and sessions of placebo PDT. The PDT group received a session of MB-light emission diode (MBLED) every 15 days for 6 months. For the procedure, 2% aqueous solution was applied to the nail bed until it was saturated, followed by a 3-min rest period. Then the nail was illuminated with noncoherent red light (630 nm, 18 J/cm^2) from an LED device with a light intensity output of 3100 mW/cm^2 and optical intensity of 100 mW/cm^2. Patients were followed and evaluated during a 6-month period. They were evaluated at the beginning and then every 4 weeks during the 6 months. Then, at the 3-, 6-, and 12-month period post treatment. Group A had a 90% cure rate, while group B responded poorly. At the 12-month post-treatment follow-up, group A had a clinical cure rate of 80%.[21]

In an open clinical trial, there are four immunocompromised patients with toenail onychomycosis. The procedure initiated with 2% aqueous MB solution was applied to the nail followed by irradiation with red light (630 nm, 36 J/cm^2) from an LED device with a light intensity output of 3100 mW/cm^2 and optical intensity of 100 mW/cm^2. Nails not penetrated by the dye had a nail abrasion. The treatment consisted of MBLED sessions for a total of 6 months. The sessions were conducted every 15 days. All the patients were cured with mycological cure.[22]

In a controlled clinical trial, 11 immunocompromised patients with severe distal-lateral subungual onychomycosis (SDSO) and 11 immunocompromised with mild-to-moderate distal and lateral subungual toenail onychomycosis (MDSO) were chosen for the study. The 22 patients had tested positive for *T. rubrum.* The patients received PDT for 6 months and they received sessions every 15 days. For the procedure, 2% aqueous MB was applied to the nail, then they received irradiation with red light (630 nm, 36 J/cm^2) from an LED device with a light intensity output of 3100 mW/cm and optical intensity of 100 mW/cm^2. If a patient had hyperkeratotic nails or dermatophytomas they were treated with an abrasive device. All the patients were cured and showed clinical improvement.[23]

A case report by da Silva and colleagues was conducted on two patients: Patient 1: Male, age 27; Patient 2: Female, age 65. Patient selection consisted of clinical diagnosis of onychomycosis by a podiatrist. The patients were diagnosed with onychomycosis for over 10 years. For the study, the PSs selected was curcumin, it was solubilized with 1% alcohol and 0.1% dimethyl sulfoxide, then the curcumin was incorporated in the 1.5% concentration into two different formulations: carbopol gel and emulsion W/O. The study consisted of initially preparing the nail plate with a 40% urea emollient 2 h before the treatment. The urea was in contact with the nail for 1 h, once the excess product was removed, PSs either gel or emulsion were applied on the nail for 1 h before LED illumination. Patients were treated for 7 days, after the treatment was complete, the patients were evaluated for their clinical response through clinical evaluation, and it was documented by weekly images. Results depicted as follows: Patient 1 was treated with gel curcumin (1.5%), six PDT sessions were conducted, and complete healing was achieved. Patient 2 was treated with emulsion (1.5%) and five PDT sessions were conducted for complete healing to be achieved.[24]

In a case study conducted by de Oliveira and colleagues, seven patients were included. For each patient, two sessions were conducted with 60-day intervals between them. The study consisted of the utilization of a fractional CO_2 laser 10.600 nm, 3rd overlap, 1.600 mJ energy, and 0.6 mm density over the affected nail area. Then, methyl aminolevulinate hydrochloride 16% was applied over the area in which it was occluded by opaque material for 2 h. Afterward, LED was applied to the area for 15 min. Both sessions were conducted following the same protocol. The patients were evaluated on three separate occasions: before the session, 30 days after the second session, and 1 year after the second session. Before the session, a mycological test and digital photograph were assessed; 30 days after the second session, only a mycological test was assessed; and 1 year after the second session, a mycological test and digital photograph were assessed. Results depicted that 7/7 had mycological cure and 5/7 clinical cure at both follow-ups.[25]

A clinical trial was conducted on 62 patients with onychomycosis. The study consisted of having the nails photographed before treatment. The nail bed was scraped with a curettage and sent to the lab for microbiological analysis. Afterwards, a 1:1 volume of the 2% MB/2% toluidine blue mixture was added between the nail plate and the nail bed. Five minutes later, a RL50 source was used to irradiate the nail initially at a 5 cm distance for 3 min at 18J/cm^2. After the procedure was complete, the site of treatment was assessed and photographed for 30 days; if necessary, the protocol was repeated. The patients attended from 1 to 22 sessions during a 1-month interval. Results indicated that there was complete clearance of 45% of the lesions and partial clearance of 40%.[26]

A randomized, placebo-controlled clinical trial was conducted on forty patients. The patients were placed in one of two study groups: (1) MAL-PDT or (2) three weekly PDT placebo sessions. In both study groups, the patients' nail plates were treated with 40% urea ointment to enhance the penetration of the PSs. The 40% urea was applied every evening for 5 days before the PDT therapy. During the PDT treatment a 635 nm LED lamp was utilized, afterwards the area was protected from light for 24 h. The protocol was then repeated once a week for 3 weeks. To determine the disease involvement, images were taken, and microbiology samples were taken at baseline and at the end of the study. Lastly, efficacy of treatment was assessed at weeks 12, 24, and 36 by analyzing the clinical photographs and microbiological samples. Results of the study indicated that there was a mycological cure of (PDT vs. Placebo) 32% versus 11% and a clinical improvement indicated (PDT vs. Placebo) 41% versus 17%.[27]

Another clinical trial was conducted by Morgado and colleagues; 16 patients participated in this study. The study protocol consisted of pretreatment with 40% urea a week before the PDT treatment in order to increase PDT penetration. During treatment, the PSs was composed of an oil-in-water gel consistency nanoemulsion (NE) that contained 65 μM of AlClPc and was applied to the affected area for 15 min. Afterward, the AlClPc-NE-PDT was illuminated with 660 nm with a light dose of 30.9 J/cm^2. The study consisted of a total of 69 total sessions (4.45 ± 1.76) at a 15-day interval. Mycological cure occurred in 50% and a clinical cure occurred in 75%.[28]

Houang and colleagues conducted a case series in which six patients participated. The study protocol included a urea ointment, nail abrasion, nail softening, or plate removal if indicated for pretreatment. The treatment consisted of the application of the rose Bengal and afterwards the illumination with 532 nm for 5 mins. This protocol was repeated every 3 weeks until both mycological and clinical clearance was achieved. Results for this study indicated that there was a clinical clearance of 6/6.[29]

Lastly, a retrospective observational study was conducted by Navarro-Bielsa and colleagues in which 20 patients were included in the study. Protocol for this study consisted of pretreatment with 40% urea for 7 days, afterwards the patient was treated every 1–2 weeks for 3 h with 16% MAL and irradiation with red-light LED lamp (37 J/cm^2). There was an average of six sessions, and the range was between 3 and 15 sessions. There were 10 patients in this study who were treated simultaneously with systemic terbinafine, and three patients received topical terbinafine during the treatment protocol. Results of the study indicated that complete clinical response in 80% of cases and microbiological cure in 60%.[16]

CONCLUSION

The effect that onychomycosis has on quality of life has been investigated in various studies.[30] Therefore appropriate treatment for this condition should be offered to patients.[30] One such treatment is PDT due to its increasing validity for the treatment of onychomycosis.[16] It has also proven to be effective in the treatment of various fungi, especially *T. rubrum*, which is the most common cause of onychomycosis.[1] More research is needed to further develop optimum protocol for the treatment of onychomycosis.[16]

REFERENCES

1. Alberdi E, Gómez C. Methylene blue vs methyl aminolevulinate photodynamic therapy in the treatment of mild-to-moderate toenail onychomycosis: short- and medium-term effects. *Dermatol Ther*. 2020;33(6):e14280. doi:10.1111/dth.14280.
2. Bhatta AK, Keyal U, Wang X, et al. A review of the mechanism of action of lasers and photodynamic therapy for onychomycosis. *Lasers Med Sci*. 2017;32(2):469–474. doi:10.1007/s10103-016-2110-9.
3. Bhatta AK, Keyal U, Wang XL. Photodynamic therapy for onychomycosis: a systematic review. *Photodiagnosis Photodyn Ther*. 2016;15:228–235. doi:10.1016/j.pdpdt.2016.07.010.
4. Megna M, Fabbrocini G, Marasca C, et al. Photodynamic therapy and skin appendage disorders: a review. *Skin Appendage Disord*. 2017;2(3–4):166–176. doi:10.1159/000453273.
5. Simmons BJ, Griffith RD, Falto-Aizpurua LA, et al. An update on photodynamic therapies in the treatment of onychomycosis. *J Eur Acad Dermatol Venereol*. 2015;29(7):1275–1279. doi:10.1111/jdv.12950.
6. Lipner SR, Scher RK. Onychomycosis: treatment and prevention of recurrence. *J Am Acad Dermatol*. 2019;80(4):853–867. doi:10.1016/j.jaad.2018.05.1260.
7. Gupta AK, Versteeg SG, Shear NH. Onychomycosis in the 21st century: an update on diagnosis, epidemiology, and treatment. *J Cutan Med Surg*. 2017;21(6):525–539. doi:10.1177/1203475417716362.
8. Lipner SR, Scher RK. Onychomycosis: clinical overview and diagnosis. *J Am Acad Dermatol*. 2019;80(4):835–851. doi:10.1016/j.jaad.2018.03.062.
9. Daggett C, Brodell RT, Daniel CR, et al. Onychomycosis in athletes. *Am J Clin Dermatol*. 2019;20(5):691–698. doi:10.1007/s40257-019-00448-4.
10. Leung AKC, Lam JM, Leong KF, et al. Onychomycosis: an updated review. *Recent Pat Inflamm Allergy Drug Discov*. 2020;14(1):32–45. doi:10.2174/1872213X13666191026090713.
11. Aggarwal R, Targhotra M, Kumar B, et al. Treatment and management strategies of onychomycosis. *J Mycol Med*. 2020;30(2):100949. doi:10.1016/j.mycmed.2020.100949.
12. Queirós C, Garrido PM, Maia Silva J, et al. Photodynamic therapy in dermatology: beyond current indications. *Dermatol Ther*. 2020;33(6):e13997. doi:10.1111/dth.13997.
13. Correia JH, Rodrigues JA, Pimenta S, et al. Photodynamic therapy review: principles, photosensitizers, applications, and future directions. *Pharmaceutics*. 2021;13(9):1332. doi:10.3390/pharmaceutics13091332.
14. Kalka K, Merk H, Mukhtar H. Photodynamic therapy in dermatology. *J Am Acad Dermatol*. 2000;42(3):389–413; quiz 414–416. doi:10.1016/s0190-9622(00)90209-3.
15. Christenson JK, Peterson GM, Naunton M, et al. Challenges and opportunities in the management of onychomycosis. *J Fungi (Basel)*. 2018;4(3):87. doi:10.3390/jof4030087.
16. Navarro-Bielsa A, Gracia-Cazaña T, Robres P, et al. Combination of photodynamic therapy and oral antifungals for the treatment of onychomycosis. *Pharmaceuticals (Basel)*. 2022;15(6):722. doi:10.3390/ph15060722.

17. Watanabe D, Kawamura C, Masuda Y, et al. Successful treatment of toenail onychomycosis with photodynamic therapy. *Arch Dermatol.* 2008;144(1):19–21. doi:10.1001/archdermatol.2007.17.
18. Sotiriou E, Koussidou-Eremonti T, Chaidemenos G, et al. Photodynamic therapy for distal and lateral subungual toenail onychomycosis caused by Trichophyton rubrum: preliminary results of a single-centre open trial. *Acta Derm Venereol.* 2010;90(2):216–217. doi:10.2340/00015555-0811.
19. Gilaberte Y, Aspiroz C, Martes MP, et al. Treatment of refractory fingernail onychomycosis caused by nondermatophyte molds with methylaminolevulinate photodynamic therapy. *J Am Acad Dermatol.* 2011;65(3):669–671. doi:10.1016/j.jaad.2010.06.008.
20. Silva AP, Kurachi C, Bagnato VS, et al. Fast elimination of onychomycosis by hematoporphyrin derivative-photodynamic therapy. *Photodiagnosis Photodyn Ther.* 2013;10(3):328–330. doi:10.1016/j.pdpdt.2013.01.001.
21. Figueiredo Souza LW, Souza SV, Botelho AC. Randomized controlled trial comparing photodynamic therapy based on methylene blue dye and fluconazole for toenail onychomycosis. *Dermatol Ther.* 2014;27(1):43–47. doi:10.1111/dth.12042.
22. Souza LW, Souza SV, Botelho AC. Endonyx toenail onychomycosis caused by *Trichophyton rubrum:* treatment with photodynamic therapy based on methylene blue dye. *An Bras Dermatol.* 2013;88(6):1019–1021. doi:10.1590/abd1806-4841.20132180.
23. Souza LW, Souza SV, Botelho AC. Distal and lateral toenail onychomycosis caused by *Trichophyton rubrum:* treatment with photodynamic therapy based on methylene blue dye. *An Bras Dermatol.* 2014;89(1):184–186. doi:10.1590/abd1806-4841.20142197.
24. da Silva AP, Carbinatto FM, Bagnato VS, et al. A promising strategy for the treatment of onychomycosis with curcumin and photodynamic therapy. David Publishing. *J Pharm Pharmacol.* 2015;3:434–437.
25. de Oliveira GB, Antonio JR, Antonio CR, et al. The association of fractional CO2 laser 10.600 nm and photodynamic therapy in the treatment of onychomycosis. *An Bras Dermatol.* 2015;90(4):468–471. doi:10.1590/abd1806-4841.20153588.
26. Tardivo JP, Wainwright M, Baptista M. Small scale trial of photodynamic treatment of onychomycosis in São Paulo. *J Photochem Photobiol B.* 2015;150:66–68. doi:10.1016/j.jphotobiol.2015.03.015.
27. Gilaberte Y, Robres MP, Frías MP, et al. Methyl aminolevulinate photodynamic therapy for onychomycosis: a multicentre, randomized, controlled clinical trial. *J Eur Acad Dermatol Venereol.* 2017;31(2):347–354. doi:10.1111/jdv.13842.
28. Morgado LF, Trávolo ARF, Muehlmann LA, et al. Photodynamic therapy treatment of onychomycosis with aluminium-phthalocyanine chloride nanoemulsions: a proof of concept clinical trial. *J Photochem Photobiol B.* 2017;173:266–270. doi:10.1016/j.jphotobiol.2017.06.010.
29. Houang J, Perrone GG, Pedrinazzi C, et al. Genetic tolerance to rose bengal photodynamic therapy and antifungal clinical application for onychomycosis. *Adv Ther (Weinh).* 2019;2(2):1800105-n/a. doi:10.1002/adtp.201800105.
30. Stewart CR, Algu L, Kamran R, et al. Effect of onychomycosis and treatment on patient-reported quality-of-life outcomes: a systematic review. *J Am Acad Dermatol.* 2021;85(5):1227–1239. doi:10.1016/j.jaad.2020.05.143.

15

Photodynamic Therapy for Antimicrobial-Resistant Microorganisms and Biofilms

Macrene Alexiades, Katerina Tsaoutou

KEY POINTS

- The rise in antimicrobial-resistant infections highlights the urgent need for innovative management strategies.
- Photodynamic therapy (PDT) has proven to be an effective method for addressing biofilms and resistant microorganisms.
- The discussion includes the mechanism of action and selectivity of PDT.
- Details on photosensitizers and PDT protocols for targeting MRSA and biofilms are provided.
- A comprehensive summary of published PDT protocols, including dosage, efficacy, and outcomes for treating MRSA, biofilms, and antimicrobial-resistant pathogens, is presented.

OBJECTIVES

- Understand the impact of antimicrobial resistance, including methicillin-resistant *Staphylococcus aureus* (MRSA) and biofilms, on disease incidence and mortality.
- Explore new treatments targeting resistant microbes, with a focus on photodynamic therapy (PDT).
- Learn the rationale, principles, and methodologic approach of PDT for treating resistant microbes.
- Acquire knowledge about approved and investigational photosensitizers utilized in PDT for combating resistant microorganisms.
- Examine in vitro and in vivo studies that demonstrate the effectiveness of PDT against MRSA and biofilms.

INTRODUCTION

The management of antibiotic-resistant microorganisms and infections linked to biofilms necessitates the creation of modern tools in the field of infectious disease management. Traditional antimicrobial approaches prove ineffective against pathogenic strains employing resistance mechanisms and are thwarted by biofilms, leading to the persistence of chronic infections. In the mid of this changing paradigm, photodynamic therapy (PDT) has surfaced as an alternative therapeutic approach.[1]

Phototherapy dates back to ancient Egypt, India, and Greece in the form of treating skin diseases with sunlight. For example, leprosy treatment included application of natural photosensitizers (PSs), such as psoralens.[2] In the late 19th century, light-induced effects on certain dyes and tissues were described. The foundational work of Oscar Raab, a medical student, in the early 20th century, followed by the breakthroughs of Von Tappeiner and Jesionek, provided the foundation of PDT by linking light, PSs, and tissue damage.[2] However, materialization of the clinical potential of PDT was first achieved during the latter half of the 20th century, primarily in the field of oncology.[2,3]

The rise of antibiotic resistance, estimated to cause approximately 5 million deaths annually worldwide, underscores the urgency for innovative antimicrobial strategies.[4] The six primary pathogens contributing to deaths linked to resistance are *Escherichia coli, Staphylococcus aureus* (especially methicillin-resistant strains, MRSA), *Klebsiella pneumoniae, Streptococcus pneumoniae, Acinetobacter baumannii,* and *Pseudomonas aeruginosa*.[4] Biofilms, communities of antimicrobial-resistant microorganisms enclosed within robust matrices, are implicated in 70% of all human microbial infections, encompassing conditions such as chronic wounds, endocarditis, periodontitis, cystic rhinosinusitis, fibrosis, meningitis, osteomyelitis, renal infections, and infections related to prostheses and implantable devices.[5] The global deterioration of biofilm-related conditions is exacerbated by the ineffectiveness of conventional antibiotic treatments. Biofilms continually alter their extracellular polymeric substances (EPS), making them resistant to various antibiotics.[5]

Therefore there is a significant emphasis on developing alternative strategies to address antimicrobial resistance and biofilms.[6,7] Among the emerging anti-biofilm agents are halimane diterpenoids, imidazole and indole derivatives, plant extracts, peptides and polysaccharides, degradation enzymes, drug delivery nanoparticles, and PDT.[8]

MECHANISM OF ACTION

The effectiveness of PDT in treating biofilms and microbial resistance is rooted in its distinctive mechanism of action. The interaction among PSs, light energy, and molecular oxygen initiates a series of photochemical reactions leading to the production of cytotoxic reactive oxygen species (ROS).[3] Numerous studies have indicated that ROS generated by PDT disrupts various targets within biofilms, including the EPS matrix, DNA, lipids, proteins, and extracellular polysaccharides.[9] PDT has been observed to impede various stages of biofilm development.[9]

Unlike conventional antibiotics that target isolated cellular components, PDT-induced ROS inflict broad-spectrum damage on microbial cells.[1,10] Disruption of cellular membranes, proteins, lipids, and nucleic acids preempts the microorganism's ability to mount effective resistance strategies. PDT's modifiable parameters, from PS selection to light parameters, endow it with the agility required to confront diverse microbial challenges with precision.[1,10]

PDT TYPE I AND II REACTIONS

The first step in PDT is the administration, either intravenous or topically, of a PS—a light-absorbing molecule that accumulates selectively within target cells or tissues.[11] PSs may be synthetic or naturally occurring compounds, selected based on their absorption spectra and targeting capabilities. PS molecules do not react with biomolecules until excited by light, which results in the formation of reactive molecules.[11,12]

The second step in PDT is illumination with a specific wavelength that matches the PS absorption peak in the presence of oxygen.[11,12] Upon light absorption, the PS is transformed from the ground state (singlet state, ^{1}PS) to an excited singlet state lasting several nanoseconds (excited singlet state, $^{1}PS^{*}$).[11] The excited singlet state is unstable and decays to the ground state, emitting the energy difference through light emission (fluorescence) or heat (internal conversion).[11] The singlet state may also progress through spin conversion of the electron in the higher-energy orbital to a more stable, long-lived, electronically excited state (triplet state, $^{3}PS^{*}$).[11] The excited triplet state persists up to tens of microseconds and decays to the ground state through several pathways: light emission (phosphorescence) or two types of reactions.

The type I reaction occurs when the excited triplet state of the PS reacts directly with a target, such as cell membrane, resulting in hydrogen atom abstraction or electron transfer and generating free radicals and radical ions. The free radicals react with molecular oxygen, producing ROS, such as superoxide radical ($O_2^{-\bullet}$), hydroxyl radical ($HO^{\bullet}$), and hydrogen peroxide (H_2O_2), which cause oxidative damage that can destroy the target.[11]

The type II reaction occurs when the excited triplet state of the PS directly transfers energy to molecular oxygen (O_2) leading to the formation of singlet oxygen ($^{1}O_2$) and the fundamental state of the PS, the type II reaction.[11] The $^{1}O_2$ is highly reactive and may interact with numerous biological substrates, inflicting oxidative damage and triggering cell death.[11]

CYTOTOXIC REACTIONS AND CELL DEATH

The cytotoxic photoproducts of PDT are highly reactive and begin a cascade of biochemical events, such as lipid peroxidation, protein cross-linking, and DNA damage which lead to compromised cell integrity and death of the target. This multifaceted attack on cellular structures minimizes the likelihood of development of resistance.[3,13–15] The presence of molecular oxygen is crucial for PDT. Hypoxic conditions due to limited oxygen availability can render PDT ineffective. Methods to enhance oxygen availability, on the contrary, can lead to improved results.[13,16]

ANTIMICROBIAL SELECTIVITY

PDT selectively targets the microbial cell as opposed to surrounding tissue through the selective uptake of a PS and pairing with a wavelength to target the photosensitized microbial cells. This selectivity largely prevents collateral damage to healthy tissues.[10]

PDT FOR MRSA

Background

The Gram-positive spherical bacterium *Staphylococcus aureus* frequently colonizes the skin and mucous membranes of humans at rates estimated at 30%; however, it is also a pathogen that can cause life-threatening infection.[17] Armed with an array of virulence factors, including toxins, enzymes, and adhesins, *S. aureus* causes diverse diseases ranging from soft skin and tissue infections to severe and life- threatening infections, such as pneumonia, osteomyelitis, endocarditis, and sepsis.[17]

The evolutionary trajectory of *S. aureus* has been characterized by the emergence of methicillin-resistant *Staphylococcus aureus* (MRSA).[18,19] MRSA exhibits resistance to beta-lactams owing to the acquisition of the mecA gene, encoding an altered penicillin-binding protein. Furthermore, MRSA demonstrates the ability to form biofilms, enhancing its resilience. In healthcare settings, MRSA can lead to outbreaks and give rise to life-threatening infections.[18,19]

The limited development of new antibiotics, coupled with the escalating prevalence of multidrug-resistant MRSA and other bacteria, has been identified by the World Health Organization (WHO) as one of the foremost global threats to human health in the 21st century.[18,20,21]

In this context, new strategies are in development aside from new, more potent antibiotics. Such approaches include phage therapy, metallic nanoparticles, cationic polymers, nanocarriers, photothermotherapy, and PDT, which is one of the most promising approaches.[22–24] PDT-based antimicrobial therapies in basic science and clinical trials have demonstrated reproducible efficacy in treating *S. aureus* infections of the skin and soft tissue.[1,21]

The selection of a protocol for the antimicrobial application of PDT is contingent on several factors, including the absorption and emission wavelengths of the PS, the intended light source, the delivery of the PS, its capacity to penetrate target tissues, and the specificity of the PS and light irradiation for targeting the pathogen, such as MRSA cells.[25] Each PS necessitates specific dosimetry and treatment protocols to attain optimal results.[1,25]

Porphyrin and Derivatives

Porphyrin and its derivatives belong to a category of organic molecules featuring a tetrapyrrole ring structure, and they represent one of the initial classes of PS employed in PDT targeting MRSA and other resistant bacteria. The metabolic pathways of porphyrin utilized by MRSA cells facilitate the accumulation of the PS in these cells.[1,11,26,27]

Chemical engineering of porphyrin derivatives is undertaken to enhance specific properties, enabling optimized antimicrobial efficacy and targeted action against MRSA. The modification of these molecules is geared toward achieving a higher affinity for MRSA cells and fostering more effective interaction with the cell's metabolic pathways.[27,28]

Hematoporphyrin (Hp), protoporphyrin IX (PpIX), Protoporphyrin arginate, novel porphyrin derivatives, commercially available porphyrin-based PSs and metalloporphyrins represent the most important types of porphyrin derivatives.

Hp is a historically significant PS that played an important role in laying the foundation for PDT.[29] While not commonly used due to systemic side effects, hematoporphyrin derivative (HPD) played a key role in the development of our understanding of the basic principles of PDT and its applications to treatment of MRSA and other infections.

PpIX is an intermediate in the heme biosynthesis pathway, a path central to hemoglobin production in red blood cells. A unique characteristic of PpIX is its selective accumulation in specific cell types, such as cancer cells and pathogens like MRSA. This phenomenon, "PpIX accumulation," is based on altered heme metabolism pathways in these cells. ALA is a precursor of PpIX that leads to the production of PpIX within cells.[10,30]

Protoporphyrin diarginate (PPArg2) is a specialized derivative of PpIX, and it incorporates two arginine residues, which are positively charged, facilitating, this way, enhanced binding to negatively charged bacterial membranes.[10]

A systematic review and critical appraisal of original research articles investigating PDT against MRSA, both in vitro and in vivo, analyzed 531 studies, with 113 meeting the inclusion criteria.[10] Porphyrin derivatives assessed in these studies included Hp, PpIX, PPArg2, and novel porphyrin derivatives such as meso-tetra (N-methyl-4-pyridyl) porphine tetratosylate salt (TMPyP), and two lanthanide derivatives with europium (EuTMPyP) and praseodymium chloride (PrTMPyP).[10]

PpIX

PpIX-mediated photodynamic inactivation (PDI) of 265 MRSA strains demonstrated a 0.01e4.51 $\log_{10}$ CFU reduction by 25 mM PpIX.[31] Responses were classified as resistant, intermediately sensitive, and sensitive when the $\log_{10}$ CFU reduction was 0.01e0.99, 1e1.99 and >2, respectively with 14% of the MRSA isolates in the study rated as sensitive.[31]

Ga(III) protoporphyrin IX Chloride (Ga-PpIX)

PpIX was chelated with the Ga3þ ion to synthesize Ga(III) protoporphyrin IX chloride (Ga-PpIX), which enhances the PDI effect of PpIX against MRSA[32] Ga-PpIX resulted in >6 $\log_{10}$ CFU reduction of MRSA at a concentration of 0.24 mM.[32]

Protoporphyrin Diarginate (PPArg2)

A PpIX derivative, PPArg2, was synthesized with the attachment of two arginine groups to improve the solubility in aqueous medium and confer amphiphilic character. The investigators reported 3.6 $\log_{10}$ CFU reductions of clinical isolates of MRSA at 10 mM.[33,34]

Meso-tetrakis(2-*N*-methylpyridyl)porphyrin (TMPyP)

TMPyP-mediated PDT at 10 mM concentration and a 40 J cm^2 fluence rate for 10 s with IPL (in both 83 ms and 100 ms) resulted in 5 $\log_{10}$ CFU reduction of two MRSA strains (ATCC 43,300 and BAA 44).[35]

A two-layer polyethylene (PE) film incorporating TMPyP produced a 3.61 $\log_{10}$ CFU reduction per square centimeter against MRSA at 0.4% (w/w). This type of anti-infective material has broad applications as a coating or cover for equipment.[36]

Meso-tetra (4-aminophenyl) Porphine (TAPP)

The cationic porphyrin, meso-tetra (4-aminophenyl) porphine (TAPP), at 5 mM TAPP combined with 0.5 x MIC of ceftriaxone and vancomycin, resulted in a potentiation of PDT with an additional 2e3 $\log_{10}$ CFU reduction compared to the antibiotic or TAPP alone at their sub-MIC levels at 5 h of irradiation.[37] The additive effect of tobramycin and chloramphenicol with 5 mM TAPP achieved an additional 2.5e3 $\log_{10}$ CFU reduction compared to the sub-MIC of the antibiotic or TAPP alone. This approach may potentially extend the efficacy of antibiotics against MRSA.[37]

Di- and Tricationic Porphyrin-based PS (XF70, XF73)

Novel di- and tricationic porphyrin-based and water-soluble PS molecules [XF70, XF73, and CTP1 were investigated for their anti-MRSA activity.[38,39] At a concentration of 0.005 mM, XF70 and XF73 demonstrated 2.9e3.3 log10 CFU reductions of MRSA strains BAA 44 and ATCC 43,300. At 10 mM, all three derivatives CTP1, XF70, and XF73 exhibited >5 $\log_{10}$ CFU reductions of the MRSA strains.[38]

Tetrahydroporphyrin-tetratosylat (THPTS)

A synthetic PS, tetrahydroporphyrin-tetratosylat (THPTS) resulted in a >6 $\log_{10}$ (CFUmL-1) reduction in MRSA with 30- and 90-min incubations at 10–100 mM THPTS.[40]

5-[4-(1-Dodecanoylpyridinium)]-10,15,20-triphenyl-porphyrinyl Chloride (TDPyP)

5-[4-(1-Dodecanoylpyridinium)]-10,15,20-triphenyl-porphyrinyl chloride (TDPyP) a neutrally charged porphyrin derivative induced a <3 $\log_{10}$ CFU reduction against a clinical MRSA isolate at 10 μM.[41]

The incorporation of TDPyP into cationic liposomes resulted in 4.5 and 6 $\log_{10}$ CFU reductions after 5 and 10 min of light exposure, respectively. This result indicates that the PS with cationic charges may be more effective against MRSA.[42] A complete eradication of MRSA USA 300 was demonstrated with 200 nm TPPS4 and 10 mM of KI. In contrast, the complete eradication by TMPy4 (200 nm) was observed when the KI concentration was considerably lower (0.1–1 mM). The observation for the tetra anionic TPPS4 is consistent with the increase in killing caused by free iodine (only possible at high KI concentration).[42]

Photofrin

Photofrin, a first-generation PS, was investigated for anti-MRSA activity in vitro and in vivo in a murine MRSA arthritis mouse model.[43] Potentiation of MRSA cidal activity at 1 and >2 $\log_{10}$ of photofrin (200 nm) was demonstrated in 10 and 25 mM of KI, respectively.[44]

Temoporfin

Nanosized liposomes, with a diameter of 136.6 ± 1.6 nm, that were modified with the antimicrobial peptide (AMP) WLBU2 demonstrated enhanced delivery of the PS temoporfin into MRSA strains, resulting in increased antibacterial activities.[45] The effectiveness of PDT using WLBU2-modified liposomes, temoporfin liposomes (foslip), and free temoporfin produced the following outcomes. WLBU2-liposomal temoporfin proved to be the most efficient, eradicating MRSA at both concentrations and time points. Free temoporfin exhibited a 2.69 $\log_{10}$ CFU reduction of MRSA after 180 min of incubation. Upon irradiation, all MRSA was eradicated at 1.25 μM (180 min of irradiation) and 12.5 μM (90- and 180-min irradiation). Foslip was the least efficient in killing MRSA, achieving its maximum CFU reduction of 2.6 $\log_{10}$ at 1.25 μM (180 min).[45]

Metalloporphyrins

The chelation of metal ions by a porphyrin ring has the potential to increase the generation of ROS. In an analysis involving four metal ions (Cu^{2+}, Fe^{2+}, Pd^{2+}, and Zn^{2+}) chelated with porphyrin, it was observed that Cu^{2+} and Fe^{2+} chelated porphyrin, followed by irradiation, had a minimal effect.[46] However, the chelation of Zn^{2+} and Pd^{2+} resulted in a 2.6 and 5.9 $\log_{10}$ CFU reduction, respectively, at a light dose of 2.5 J cm^{-2}. This suggests that these two di-cationic metal ions could be suitable for chelation with organic PSs.[46]

Phenothiazine Derivatives

Phenothiazine derivatives are the second major PS class following porphyrins.[10] Molecules from this category have tricyclic structures containing nitrogen atoms, that give them certain useful photophysical properties. The category is mainly represented by methylene blue (MB) and toluidine blue O (TBO), a hydrophilic cationic PS of phenothiazine dyes with a high $1O_2$ quantum yield and strong absorption bands in the 620–660 nm region.[22]

In various studies, PDT employing MB has been demonstrated to disrupt biofilms and facilitate the accumulation of neutrophils within the biofilm to eliminate bacteria. In a murine model of MRSA abrasion wound infection, PDT utilizing NorA Efflux Pump Inhibitors (EPIs) linked to MB exhibited efficacy against MRSA. Among the 16 hybrid compounds tested, INF55-(Ac) enMB 12 emerged as a lead compound, displaying increased uptake into MRSA cells and enhanced PDI and wound healing effects compared to MB.[47]

Phthalocyanine Derivatives

The chemical structure of phthalocyanines (Pc) is similar to the porphyrins and requires chelation with a metal ion to exert PDT effects.[10] Their macrocyclic structure is composed of four isoindole units linked by nitrogen atoms, and imparts strong absorption in the red and near-infrared regions, aligning with tissue-penetrating wavelengths.[23,31,32]

Aluminum disulfonated Pc ($AlPcS_2$)-mediated PDT against 16 epidemic MRSA (EMRSA) strains demonstrated a 5.48 $\log_{10}$ CFU reduction with 11 J cm^{-2} of laser light at 6.25 mgL^{-1}.[48]

Chloroaluminum phthalocyanine (ClAlPc) encapsulated in both positively and negatively charged nanoemulsions was evaluated in the context of PDT for MRSA.[49] Cationic NE-ClAlPc and free ClAlPc (ClAlPc dissolved in DMSO) produced a 6–7 $\log_{10}$ CFU reduction of MRSA, whereas anionic NE-ClAlPc did not reveal efficacy. It appears that there is a greater affinity of the negatively charged thick peptidoglycan bi-layer of MRSA for cationic PSs that may facilitate the active transport of these compounds into the bacterial cells.[49]

Zn(II) chelated Pcs were investigated for PDT-mediated anti-MRSA activity in vitro and in vivo.[50] Six different mono and di-cationic Zinc (II) Pc (ZnPc) compounds demonstrated a 3.2–5.5 log_{10} CFU reduction at a 2.5 μM concentration; two tetracationic Pcs, RLP068 and MRLP164, demonstrated 2.7–3.6 log_{10} reduction at 0.1 μM upon irradiation without cytotoxicity to human fibroblasts or keratinocyte cell lines. Ultra-short (1–5 min) irradiation times were employed to achieve the CFU reduction, which is advantageous in clinical applications.[50] Several ZnPc compounds conjugated with oligolysine groups and tri-amino phthalonitrile exhibited a 4 log_{10} CFU reduction at 12–39 nm against four different MRSA strains, including MRSA ATCC BAA43.[51] Tricationic ZnPc-mediated aPDT (N-methylamine) exhibited similar efficacy at 7–13 nm.[52] RLP068/Cl (tetracationic ZnPc chloride derivative) in a gel formulation (0.01%–0.5% w/w) was studied in mediating PDT in vivo with MRSA-infected surgical wounds in mice.[53] Illumination was conducted 24 h after the infection and CFU was performed immediately and at 7 days intervals. 0.3% w/w RLP068/Cl yielded mediated MRSA killing by approximately a 3 log_{10} CFU reduction, while the positive control (TBO) produced only a 1 log_{10} CFU reduction.[53] The efficacy of α-d-galactopyranosyl ZnPc (T1–T4)-mediated PDT of MRSA varied in the order of T1 > T2 > T3 > T4 and showed a >99.9% CFU reduction after treatment with a concentration range of 12–50 μM. T1 was the most efficient (>99.9%) CFU reduction at 12 μM in treating superficial skin abrasion wounds.[54]

Chlorin e6 Derivatives

Chlorin e6 derivatives share structural similarities with porphyrins, differing only in the presence of a double bond. They derive their name from their concurrent resemblance to natural chlorophyll. These derivatives display robust light absorption in the red and near-infrared regions, rendering them well-suited for light sources commonly employed in clinical settings and facilitating deeper skin penetration.[10]

In the mouse model, chlorin(e6) covalently linked to the basic polymer, polyethylenimine (PEI)–ce6 followed by red light was effective in treating MRSA.[55] In vivo antibacterial activity of SnCe6 conjugated with polyethylene amine (PEI-SnCe6) demonstrated a 99% CFU reduction of the bioluminescent MRSA Xen31 upon illumination with 240 J cm^{-2} of light and treatment with 400 μM Ce6. In a mouse wound model, wound healing was accelerated by an average of 8.6 days as compared to the untreated wound ($P = .0009$).[55]

Natural Derivatives

Curcumin

Curcumin, a yellow pigment isolated from the rhizomes of the plant *Curcuma longa* is a natural PS.[34] Several studies have demonstrated the efficacy of curcumin in the killing of MRSA cells in vitro, in vivo, and ex vivo.[10,35]

The light-activated anti-MRSA activity of free curcumin was demonstrated both in vitro and in vivo in a mouse model, as well as against biofilm in an artificial bone cavity created in bovine ribs (ex vivo). To enhance stability, nanoparticles conjugated with curcumin (UCNPs-curcumin) have been synthesized.[1,10,35]

Hypericin

Another naturally derived PS tested in vitro and in vivo is hypericin (HY), a polycyclic quinine extracted from *Hypericum perforatum*.[1,22] The herb, St. John's wort is known for its antidepressant effects. It has several desirable properties as a high singlet oxygen quantum yield, a high extinction coefficient close to 600 nm, and cytoplasmic membrane localization, make it suitable for use as a PS in PDT.[22] HY-laden nanoparticles at 0.03 μM inhibited the growth of MRSA biofilms by 60%–120% as compared to 55%–75% for planktonic MRSA cells. The growth inhibition of the latter approached 40%, whereas a near 100% growth inhibition was observed in the MRSA biofilms.[56]

Riboflavin

Riboflavin, vitamin B2, has served as a PS in PDT for MRSA.[10] Riboflavin and a blue 412 nm low-level (5.4 J cm^{-2}) light source resulted in a 44%–55% reduction in MRSA count in a 400 μm layer as compared to 89% for UVA-mediated PDT.[57]

Chlorophyll

Pheophorbide a (Phde a), a PS derived from chlorophyll, was modified into a water-soluble form as a sodium salt, known as Na-Phde a, to address its hydrophobic nature. In treating MRSA, four light sources and Na-Phde (at a concentration of 280 μM) were tested.[58] The light sources included a GaA1P semiconductor laser (power: 300 mW, wavelength: 670 nm, approximate fluence: 7.2 J cm^{-2}), a halogen lamp (power: 75 W, approximate fluence: 15.8 J cm^{-2}), a xenon lamp (power: 300 W, approximate fluence: 68.6 J cm^{-2}), and a fluorescent lamp (power: 27 W, approximate fluence: 19.6 J cm^{-2}). The MRSA inoculum was preincubated with Na-Phde a for 60 min and then irradiated for 30 min. The PDT groups using the semiconductor laser and halogen lamp demonstrated bactericidal effects.[58]

Fullerenes

Fullerene (C_{60}), a closed molecule composed of SP^2 hybridized carbon atoms, is produced when one s orbital and two p orbitals are combined. This delocalized π electron system exhibits a strong absorption of visible light and a sizable quantum yield of a long-lived triplet electron excited state.[59]

To overcome its hydrophobicity, a hydrophilic functional group is added and three such functionalized fullerenes (LC 14–16) were studied.[60] When tested against MRSA at a 10 μM concentration followed by light exposure (10–40 J cm^{-2} for UV light and 50–200 J cm^{-2} for white light), an 8 log_{10} CFU reduction was observed with 40 J cm^{-2} and 200 J cm^{-2} UVA and white light, respectively.[60] The order of effectiveness was LC 16 > LC 15 > LC 14. For LC 15, the inclusion of a "light-harvesting antenna," namely the addition of fluorene-triphenyl moiety, extended the light absorption into visible range (red shifting).[60] Red shifting improves penetration into tissues and reduces harmful effects of shorter UV wavelengths. Additional studies have confirmed the efficacy of the fullerenes as PDT-mediated antimicrobial agents.[61]

Aza-borondipyrromethene (aza-BODIPY) Compounds

Aza-boron dipyrromethenes (aza-BODIPYs) derivatives, where the mesomethine group is replaced with a nitrogen atom, have been investigated for their potential as antimicrobial agents mediated by PDT.[62,63] The extended π – π conjugation system in aza-BODIPY compounds leads to an inherent bathochromic shift in absorption maxima. These compounds exhibit robust fluorescence emission, high solubility, and stability across various solvent systems, along with ease of chemical modification. These features render aza-BODIPY compounds highly appealing as near-infrared-absorbing dyes for antimicrobial applications. Aza-BODIPY 6, at a concentration of 5 μg mL^{-1} and a fluence of 16 J cm^{-2}, demonstrated significant reductions of 6.8 and 3.4 log_{10} CFU for MSSA and MRSA strains, respectively. In contrast, its non-brominated counterpart was entirely ineffective at the same concentration, even with an increased fluence of 25 J cm^{-2}.[62] Another derivative of aza-BODIPY, known as DIMPy-BODIPY, exhibited a broad spectrum of antibacterial activity against viruses, fungi, and bacteria.[63] DIMPy-BODIPY achieved a 5–6 log_{10} CFU reduction of MRSA ATCC-44 at concentrations as low as 0.1 μM.[63]

Porphycenes

Porphycene, a structural isomer of porphyrin, was the focus of investigation for the light-activated anti-MRSA activities of two aryl tricationic porphycene derivatives, both in vitro and in vivo.[64,65] In vitro, low concentrations of porphycene (<2 μM) and low light intensities (<30 J cm^{-2}) were found to be sufficient for the complete inhibition of MRSA. Moreover, a tricationic water-soluble porphycene derivative demonstrated a 2.6 log10 CFU reduction in an energy-dependent manner upon irradiation with 180 J cm^{-2} at a porphycene concentration of 100 μM.[64] Similarly, a second tricationic derivative achieved a >6 log10 CFU reduction of MRSA at concentrations <750 nm, maintaining a constant fluence rate of 22.5 J cm^{-2}.[65] Both compounds are tricationic and exhibit strong binding to bacterial membranes, rendering them highly active against MRSA.

Rose Bengal (RB)

RB is a halogenated xanthene dye that is used to mediate antimicrobial PDT. RB-loaded silica (SiO_2–NH2–RB) nanoparticles displayed greater efficacy in PDT against MRSA as compared to free RB.[66]

Indocyanine Green (ICG)

Indocyanine green (ICG) is an FDA-approved dye utilized in various medical applications. It exhibits characteristic absorption in the NIR spectrum at around 800 nm, with high absorption capacity, making it a suitable PS. In a rat abrasion wound model, a 90% reduction in CFU of MRSA was observed following ICG-mediated PDT with NIR light.[67] Another study reported a 5 log10 CFU reduction at a high concentration of ICG upon illumination with high-intensity light.[68]

PDT FOR BIOFILMS

Background

Biofilms are structured and well-organized communities of microorganisms, predominantly bacteria, enveloped within a matrix of EPS that adhere to surfaces and to each other.[69] This formation is a result of the secretion of a self-produced matrix consisting of polysaccharides, proteins, and other materials. Biofilms can develop on a variety of surfaces, both biotic and abiotic, including medical devices, pipes, teeth, and even in natural environments.[69]

The EPS matrix plays a crucial role in protecting microorganisms within biofilms from adverse external factors, such as antibiotics, immune system responses, and physical stresses. Additionally, it serves as a reservoir for nutrients and establishes a stable microenvironment that fosters the growth and survival of pathogens within the biofilm. Another vital characteristic of the EPS matrix is its adhesive properties. These properties enable microorganisms to firmly attach to surfaces, providing stability to the biofilm structure.[70]

Biofilms are often linked to chronic infections because bacteria encased within biofilms typically exhibit resistance to antibiotic therapy and the host's immune responses. Several factors contribute to this resistance. For instance, the EPS matrix obstructs the penetration of antibiotics into biofilms, making it challenging to achieve high concentrations and acting as an impermeable barrier. Additionally, the slow metabolic activity of microorganisms within the biofilm significantly diminishes the efficacy of antibiotics that target active metabolic pathways of the pathogens.[71]

The diminishing efficacy of conventional antibiotics in combating biofilms underscores the urgency of exploring alternative approaches. Strategies such as surface modifiers, small molecule inhibitors, bacteriophage therapy, ultrasound, and nanoparticles are being investigated. Additionally, PDT appears to be a valuable tool in the ongoing antimicrobial battle against biofilms.[72]

Mechanism of Action

The general principles of PDT protocols for biofilms do not differ significantly from those applied in PDT protocols for the treatment of MRSA.[73] The common steps involve the application of PSs, their activation by specific wavelength light, and the subsequent generation of ROS, leading to oxidative stress and cytotoxicity.

The main mechanisms through which PDT eradicates biofilms, depending on the localization of the PS, include:

- Biofilm matrix destruction
- Damage to the cell surface
- Oxidation of lipids
- Change in permeability of the outer membrane
- Penetration and the self-promoted uptake pathway
- Intracellular damage

Gram–Negative Bacterial Biofilms

PDT has been used for the treatment of various Gram-negative bacterial biofilms, but the most frequently studied and treated biofilms include those formed by *Pseudomonas aeruginosa* and *Escherichia coli*.[74–76] These two bacterial species are highly associated with biofilm-related infections and have been the target of numerous PDT studies due to their clinical relevance and prevalence.[74–76] Reports of killing efficiency of about 7.0 $\log_{10}$ in treating *P.aeruginosa* have been published.[38] PSs that have been used in treating Gram-negative bacteria include Polyethylenimine chlorine (e6), Poly-l-lysine chlorine (e6), δ-ALA, Erythrosine, MB, and more.[74–76]

Gram-Positive Bacterial Biofilms

The Gram-positive bacteria classification is primarily represented by *S. aureus, E. faecalis*, and *Streptococcus*. There are reports indicating killing efficiency of up to 7.0 $\log_{10}$ in treating *S. aureus*.[77] PSs employed against *S. aureus* biofilms include MB, TBO, and erythrosine, among others. MB and TBO have also been employed as PSs in treating other Gram-positive bacteria, including *Staphylococcus epidermidis, Streptococcus sobrinus*, and *Streptococcus sanguinis*.[18,73,78]

Yeast Biofilms

PDT's therapeutic potential extends beyond bacterial infections to address biofilms formed by yeast species, including *Candida albicans* and other *Candida* species.[38] Yeast biofilms are implicated in various medical conditions, for example, oral and vaginal candidiasis, catheter-associated infections, and invasive candidiasis. PDT appears to be a promising alternative therapy to eradicate these resilient biofilm-forming yeasts. MB and Toluidine have been used as PSs in treating *C. albicans* biofilms, and the results show that they seem to control them.[79,80]

The therapeutic potential of PDT extends beyond bacterial infections to include the treatment of biofilms formed by yeast species, including *C. albicans* and other *Candida* species.[38] Yeast biofilms are implicated in various medical conditions such as oral and vaginal candidiasis, catheter-associated infections, and invasive candidiasis. PDT presents itself as a promising alternative therapy to eradicate these resilient biofilm-forming yeasts. MB and TBO have been utilized as PSs in treating *C. albicans* biofilms, with results indicating their potential to control these biofilms.[79,80]

Other PDT Antimicrobial Applications

PDT exhibits a broad spectrum of antimicrobial applications that extend beyond treating MRSA and biofilms. Here are some additional applications:

1. Bacterial infections: PDT has been utilized to treat various bacterial infections caused by bacteria such as *Pseudomonas aeruginosa, Acinetobacter baumannii, Klebsiella pneumoniae*, and others.[1,81]
2. Fungal infections: PDT has shown success in treating fungal infections caused by different *Candida* species, Aspergillus species, *Cryptococcus neoformans, Microsporum* species, and more. The mechanism of action against fungi is similar to that in treating bacteria and MRSA.[82,83]
3. Viral deactivation: Although information in this field is limited, PDT has been explored for viral deactivation. Certain viruses, including HIV, HCV, and HSV, have been targeted by PDT. The outer lipid envelopes of viruses are susceptible to ROS generated by activated PSs, leading to reduced infectivity and prevention of transmission.[84,85]
4. Wound care: PDT contributes to wound healing by reducing bacterial load and preventing wound infection. Additionally, the activation of PSs to generate ROS in PDT promotes wound healing by stimulating skin resident cells and recruiting immune cells.[72,86–88]
5. Water and air purification: PDT can be applied for the deactivation of microorganisms in water and air. This provides an alternative to conventional chemical disinfection methods, demonstrating the versatility of PDT in environmental applications.[89]

CONCLUSION

PDT provides a highly promising strategy for efficient therapy against resistant microbial infections, including MRSA, biofilms, and others. The combination of PDT with conventional antimicrobial agents, such as antibiotics, holds the potential for potent synergistic effects. This synergy has been investigated in conjunction with certain antibiotics like gentamicin and linezolid, yielding promising outcomes.[30–36] This strategic combination has the capacity to amplify the antimicrobial efficacy of each therapy individually, offering a potential solution to counteract resistance mechanisms that have developed against single-agent therapies. The diverse applications described in this chapter highlight the utility of PDT as a versatile and innovative intervention, offering solutions to a range of antimicrobial challenges.

REFERENCES

1. Ghorbani J, Rahban D, Aghamiri S, Teymouri A, Bahador A. PSs in antibacterial photodynamic therapy: an overview. *Laser Ther.* 2018;27(4):293–302. doi:10.5978/islsm.27_18-RA-01.
2. Daniell MD, Hill JS. A history of photodynamic therapy. *Aust N Z J Surg.* 1991;61(5):340–348. doi:10.1111/j.1445-2197.1991.tb00230.x.
3. Kang K, Bacci S. Photodynamic therapy. *Biomedicines.* 2022;10(11):2701. doi:10.3390/biomedicines10112701.
4. Antimicrobial Resistance Collaborators. Global burden of bacterial antimicrobial resistance in 2019: a systematic analysis. *Lancet.* 2022;399(10325):629–655. doi:10.1016/S0140-6736(21)02724-0.
5. Sharma S, Mohler J, Mahajan SD, Schwartz SA, Bruggemann L, Aalinkeel R. Microbial biofilm: a review on formation, infection, antibiotic resistance, control measures, and innovative treatment. *Microorganisms.* 2023;11(6):1614. doi:10.3390/microorganisms11061614.
6. Ciofu O, Moser C, Jensen PØ, Høiby N. Tolerance and resistance of microbial biofilms. *Nat Rev Microbiol.* 2022;20(10):621–635. doi:10.1038/s41579-022-00682-4.
7. Roy R, Tiwari M, Donelli G, Tiwari V. Strategies for combating bacterial biofilms: a focus on anti-biofilm agents and their mechanisms of action. *Virulence.* 2018;9(1):522–554. doi:10.1080/21505594.2017.1313372.
8. Mirghani R, Saba T, Khaliq H, et al. Biofilms: formation, drug resistance and alternatives to conventional approaches. *AIMS Microbiol.* 2022;8(3):239–277. doi:10.3934/microbiol.2022019.
9. Martins Antunes de Melo WC, Celiešiūtė-Germanienė R, Šimonis P, Stirkė A. Antimicrobial photodynamic therapy (aPDT) for biofilm treatments. Possible synergy between aPDT and pulsed electric fields. *Virulence.* 2021;12(1):2247–2272. doi:10.1080/21505594.2021.1960105.
10. Dharmaratne P, Sapugahawatte DN, Wang B, et al. Contemporary approaches and future perspectives of antibacterial photodynamic therapy (aPDT) against methicillin-resistant Staphylococcus aureus (MRSA): a systematic review. *Eur J Med Chem.* 2020;200:112341. doi:10.1016/j.ejmech.2020.112341.
11. Correia JH, Rodrigues JA, Pimenta S, Dong T, Yang Z. Photodynamic therapy review: principles, PSs, applications, and future directions. *Pharmaceutics.* 2021;13(9):1332. doi:10.3390/pharmaceutics13091332.
12. Kwiatkowski S, Knap B, Przystupski D, et al. Photodynamic therapy - mechanisms, PSs and combinations.

Biomed Pharmacother. 2018;106:1098–1107. doi:10.1016/j.biopha.2018.07.049.

13. Zhou Z, Song J, Nie L, Chen X. Reactive oxygen species generating systems meeting challenges of photodynamic cancer therapy. *Chem Soc Rev*. 2016;45(23):6597–6626. doi:10.1039/c6cs00271d.
14. Girotti AW, Korytowski W. Nitric oxide inhibition of chain lipid peroxidation initiated by photodynamic action in membrane environments. *Cell Biochem Biophys*. 2020;78(2):149–156. doi:10.1007/s12013-020-00909-2.
15. Benov L. Photodynamic therapy: current status and future directions. *Med Princ Pract*. 2015;24(Suppl 1):14–28. doi:10.1159/000362416.
16. Du Y, Han J, Jin F, Du Y. Recent strategies to address hypoxic tumor environments in photodynamic therapy. *Pharmaceutics*. 2022;14(9):1763. doi:10.3390/pharmaceutics14091763.
17. Laux C, Peschel A, Krismer B. *Staphylococcus aureus* colonization of the human nose and interaction with other microbiome members. *Microbiol Spectr*. 2019;7(2):1–10. doi:10.1128/microbiolspec.GPP3-0029-2018.
18. Craft KM, Nguyen JM, Berg LJ, Townsend SD. Methicillin-resistant Staphylococcus aureus (MRSA): antibiotic-resistance and the biofilm phenotype. *Medchemcomm*. 2019;10(8):1231–1241. doi:10.1039/c9md00044e.
19. Siddiqui AH, Koirala J. *Methicillin-Resistant Staphylococcus Aureus*. StatPearls Publishing; 2023. https://www.ncbi.nlm.nih.gov/books/NBK482221/.
20. Aslam B, Wang W, Arshad MI, et al. Antibiotic resistance: a rundown of a global crisis. *Infect Drug Resist*. 2018;11:1645–1658. doi:10.2147/IDR.S173867.
21. Pérez C, Zúñiga T, Palavecino CE. Photodynamic therapy for treatment of Staphylococcus aureus infections. *Photodiagnosis Photodyn Ther*. 2021;34:102285. doi:10.1016/j.pdpdt.2021.102285.
22. Pérez C, Zúñiga T, Palavecino CE. Photodynamic therapy for treatment of Staphylococcus aureus infections. *Photodiagnosis Photodyn Ther*. 2021;34:102285. doi:10.1016/j.pdpdt.2021.102285.
23. Mahmoudi H, Bahador A, Pourhajibagher M, Alikhani MY. Antimicrobial photodynamic therapy: an effective alternative approach to control bacterial infections. *J Lasers Med Sci*. 2018;9(3):154–160. doi:10.15171/jlms.2018.29.
24. Suresh MK, Biswas R, Biswas L. An update on recent developments in the prevention and treatment of Staphylococcus aureus biofilms. *Int J Med Microbiol*. 2019;309(1):1–12. doi:10.1016/j.ijmm.2018.11.002.
25. Li X, Lee S, Yoon J. Supramolecular PSs rejuvenate photodynamic therapy. *Chem Soc Rev*. 2018;47(4):1174–1188. doi:10.1039/c7cs00594f.
26. Abrahamse H, Hamblin MR. New PSs for photodynamic therapy. *Biochem J*. 2016;473(4):347–364. doi:10.1042/BJ20150942.
27. Amos-Tautua BM, Songca SP, Oluwafemi OS. Application of porphyrins in antibacterial photodynamic therapy. *Molecules*. 2019;24(13):2456. doi:10.3390/molecules24132456.
28. Imran M, Ramzan M, Qureshi AK, Khan MA, Tariq M. Emerging applications of porphyrins and metalloporphyrins in biomedicine and diagnostic magnetic resonance imaging. *Biosensors (Basel)*. 2018;8(4):95. doi:10.3390/bios8040095.
29. Yoon I, Li JZ, Shim YK. Advance in PSs and light delivery for photodynamic therapy. *Clin Endosc*. 2013;46(1):7–23. doi:10.5946/ce.2013.46.1.7.
30. Morales-de-Echegaray AV, Maltais TR, Lin L, et al. Rapid uptake and photodynamic inactivation of staphylococci by Ga(III)-protoporphyrin IX. *ACS Infect Dis*. 2018;4(11):1564–1573. doi:10.1021/acsinfecdis.8b00125.
31. Grinholc M, Rapacka-Zdonczyk A, Rybak B, Szabados F, Bielawski KP. Multiresistant strains are as susceptible to photodynamic inactivation as their naïve counterparts: protoporphyrin IX-mediated photoinactivation reveals differences between methicillin-resistant and methicillin-sensitive Staphylococcus aureus strains. *Photomed Laser Surg*. 2014;32:121–129. doi:10.1089/pho.2013.3663.
32. Morales-De-Echegaray AV, Maltais TR, Lin L, et al. Rapid uptake and photodynamic inactivation of staphylococci by Ga(III)-protoporphyrin IX. *ACS Infect Dis*. 2018;4:1564–1573. doi:10.1021/acsinfecdis.8b00125.
33. Grinholc M, Kawiak A, Kurlenda J, Graczyk A, Bielawski KP. Photodynamic effect of protoporphyrin diarginate (PPArg2) on methicillin-resistant Staphylococcus aureus and human dermal fibroblasts. *Acta Biochim Pol*. 2008;55:85–90.
34. Grinholc M, Zawacka-Pankau J, Gwizdek-Wisniewska A, Bielawski KP. Evaluation of the role of the pharmacological inhibition of *Staphylococcus aureus* multidrug resistance pumps and the variable levels of the uptake of he sensitizer in the strain-dependent response of Staphylococcus aureus to PPArg2-based photodynamic ina. *Photochem Photobiol*. 2010;86:1118–1126. doi:10.1111/j.1751-1097.2010.00772.x.
35. Maisch T, Spannberger F, Regensburger J, Felgenträger A, Bäumler W. Fast and effective: intense pulse light photodynamic inactivation of bacteria. *J Ind Microbiol. Biotechnol*. 2012;39:1013–1021. doi:10.1007/s10295-012-1103-3.
36. Mccoy CP, O'Neil EJ, Cowley JF, et al. Photodynamic antimicrobial polymers for infection control. *PLoS One*. 2014;9:e108500. doi:10.1371/journal.pone.0108500.

37. Dastgheyb SS, Eckmann DM, Composto RJ, Hickok NJ. Photo-activated porphyrin in combination with antibiotics: therapies against Staphylococci. *J Photochem Photobiol B Biol*. 2013;129:27–35. doi:10.1016/j.jphotobiol.2013.09.006.
38. Maisch T, Bosl C, Szeimies R-M, Lehn N, Abels C. Photodynamic effects of novel XF porphyrin derivatives on prokaryotic and eukaryotic cells. *Antimicrob Agents Chemother*. 2005;49:1542–1552. doi:10.1128/aac.49.4.1542-1552.2005.
39. Maisch T, Bosl C, Szeimies R-M, Love B. Abels C. Determination of the antibacterial efficacy of a new porphyrin-based photosensitizer against MRSA ex vivo. *Photochem Photobiol Sci*. 2007;6:545. doi:10.1039/b614770d.
40. Schastak S, Ziganshyna S, Gitter B, Wiedemann P, Claudepierre T. Efficient photodynamic therapy against gram-positive and gram-negative bacteria using THPTS, a cationic photosensitizer excited by infrared wavelength. *PLoS One*. 2010;5:e11674. doi:10.1371/journal.pone.0011674.
41. Ferro S, Ricchelli F, Monti D, Mancini G, Jori G. Efficient photoinactivation of methicillin-resistant Staphylococcus aureus by a novel porphyrin incorporated into a poly-cationic liposome. *Int J Biochem Cell Biol*. 2007;39:1026–1034. doi:10.1016/j.biocel.2007.02.001.
42. Huang L, El-Hussein A, Xuan W, Hamblin MR. Potentiation by potassium iodide reveals that the anionic porphyrin TPPS4 is a surprisingly effective photosensitizer for antimicrobial photodynamic inactivation. *J Photochem Photobiol B Biol*. 2018;178:277–286. doi:10.1016/j.jphotobiol.2017.10.036.
43. Tanaka M, Kinoshita M, Yoshihara Y, et al. Photodynamic therapy using intra-articular photofrin for murine MRSA arthritis: biphasic light dose response for neutrophil-mediated antibacterial effect. *Laser Surg Med*. 2011;43:221–229. doi:10.1002/lsm.21037.
44. Huang L, Szewczyk G, Sarna T, Hamblin MR. Potassium iodide potentiates broad-spectrum antimicrobial photodynamic inactivation using photofrin. *ACS Infect Dis*. 2017;3:320–328. doi:10.1021/acsinfecdis.7b00004.
45. Yang K, Gitter B, Rüger R, et al. Antimicrobial peptide-modified liposomes for bacteria targeted delivery of temoporfin in photodynamic antimicrobial chemotherapy. *Photochem Photobiol Sci*. 2011;10:1593. doi:10.1039/c1pp05100h.
46. Skwor TA, Klemm S, Zhang H, Schardt B, Blaszczyk S, Bork MA. Photo-dynamic inactivation of methicillin-resistant *Staphylococcus aureus* and *Escherichia coli*: a metalloporphyrin comparison. *J Photochem Photobiol B Biol*. 2016;165:51–57. doi:10.1016/j.jphotobiol.2016.10.016.
47. Rineh A, Dolla NK, Ball AR, et al. Attaching the NorA efflux pump inhibitor INF55 to methylene blue enhances antimicrobial photodynamic inactivation of methicillin-resistant *Staphylococcus aureus* in vitro and in vivo. *ACS Infect Dis*. 2017;3:756–766. doi:10.1021/acsinfecdis.7b00095.
48. Griffiths M. Killing of methicillin-resistant *Staphylococcus aureus* in vitro using aluminium disulphonated phthalocyanine, a light-activated antimicrobial agent. *J Antimicrob Chemother*. 1997;40:873–876. doi:10.1093/jac/40.6.873.
49. Ribeiro APD, Andrade MC, Bagnato VS, et al. Antimicrobial photodynamic therapy against pathogenic bacterial suspensions and biofilms using chloro-aluminum phthalocyanine encapsulated in nanoemulsions. *Laser Med Sci*. 2013;30:549–559. doi:10.1007/s10103-013-1354-x.
50. Soncin M, Fabris C, Busetti A, et al. Approaches to selectivity in the Zn(ii)ephthalocyanine-photosensitized inactivation of wild-type and antibiotic-resistant *Staphylococcus aureus*. *Photochem Photobiol Sci*. 2002;1:815–819. doi:10.1039/b206554a.
51. Ke M-R, Eastel JM, Ngai KL, et al. Photodynamic inactivation of bacteria and viruses using two monosubstituted zinc(II) phthalocyanines. *Eur J Med Chem*. 2014;84:278–283. doi:10.1016/j.ejmech.2014.07.022.
52. Ke M-R, Eastel JM, Ngai KLK, et al. Oligolysine-conjugated zinc(II) phthalocyanines as efficient photosensitizers for antimicrobial photodynamic therapy. *Chem Asian J*. 2014;9:1868–1875. doi:10.1002/asia.201402025.
53. Simonetti O, Cirioni O, Orlando F, et al. Effectiveness of antimicrobial photodynamic therapy with a single treatment of RLP068/Cl in an experimental model of Staphylococcus aureus wound infection. *Br J Dermatol*. 2011;164:987–995. doi:10.1111/j.13652133.2011.10232.x.
54. Zhao Z, Li Y, Meng S, Li S, Wang Q, Liu T. Susceptibility of methicillin- resistant *Staphylococcus aureus* to photodynamic antimicrobial chemo- therapy with a-d-galactopyranosyl zinc phthalocyanines: in vitro study. *Laser Med Sci*. 2013;29:1131–1138. doi:10.1007/s10103-013- 1488-x.
55. Dai T, Tegos GP, Zhiyentayev T, Mylonakis E, Hamblin MR. Photodynamic therapy for methicillin-resistant *Staphylococcus aureus* infection in a mouse skin abrasion model. *Lasers Surg Med*. 2010;42(1):38–44. doi:10.1002/lsm.20887.
56. Nafee N, Youssef A, El-Gowelli H, Asem H, Kandil S. Antibiotic-free nanotherapeutics: hypericin nanoparticles thereof for improved in vitro and in vivo antimicrobial photodynamic therapy and wound healing. *Int J Pharm*. 2013;454:249–258. doi:10.1016/j.ijpharm.2013.06.067.

57. Makdoumi K, Bäckman A. Photodynamic UVA-riboflavin bacterial elimination in antibiotic-resistant bacteria. *Clin Exp Ophthalmol.* 2016;44:582–586. doi:10.1111/ceo.12723.
58. Yamamoto T, Iriuchishima T, Aizawa S, et al. Bactericidal effect of photodynamic therapy using Na-pheophorbide a: evaluation of adequate light source. *Photomed Laser Surg.* 2009;27:849–853. doi:10.1089/pho.2008.2319.
59. Wang H, He Y, Li Y, Su H. Photophysical and electronic properties of five PCBM-like C60 derivatives: spectral and quantum chemical view. *J Phys Chem.* 2011;116:255–262. doi:10.1021/jp208520v.
60. Yin R, Wang M, Huang Y-Y, et al. Antimicrobial photodynamic inactivation with decacationic functionalized fullerenes: oxygen-independent photokilling in presence of azide and new mechanistic insights. *Free Radic Biol Med.* 2015;79:14–27. doi:10.1016/j.freeradbiomed.2014.10.514.
61. Zhang Y, Dai T, Wang M, Vecchio D, Chiang LY, Hamblin MR. Potentiation of antimicrobial photodynamic inactivation mediated by a cationic fullerene by added iodide: in vitro and in vivo studies. *Nanomedicine.* 2015;10:603–614. doi:10.2217/nnm.14.131.
62. Frimannsson DO, Grossi M, Murtagh J, Paradisi F, O'Shea DF. Light induced antimicrobial properties of a brominated boron difluoride (BF2) chelated tetraarylazadipyrromethene photosensitizer. *J Med Chem.* 2010;53:7337–7343. doi:10.1021/jm100585j.
63. Carpenter B, Situ X, Scholle F, Bartelmess J, Weare W, Ghiladi R. Antiviral, antifungal and antibacterial activities of a BODIPY-based photosensitizer. *Molecules.* 2015;20:10604–10621. doi:10.3390/molecules200610604.
64. Ragàs X, Sánchez-García D, Ruiz-González R, et al. Cationic porphycenes as potential photosensitizers for antimicrobial photodynamic therapy. *J Med Chem.* 2010;53:7796–7803. doi:10.1021/jm1009555.
65. Ruiz-Gonzalez R, Agut M, Reddi E, Nonell S. A comparative study on two cationic porphycenes: photophysical and antimicrobial photoinactivation evaluation. *Int J Mol Sci.* 2015;16:27072–27086. doi:10.3390/ijms161125999.
66. Guo Y, Rogelj S, Zhang P. Rose Bengal-decorated silica nanoparticles as photosensitizers for inactivation of gram-positive bacteria. *Nanotechnology.* 2010;21:065102. doi:10.1088/0957-4484/21/6/065102.
67. Topaloglu N, Güney M, Yuksel S, Gülsoy M. Antibacterial photodynamic therapy with 808-nm laser and indocyanine green on abrasion wound models. *J Biomed Opt.* 2015;20:28003. doi:10.1117/1.jbo.20.2.028003.
68. Wong T-W, Wu E-C, Ko W-C, Lee C-C, Hor L-I, Huang I-H. Photodynamic inactivation of methicillin-resistant *Staphylococcus aureus* by indocyanine green and near infrared light. *Dermatol Sin.* 2018;36:8–15. doi:10.1016/j.dsi.2017.08.003.
69. Donlan RM. Biofilms: microbial life on surfaces. *Emerg Infect Dis.* 2002;8(9):881–890. doi:10.3201/eid0809.020063.
70. Samrot AV, Abubakar Mohamed A, Faradjeva E, et al. Mechanisms and impact of biofilms and targeting of biofilms using bioactive compounds-a review. *Medicina (Kaunas).* 2021;57(8):839. doi:10.3390/medicina57080839.
71. Khan J, Tarar SM, Gul I, Nawaz U, Arshad M. Challenges of antibiotic resistance biofilms and potential combating strategies: a review. *3 Biotech.* 2021;11(4):169. doi:10.1007/s13205-021-02707-w.
72. Hu X, Huang YY, Wang Y, Wang X, Hamblin MR. Antimicrobial photodynamic therapy to control clinically relevant biofilm infections. *Front Microbiol.* 2018;9:1299. doi:10.3389/fmicb.2018.01299.
73. Garcez AS, Núñez SC, Jr Azambuja N, et al. Effects of photodynamic therapy on gram-positive and gram-negative bacterial biofilms by bioluminescence imaging and scanning electron microscopic analysis. *Photomed Laser Surg.* 2013;31(11):519–525. doi:10.1089/pho.2012.3341.
74. Tan Y, Cheng Q, Yang H, et al. Effects of ALA-PDT on biofilm structure, virulence factor secretion, and QS in Pseudomonas aeruginosa. *Photodiagnosis Photodyn Ther.* 2018;24:88–94. doi:10.1016/j.pdpdt.2018.07.005.
75. Warrier A, Mazumder N, Prabhu S, Satyamoorthy K, Murali TS. Photodynamic therapy to control microbial biofilms. *Photodiagnosis Photodyn Ther.* 2021;33:102090. doi:10.1016/j.pdpdt.2020.102090.
76. Sperandio FF, Huang YY, Hamblin MR. Antimicrobial photodynamic therapy to kill Gram-negative bacteria. *Recent Pat Antiinfect Drug Discov.* 2013;8(2):108–120. doi:10.2174/1574891x113089990012.
77. Lin HY, Chen CT, Huang CT. Use of merocyanine 540 for photodynamic inactivation of *Staphylococcus aureus* planktonic and biofilm cells. *Appl Environ Microbiol.* 2004;70(11):6453–6458. doi:10.1128/AEM.70.11.6453-6458.2004.
78. Iluz N, Maor Y, Keller N, Malik Z. The synergistic effect of PDT and oxacillin on clinical isolates of Staphylococcus aureus. *Lasers Surg Med.* 2018;50(5):535–551. doi:10.1002/lsm.22785.
79. Lopes M, Alves CT, Rama Raju B, et al. Application of benzo[a]phenoxazinium chlorides in antimicrobial photodynamic therapy of Candida albicans biofilms. *J Photochem Photobiol B.* 2014;141:93–99. doi:10.1016/j.jphotobiol.2014.09.006.
80. Ribeiro AP, Andrade MC, da Silva Jde F, et al. Photodynamic inactivation of planktonic cultures and biofilms of *Candida albicans* mediated by aluminum-chloride-phthalocyanine entrapped in nanoemulsions.

Photochem Photobiol. 2013;89(1):111–119. doi:10.1111/j.1751-1097.2012.01198.x.

81. Liu Y, Qin R, Zaat SAJ, Breukink E, Heger M. Antibacterial photodynamic therapy: overview of a promising approach to fight antibiotic-resistant bacterial infections. *J Clin Transl Res.* 2015;1(3):140–167.
82. Ziental D, Mlynarczyk DT, Czarczynska-Goslinska B, Lewandowski K, Sobotta L. PSs mediated photodynamic inactivation against fungi. *Nanomaterials (Basel).* 2021;11(11):2883. doi:10.3390/nano11112883.
83. Donnelly RF, McCarron PA, Tunney MM. Antifungal photodynamic therapy. *Microbiol Res.* 2008;163(1):1–12. doi:10.1016/j.micres.2007.08.001.
84. Willis JA, Cheburkanov V, Kassab G, et al. Photodynamic viral inactivation: recent advances and potential applications. *Appl Phys Rev.* 2021;8(2):021315. doi:10.1063/5.0044713.
85. Sadraeian M, Bahou C, da Cruz EF, et al. Photoimmunotherapy using cationic and anionic PS-antibody conjugates against HIV env-expressing cells. *Int J Mol Sci.* 2020;21(23):9151. doi:10.3390/ijms21239151.
86. Sun Y, Ogawa R, Xiao BH, et al. Antimicrobial photodynamic therapy in skin wound healing: a systematic review of animal studies. *Int Wound J.* 2020;17(2):285–299. doi:10.1111/iwj.13269.
87. Pariser DM, Eichenfield LF, Bukhalo M, Waterman G, Jarratt M, Study Group PDT. Photodynamic therapy with methyl aminolaevulinate 80 mg g(-1) for severe facial acne vulgaris: a randomized vehicle-controlled study. *Br J Dermatol.* 2016;174(4):770–777. doi:10.1111/bjd.14345.
88. Ning X, He G, Zeng W, Xia Y. The PS-based therapies enhance the repairing of skin wounds. *Front Med (Lausanne).* 2022;9:915548. doi:10.3389/fmed.2022.915548.
89. Almeida A, Faustino MAF, Neves MGPMS. Antimicrobial photodynamic therapy in the control of COVID-19. *Antibiotics (Basel).* 2020;9(6):320. doi:10.3390/antibiotics9060320.

INDEX

Note: Page numbers followed by "*f*" indicate figures, "*t*" indicate tables, and "*b*" indicate boxes.